Anticancer Drugs

Anticancer Drugs

Special Issue Editors

Mary J. Meegan
Niamh M. O'Boyle

MDPI • Basel • Beijing • Wuhan • Barcelona • Belgrade

Special Issue Editors
Mary J. Meegan
Trinity College Dublin
Ireland

Niamh M. O'Boyle
Trinity College Dublin
Ireland

Editorial Office
MDPI
St. Alban-Anlage 66
4052 Basel, Switzerland

This is a reprint of articles from the Special Issue published online in the open access journal *Pharmaceuticals* (ISSN 1424-8247) from 2018 to 2019 (available at: https://www.mdpi.com/journal/pharmaceuticals/special_issues/Anticancer_Drugs)

For citation purposes, cite each article independently as indicated on the article page online and as indicated below:

LastName, A.A.; LastName, B.B.; LastName, C.C. Article Title. *Journal Name* **Year**, *Article Number*, Page Range.

ISBN 978-3-03921-586-7 (Pbk)
ISBN 978-3-03921-587-4 (PDF)

Contents

About the Special Issue Editors vii

Mary J. Meegan and Niamh M. O'Boyle
Special Issue "Anticancer Drugs"
Reprinted from: *Pharmaceuticals* **2019**, *12*, 134, doi:10.3390/ph12030134 1

Sami A. Makharza, Giuseppe Cirillo, Orazio Vittorio, Emanuele Valli, Florida Voli, Annafranca Farfalla, Manuela Curcio, Francesca Iemma, Fiore Pasquale Nicoletta, Ahmed A. El-Gendy, Gerardo F. Goya and Silke Hampel
Magnetic Graphene Oxide Nanocarrier for Targeted Delivery of Cisplatin: A Perspective for Glioblastoma Treatment
Reprinted from: *Pharmaceuticals* **2019**, *12*, 76, doi:10.3390/ph12020076 7

Amy M. Buckley, Becky AS. Bibby, Margaret R. Dunne, Susan A. Kennedy, Maria B. Davern, Breandán N. Kennedy, Stephen G. Maher and Jacintha O'Sullivan
Characterisation of an Isogenic Model of Cisplatin Resistance in Oesophageal Adenocarcinoma Cells
Reprinted from: *Pharmaceuticals* **2019**, *12*, 33, doi:10.3390/ph12010033 22

Shu Wang, Azizah M. Malebari, Thomas F. Greene, Niamh M. O'Boyle, Darren Fayne, Seema M. Nathwani, Brendan Twamley, Thomas McCabe, Niall O. Keely, Daniela M. Zisterer and Mary J. Meegan
3-Vinylazetidin-2-Ones: Synthesis, Antiproliferative and Tubulin Destabilizing Activity in MCF-7 and MDA-MB-231 Breast Cancer Cells
Reprinted from: *Pharmaceuticals* **2019**, *12*, 56, doi:10.3390/ph12020056 42

Charlotte M. Miller, Elaine C. O'Sullivan and Florence O. McCarthy
Novel 11-Substituted Ellipticines as Potent Anticancer Agents with Divergent Activity against Cancer Cells
Reprinted from: *Pharmaceuticals* **2019**, *12*, 90, doi:10.3390/ph12020090 91

João Antônio Leal de Miranda, João Erivan Façanha Barreto, Dainesy Santos Martins, Paulo Vitor de Souza Pimentel, Deiziane Viana da Silva Costa, Reyca Rodrigues e Silva, Luan Kelves Miranda de Souza, Camila Nayane de Carvalho Lima, Jefferson Almeida Rocha, Ana Paula Fragoso de Freitas, Durcilene Alves da Silva, Ariel Gustavo Scafuri, Renata Ferreira de Carvalho Leitão, Gerly Anne de Castro Brito, Jand Venes Rolim Medeiros and Gilberto Santos Cerqueira
Protective Effect of Cashew Gum (*Anacardium occidentale* L.) on 5-Fluorouracil-Induced Intestinal Mucositis
Reprinted from: *Pharmaceuticals* **2019**, *12*, 51, doi:10.3390/ph12020051 106

Mónica Fernández-Cancio, Núria Camats, Christa E. Flück, Adam Zalewski, Bernhard Dick, Brigitte M. Frey, Raquel Monné, Núria Torán, Laura Audí and Amit V. Pandey
Mechanism of the Dual Activities of Human CYP17A1 and Binding to Anti-Prostate Cancer Drug Abiraterone Revealed by a Novel V366M Mutation Causing 17,20 Lyase Deficiency
Reprinted from: *Pharmaceuticals* **2018**, *11*, 37, doi:10.3390/ph11020037 123

Hazel O'Neill, Vinod Malik, Ciaran Johnston, John V Reynolds and Jacintha O'Sullivan
Can the Efficacy of [^{18}F]FDG-PET/CT in Clinical Oncology Be Enhanced by Screening Biomolecular Profiles?
Reprinted from: *Pharmaceuticals* **2019**, *12*, 16, doi:10.3390/ph12010016 147

Alessandra Pannunzio and Mauro Coluccia
Cyclooxygenase-1 (COX-1) and COX-1 Inhibitors in Cancer: A Review of Oncology and Medicinal Chemistry Literature
Reprinted from: *Pharmaceuticals* **2018**, *11*, 101, doi:10.3390/ph11040101 . . . . **162**

Nirnoy Dan, Saini Setua, Vivek K. Kashyap, Sheema Khan, Meena Jaggi, Murali M. Yallapu and Subhash C. Chauhan
Antibody-Drug Conjugates for Cancer Therapy: Chemistry to Clinical Implications
Reprinted from: *Pharmaceuticals* **2018**, *11*, 32, doi:10.3390/ph11020032 . . . . **182**

About the Special Issue Editors

Mary J. Meegan, Dr., Professor, completed her Ph.D. degree in University College Dublin under the direction of Professor Dervilla Donnelly in the area of natural product chemistry and subsequently carried out postdoctoral research at the University Chemical Laboratory, Cambridge University in the research group of Professor Alan Battersby in the area of porphyrin synthesis and biosynthesis. Following further research appointments at University College Dublin and CNRS Gif-sur-Yvette, she was appointed as Lecturer in Pharmaceutical Chemistry at the School of Pharmacy and Pharmaceutical Sciences in Trinity College Dublin. Her research experience is in the general area of pharmaceutical and medicinal chemistry, with over 100 peer-reviewed scientific papers covering topics such as (i) novel ligands for nuclear receptor (ER&AR), HSP90, and tubulin; (ii) synthesis of small molecule inhibitors of the enzymes involved in metastasis of breast tumours; (iii) the design and evaluation of dual targeting agents for tubulin and aromatase; and (iv) the design of drugs which target proliferation of chronic lymphocytic leukaemia (CLL), Burkitt lymphoma, and related malignancies. Research collaborations have been established within Trinity College with Dr. Niamh O'Boyle (School of Pharmacy and Pharmaceutical Sciences), Dr. D. Zisterer, Dr. D. Fayne in the School of Biochemistry and Immunology and also with many European research centres. She is a member of the Royal Society of Chemistry and the Irish and European Associations for Cancer Research.

Niamh M. O'Boyle, Dr., Assistant Professor, is a qualified pharmacist and a member of the Pharmaceutical Society of Ireland. She received her B.Sc. (Pharm) and Ph.D. degree from Trinity College Dublin, and was subsequently awarded a postdoctoral scholarship at University of Göteborg in Sweden investigate the allergenic activity of epoxides and epoxy resins. Niamh was awarded a Government of Ireland Postdoctoral Research Fellowship at the School of Biochemistry & Immunology, TCD, working on 'Cancer, Tubulin and Free Radicals: New Therapy'. Following a period as Assistant Lecturer at the School of Chemical and Pharmaceutical Sciences at Dublin Institute of Technology, she was appointed as Assistant Professor at the School of Pharmacy and Pharmaceutical Sciences at TCD in 2017. She is a member of the Irish and European Associations for Cancer Research, and the Royal Society of Chemistry. She is part of the COST action MuTaLig (15135). Her main research interest is in the development of new treatments for cancer. Drug targets of interest include the protein tubulin, the oestrogen and progesterone receptors, and the role of reactive oxygen species. She is also interested in developing novel chemotherapeutics from natural products.

pharmaceuticals

Editorial

Special Issue "Anticancer Drugs"

Mary J. Meegan * and Niamh M. O'Boyle *

School of Pharmacy and Pharmaceutical Sciences, Trinity College Dublin, Trinity Biomedical Sciences Institute, 152-160 Pearse Street, 2 DO2R590 Dublin, Ireland
* Correspondence: mmeegan@tcd.ie (M.J.M.); niamh.oboyle@tcd.ie (N.M.O.)

Received: 6 September 2019; Accepted: 6 September 2019; Published: 16 September 2019

Abstract: The focus of this Special Issue of *Pharmaceuticals* is on the design, synthesis, and molecular mechanism of action of novel antitumor, drugs with a special emphasis on the relationship between the chemical structure and the biological activity of the molecules. This Special Issue also provides an understanding of the biologic and genotypic context in which targets are selected for oncology drug discovery, thus providing a rationalization for the biological activity of these drugs and guiding the design of more effective agents. In this Special Issue of *Pharmaceuticals* dedicated to anticancer drugs, we present a selection of preclinical research papers including both traditional chemotherapeutic agents and newer more targeted therapies and biological agents. We have included articles that report the design of small molecules with promising anticancer activity as tubulin inhibitors, vascular targeting agents, and topoisomerase targeting agents, alongside a comprehensive review of clinically successful antibody-drug conjugates used in cancer treatment.

Keywords: snticancer drugs; cancer drug design; cancer immunotherapy; conjugate and hybrid drugs, cisplatin resistance, topoisomerase inhibitors; microtubule targeted drugs

---

We have great pleasure in accepting the invitation to be guest editors for this Special Issue of "Pharmaceuticals". This volume presents reviews and original research papers by experts on a wide range of topics relevant to the topic of "Anticancer Drugs" and includes contributions relevant to both traditional chemotherapeutic agents and newer targeted therapies and biological therapeutics.

The global cancer burden is estimated by the World Health Organization at 18.1 million new cases and 9.6 million deaths in 2018 [1]. One in five men and one in six women worldwide are predicted to develop cancer during their lifetime, while one in 8 men and one in 11 women will die from the disease. The leading types of cancer worldwide in terms of the number of new cases are cancers of the lung and female breast; the largest number of deaths annually is from lung cancer (1.8 million deaths, 18.4% of the total), attributed to the poor prognosis for this cancer, followed by colorectal cancer (881,000 deaths, 9.2%), stomach cancer (783,000 deaths, 8.2%), and liver cancer (782,000 deaths, 8.2%).

This is an exciting era for cancer drug discovery and development and presents enormous opportunities for medicinal chemists, chemical biologists, and molecular biologists. In this Special Issue, we highlight both the opportunities and challenges available in the discovery and design of innovative cancer therapies, novel small-molecule cancer drugs, and antibody–drug conjugates. We hope to demonstrate the potential for future research in these areas. The transition from traditional cytotoxic chemotherapy to more targeted cancer drug discovery has resulted in an increasing selection of tools available to oncologists for cancer treatment. Continued research on the design of effective oncology drugs for application in chemotherapy has improved our understanding of the mechanism of the action of these drugs, expanded their activity/function spectrum, and unlocked new applications for improved patient outcomes. Chemotherapy is one of the most powerful tools available for treating cancer, and research continues to find new chemotherapy drugs, as well as new uses for existing ones. Newer types of drugs are being developed that attack cancer cells in different ways. These drugs include targeted therapies that are designed to attack cancer cells while demonstrating less damage to normal cells. Immunotherapies use the body's own immune system to find and destroy cancer cells.

The development and availability of new effective oncology drugs is encouraging. The FDA (U.S. Food and Drug Administration) approved 8 drugs for orphan cancer indications in 2017 and 12 cancer drugs (26% of the total approvals), including 2 landmark approvals, to the first Chimeric Antigen Receptor (CAR)-T cell therapies. The approval of the IDH2 inhibitor enasidenib is also noteworthy, demonstrating that drugs can target cancer cells by blocking cancer-specific metabolic pathways. In 2018, the FDA approved 19 applications for new cancer drug and biologics, as well as 38 supplemental indications and 4 biosimilars [2]. In 2018, the FDA granted its second-ever approval for a 'tissue-agnostic' drug to treat tumors with a specific genetic change regardless of cancer type, and a second-ever biosimilar drug to treat cancer was approved. In 2018, 8 of 10 of the top selling pharmaceuticals were large molecules, and 6 out of 10 have cancer-related indications. Among the cancer drugs approved to date by the FDA in 2019 are selinexor, a first-in-class selective inhibitor of nuclear export for treating adult patients with relapsed or refractory multiple myeloma (RRMM). However, despite intense efforts and the discovery of many effective targeted therapies, oncology drug development remains challenging; combination therapy may be the future for oncology patients.

It is recognized that cancer is a multifactorial disease and the genesis and progression of the disease are extremely complex. One of the major problems in the development of anticancer drugs is the emergence of multidrug resistance and relapse. Classical chemotherapeutic drugs directly target the DNA of the cell, but mutations enable the cell to develop resistance. More recent developments in the availability of anticancer drugs include molecular-targeted therapy such as targeting the proteins with abnormal expression inside the cancer cells, and the design and subsequent development of new anticancer small molecule agents. In recent years, many promising drug targets have been identified for effective exploitation in the treatment of cancer. Targeted chemotherapies are successful in certain malignancies; however the effectiveness has often been limited by drug resistance and side effects on normal tissues and cells. Their often high cost also precludes access to these agents by many patients who could potentially benefit.

Many types of cancers are responsive to the "traditional" chemotherapy drug treatments, for example, alkylating agents, intercalating dugs, topoisomerase inhibitors, antimetabolites, and antimitotic drugs, as well as the more recently identified targeted therapies such as various kinase inhibitors. The targeted monoclonal antibodies have been proven to be spectacularly successful in specific cancers. A limited number of cancers can be completely cured using these treatment approaches. However, the success of cancer treatments varies enormously depending on the specific type of cancer diagnosed and stage of diagnosis.

Resistance exists against every effective anticancer drug and can develop by numerous mechanisms. Many patients exhibit intrinsic and acquired resistance to treatment with chemotherapeutic anticancer drugs and become refractory to treatment. Drug resistance can be caused by different mechanisms depending on the structure and action of the drug, including multi-drug resistance (MDR), cell death inhibition (apoptosis suppression), alterations in drug metabolism, epigenetic and drug targets, enhancement of DNA repair, and gene amplification. The development of MDR to chemotherapy remains a major challenge in treating cancer.

With the development of genomic profiling technologies and selective molecular targeted therapies, the use of biomarkers plays an increasingly important role in the clinical management of cancer patients. To achieve a more comprehensive understanding of current research activities in the area of anticancer drugs, contributions of reviews and original research articles covering the different facets of anticancer drug research are now collected in this *Pharmaceuticals* Special Issue on "Anticancer Drugs". The focus of this Special Issue is on the design, synthesis, and molecular mechanism of action of novel antitumor drugs and on the relationship between the chemical structure and biochemical reactivity of the molecules. This Special Issue provides an understanding of the biologic and genotypic context in which targets are selected for oncology drug discovery, thus allowing rationalization of the activity of these drugs and guiding the design of more effective agents. This Special Issue of *Pharmaceuticals* on "Anticancer Drugs" addresses a varied selection of preclinical research areas, including both traditional chemotherapeutic agents and newer more targeted therapies and biological agents. We have included articles describing the design of small molecules with promising anticancer activity as tubulin inhibitors, vascular targeting agents, and topoisomerase targeting agents, alongside a comprehensive review of antibody–drug conjugates. In addition, promising drug candidates under various phases of preclinical clinical trials are also described. Multi-acting drugs that simultaneously target different cancer cell signaling pathways may facilitate the design of effective anti-cancer drug therapies. The specific topics include synthesis and evaluation of novel small molecules targeting biomolecules such as tubulin and topoisomerase; development of novel nanocarrier drug delivery systems for cytotoxic cisplatin, cisplatin resistance in oesophageal cancer, approaches to treatment of 5-fluorouracil-induced intestinal mucositis; mechanism of action of the anti-prostate cancer drug abiraterone; a study of [^{18}F]FDG-PET/CT in clinical oncology; cyclooxygenase-1 (COX-1) and COX-1 inhibitors in cancer; and chemistry and clinical implications of antibody–drug conjugates for cancer therapy.

Chemotherapy is widely used to treat cancer, which is the second leading cause of death worldwide. Nonspecific distribution and uncontrollable release of drugs in conventional drug delivery systems have led to the development of smart nanocarrier-based drug delivery systems, which are also known as smart drug delivery systems (SSDS) as an alternative to chemotherapy. SDDSs can deliver drugs to the target sites with reduced dosage frequency and in a controlled manner to reduce the side effects experienced in conventional drug delivery systems. Makharza et al. describe selective delivery of the widely used chemotherapeutic drug cisplatin to glioblastoma U87 cells by the design of a hybrid nanocarrier composed of magnetic γ-Fe_2O_3 nanoparticles and nanographene oxide [3]. They demonstrated negligible toxicity for the nanoparticle system; the anticancer activity of cisplatin was retained with loading onto the carrier, together with control of drug delivery at the target site. Although cisplatin is one of the most widely used chemotherapeutic drugs for the treatment of solid tumors, the development of resistance hinders the success of this drug in the clinic.

The study by Buckley et al. provides novel insights into the molecular and phenotypic changes in an isogenic oesophageal adenocarcinoma model of acquired cisplatin resistance in oesophageal adenocarcinoma [4]. Key differences that could be targeted to overcome cisplatin resistance are identified in this study, including differences in treatment sensitivity, gene expression, inflammatory protein secretions, and metabolic rate in their model. It is of interest that cisplatin resistant cells have an altered metabolic profile under normal and low oxygen conditions. The molecular differences identified in this study, for example, increased sensitivity to radiation and 5-fluorouracil of cisplatin resistant cells, provide novel insight into cisplatin resistance in oesophageal adenocarcinoma. The authors have identified potential molecular processes that could be targeted to overcome cisplatin resistance and improve therapeutic outcomes for oesophageal adenocarcinoma patients.

Even with the emergence of targeted therapies for cancer treatment, natural products and their derivatives that target microtubules are some of the most effective drugs used in the clinical treatment of solid tumors and hematological malignancies. Many natural products have been discovered that bind to tubulin/microtubules and disrupt microtubule function. Although these drugs inhibit mitosis, emerging evidence indicates that their actions are complex and inhibit signaling events important for carcinogenesis. Microtubule-targeted drugs are essential chemotherapeutic agents for various types of cancer, for example, taxol and the vinca alkaloids such as vincristine and vinblastine. The design and evaluation of novel small molecules that target mitosis continues to attract the interest of medicinal chemists. Microtubules are an important target for structurally diverse natural products, and a fuller understanding of the mechanisms of action of these drugs will promote their optimal use. A series of 3-vinyl-β-lactams (2-azetidinones) was designed, synthesized, and evaluated as potential tubulin polymerization inhibitors in breast cancer cells by Wang et al [5]. The compounds inhibited the polymerization of tubulin, and were shown to interact at the colchicine-binding site on tubulin, resulting in significant G_2/M phase cell cycle arrest and mitotic catastrophe. These compounds are promising candidates for development as antiproliferative microtubule-disrupting agents. Continued efforts to identify the effects of microtubule targeting agents on oncogenic signaling pathways will provide opportunities to discover therapeutic uses for these drugs.

Ellipticines have well documented anticancer activity, based on the structure of the alkaloid ellipticine, which inhibits the enzyme topoisomerase II via intercalative binding to DNA in particular. The anti-tumor alkaloid ellipticine and its derivatives act as potent anticancer agents via a combined mechanism involving cell cycle arrest and induction of apoptosis. The prevalent DNA-mediated mechanisms of anti-tumor, mutagenic, and cytotoxic activities of ellipticine are DNA intercalation, inhibition of DNA topoisomerase II activity, and covalent binding to DNA. However, owing to limitations in synthesis and coherent screening methodology, it has not been possible to achieve the full structure-activity relationship (SAR) profile of this important anticancer class to date. Miller et al. have addressed this issue, and have explored the anticancer activity of this potent natural product by a series of substitutions on the heterocyclic structure [6]. The synthesis of a panel of novel 11-substituted ellipticines is described, with two specific derivatives showing potency and diverging cellular growth effects on cancer cell lines on a panel of 60 National Cancer Institute (NCI) cell lines.

Side effects of chemotherapy can limit its usefulness. Intestinal mucositis is a common complication associated with 5-fluorouracil (5-FU) treatment, a chemotherapeutic agent used for colon, oesophageal, stomach, breast, pancreatic, and cervical cancers. Miranda et al. have evaluated the effects of Cashew gum (bark exudate from *Anacardium occidentale* L.) as a potent anti-inflammatory agent on experimental intestinal mucositis induced by 5-FU [7]. Use of Cashew gum, as a versatile polymer scaffold material in formulating pharmaceuticals, is of considerable interest owing to the polymer's biocompatibility, low toxicity, and biodegradability. The authors report that Cashew gum prevented 5-FU-induced histopathological changes and decreased oxidative stress through decrease of malondialdehyde levels and increase of glutathione concentration. The authors suggest that Cashew gum reverses the effects of 5-FU-induced intestinal mucositis. Cashew gum decreases inflammation, oxidative stress, and intestinal injury induced by 5-fluorouracil in the duodenum. The effects of Cashew gum were found to be related to the cyclooxygenase-2 (COX-2) pathway. Cashew gum attenuated an inflammatory process by decreasing myeloperoxidase activity, intestinal mastocytosis, and interleukin (IL)-1β and cyclooxygenase-2 (COX-2) expression. The co-administration of Cashew gum and celecoxib completely reversed COX-2 and IL-1β expression and the intestinal injury induced by 5-FU. It is suggested that Cashew gum has potential application in the development of novel treatments for intestinal mucositis owing to 5-FU and other antineoplastic agents.

Knowledge about the specificity of the cytochrome P450 CYP17A1 enzyme activities is of importance for the development of treatments for the polycystic ovary syndrome and inhibitors for prostate cancer therapy. Androgens have an important role in the development of both normal prostate epithelium and prostate cancer and variants of genes involved in androgen metabolism may be linked to an increased risk of prostate cancer. Cytochrome P450 17α-hydroxylase/17,20-lyase (CYP17A1) is a key regulatory enzyme in the steroid metabolism; it catalyses both 17,20-lyase and 17α-hydroxylase transformations and is essential for the biosynthesis of androgens and glucocorticoids. Fernández-Cancio et al. discuss the mechanism of the dual activities of human CYP17A1 and the interaction of this enzyme with the anti-prostate cancer drug abiraterone [8]. These results are presented in their studies of a novel V366M mutation causing 17,20 lyase deficiency. Molecular dynamics simulations are effectively used to demonstrate how the V366M mutation facilitates a mechanism for dual activities of human CYP17A1 requiring the conversion of pregnenolone to 17OH-pregnenolone, which re-enters the active site for conversion to dehydroepiandrosterone. The effectiveness of the anti-prostate cancer drug abiraterone as a potent inhibitor of CYP17A1 is rationalized.

Positron emission tomography (PET) is a functional imaging modality widely used in clinical oncology. Over the years, the sensitivity and specificity of PET has improved with the advent of specific radiotracers, increased technical accuracy of PET scanners, and incremental experience of radiologists. The potential influence of individual molecular markers of glucose transport, glycolysis, hypoxia, and angiogenesis, in addition to the relationships between these key cellular processes and their influence on fluorodeoxyglucose (FDG) uptake, is reviewed by O'Neill et al [9]. The potential role for biomolecular profiling of individual tumors to predict positivity on ^{18}F-fluorodeoxyglucose (^{18}F-FDG) positron emission tomography/computed tomography (PET/CT) imaging is discussed with a view of enhancing accuracy and clinical utility.

Cancer may originate in the chronic inflammation setting associated with persistent infections, immune-mediated damage, or prolonged exposure to irritants. Prostaglandins and thromboxane are lipid signalling molecules produced from arachidonic acid by the action of the cyclooxygenase isoenzymes COX-1 and COX-2. Pannunzio and Coluccia review the role of cyclooxygenase-1 (COX-1) and cyclooxygenase-2 (COX-2) inhibitors in cancer [10]. The role of cyclooxygenases (particularly COX-2) and prostaglandins (particularly PGE_2) in cancer-related inflammation has been extensively investigated. Although COX-1 expression increases in several human cancers, the contribution of COX-1 remains much less explored. COX-1 and COX-2 isoforms seem to operate in a coordinated manner in cancer pathophysiology. In some cases, such as serous ovarian carcinoma, COX-1 plays a significant role. The precise genetic and molecular defects underlying epithelial ovarian cancer remain largely unknown, and treatment options for patients with advanced disease are limited. Human epithelial ovarian tumors have increased levels of COX-1, but not COX-2. The authors discuss the choice of the most appropriate tumor cell models for investigation of the role of COX-1 in the context of arachidonic acid metabolic network and review the in vitro and in vivo antitumor properties of COX-1-selective inhibitors.

Antibody–drug conjugates (ADCs) are highly targeted biopharmaceutical drugs that combine monoclonal antibodies specific to surface antigens present on particular tumour cells with highly potent anti-cancer agents linked *via* a chemical linker. ADCs have become a powerful class of therapeutic agents in oncology and hematology, with five approved drugs on the market, namely, Ado-trastuzumab emtansine, Brentuximab Vedotin, Gemtuzumab Ozogamicin, Inotuzumab Ozogamicin, and Polatuzumab Vedotin-piiq. This targeted approach can improve the tumour-to-normal tissue selectivity and specificity in chemotherapy. The continuing developments in the therapeutic use of antibody-drug conjugates for cancer therapy is discussed by Dan et al., where they consider the chemistry aspects of the conjugate design and stability together with the drug-linker targeting [11]. This review focuses on site-specific conjugation methods for producing homogenous ADCs with a constant drug–antibody ratio (DAR) and discusses the major challenges in conventional conjugation methods.

The past forty years have seen major developments in the understanding of the cellular and molecular biology of cancer. Significant increases have been achieved in long-term survival for many cancers, such as the use of tamoxifen touted as one of the game-changers for breast cancer, treatment of chronic myeloid leukemia with imatinib, and the success of biological drugs. The overall success rate for oncology drugs in clinical development estimated at ~10%, while the cost in introducing a new drug to market is estimated at greater than 1 billion US$. A number of factors are to be considered in the development of effective anticancer drugs. These include the role of the target identified in the pathogenesis of specific human cancers, target overexpression in a specific malignancy, interactions among the cellular components of malignant tissues, choice of preclinical cancer models of drug effects, balance between drug safety and efficacy in cancer patients, and the benefits of biomarkers in achieving a personalized approach to cancer drug development [12]. Unfortunately, resistance to treatment continues to be challenging, and contributes to mortality and morbidity. However, as is evident from the research and review papers presented in this *Pharmaceuticals* Special Issue on "Anticancer Drugs", significant efforts are being made to develop and improve cancer treatments and to translate basic research findings into clinical use, resulting in improvements in survival rates and quality of life for cancer patients.

Author Contributions: M.J.M. and N.M.O. compiled the editorial manuscript and M.J.M. submitted the manuscript

Funding: This research received no external funding.

Acknowledgments: We thank the authors for their hard work to produce an up-to-date and comprehensive issue on anticancer drugs. We also thank the Editor-in-Chief of *Pharmaceuticals*, Vanden Eynde, for giving us the opportunity to edit this special issue. The editorial assistance of Fendy Fan is also acknowledged.

Conflicts of Interest: The authors declare no conflict of interest.

References

1. The International Agency for Research on Cancer. Available online: https://www.who.int/cancer/PRGlobocanFinal.pdf (accessed on 11 September 2019).
2. 2018 New Drug Therapy Approvals Impact. Available online: https://www.fda.gov/files/drugs/published/New-Drug-Therapy-Approvals-2018_3.pdf (accessed on 11 September 2019).
3. Makharza, S.A.; Cirillo, G.; Vittorio, O.; Valli, E.; Voli, F.; Farfalla, A.; Curcio, M.; Iemma, F.; Nicoletta, F.P.; El-Gendy, A.A.; et al. Magnetic Graphene Oxide Nanocarrier for Targeted Delivery of Cisplatin: A Perspective for Glioblastoma Treatment. *Pharmaceuticals* **2019**, *12*, 76. [CrossRef] [PubMed]
4. Buckley, A.M.; Bibby, B.A.; Dunne, M.R.; Kennedy, S.A.; Davern, M.B.; Kennedy, B.N.; Maher, S.G.; O'Sullivan, J. Characterisation of an Isogenic Model of Cisplatin Resistance in Oesophageal Adenocarcinoma Cells. *Pharmaceuticals* **2019**, *12*, 33. [CrossRef] [PubMed]
5. Wang, S.; Malebari, A.M.; Greene, T.F.; O'Boyle, N.M.; Fayne, D.; Nathwani, S.M.; Twamley, B.; McCabe, T.; Keely, N.O.; Zisterer, D.M.; et al. 3-Vinylazetidin-2-Ones: Synthesis, Antiproliferative and Tubulin Destabilizing Activity in MCF-7 and MDA-MB-231 Breast Cancer Cells. *Pharmaceuticals* **2019**, *12*, 56. [CrossRef] [PubMed]
6. Miller, C.M.; O'Sullivan, E.C.; McCarthy, F.O. Novel 11-Substituted Ellipticines as Potent Anticancer Agents with Divergent Activity against Cancer Cells. *Pharmaceuticals* **2019**, *12*, 90. [CrossRef] [PubMed]
7. De Miranda, J.A.L.; Barretto, J.E.F.; Martins, D.S.; de Souza Pimentel, P.V.; da Silva Costa, D.V.; Silva, R.R.; de Souza, L.K.M.; de Lima, C.N.; Rocha, J.A.; de Freitas, A.P.F.; et al. Protective Effect of Cashew Gum (*Anacardium occidentale* L.) on 5-Fluorouracil-Induced Intestinal Mucositis. *Pharmaceuticals* **2019**, *12*, 51. [CrossRef] [PubMed]
8. Fernández-Cancio, M.; Camats, N.; Flück, C.E.; Zalewski, A.; Dick, B.; Frey, B.M.; Monné, R.; Torán, N.; Audí, L.; Pandey, A.V. Mechanism of the Dual Activities of Human CYP17A1 and Binding to Anti-Prostate Cancer Drug Abiraterone Revealed by a Novel V366M Mutation Causing 17,20 Lyase Deficiency. *Pharmaceuticals* **2018**, *11*, 37. [CrossRef] [PubMed]
9. O'Neill, H.; Malik, V.; Johnston, C.; Reynolds, J.V.; O'Sullivan, J. Can the Efficacy of [^{18}F]FDG-PET/CT in Clinical Oncology Be Enhanced by Screening Biomolecular Profiles? *Pharmaceuticals* **2019**, *12*, 16. [CrossRef] [PubMed]
10. Pannunzio, A.; Coluccia, M. Cyclooxygenase-1 (COX-1) and COX-1 Inhibitors in Cancer: A Review of Oncology and Medicinal Chemistry Literature. *Pharmaceuticals* **2018**, *11*, 101. [CrossRef] [PubMed]
11. Dan, N.; Setua, S.; Kashyap, V.K.; Khan, S.; Jaggi, M.; Yallapu, M.M.; Chauhan, S.C. Antibody-Drug Conjugates for Cancer Therapy: Chemistry to Clinical Implications. *Pharmaceuticals* **2018**, *11*, 32.
12. Goossens, N.; Nakagawa, S.; Sun, X.; Hoshida, Y. Cancer biomarker discovery and validation. *Transl. Cancer Res.* **2015**, *4*, 256–269. [PubMed]

pharmaceuticals

MDPI

Article

Magnetic Graphene Oxide Nanocarrier for Targeted Delivery of Cisplatin: A Perspective for Glioblastoma Treatment

Sami A. Makharza [1,2], Giuseppe Cirillo [1,3,*], Orazio Vittorio [4,5,6], Emanuele Valli [4,6], Florida Voli [4], Annafranca Farfalla [3], Manuela Curcio [3], Francesca Iemma [3], Fiore Pasquale Nicoletta [3], Ahmed A. El-Gendy [7], Gerardo F. Goya [8] and Silke Hampel [1]

1. Leibniz Institute of Solid State and Material Research Dresden, 01069 Dresden, Germany; samim@hebron.edu (S.A.M.); s.hampel@ifw-dresden.de (S.H.)
2. College of Pharmacy and Medical Sciences, Hebron University, Hebron 00970, Palestine
3. Department of Pharmacy, Health and Nutritional Sciences, University of Calabria, Rende (CS), 87036 Rende, Italy; annafranca.farfalla@gmail.com (A.F.); manuela.curcio@unical.it (M.C.); francesca.iemma@unical.it (F.I.); fiore.nicoletta@unical.it (F.P.N.)
4. Children's Cancer Institute, Lowy Cancer Research Centre, UNSW Sydney, Sydney 2031, Australia; OVittorio@ccia.org.au (O.V.); EValli@ccia.org.au (E.V.); FVoli@ccia.org.au (F.V.)
5. ARC Centre of Excellence for Convergent BioNano Science and Technology, Australian Centre for NanoMedicine, UNSW Sydney, Sydney 2052, Australia
6. School of Women's and Children's Health, Faculty of Medicine, UNSW Sydney, Sydney 2052, Australia
7. Department of Physics, University of Texas at El Paso, El Paso, TX 79968, USA; aelgendy@utep.edu
8. Institute of Nanoscience of Aragon (INA) & Department of Condensed Matter Physics, University of Zaragoza, 50018 Zaragoza, Spain; goya@unizar.es

* Correspondence: giuseppe.cirillo@unical.it; Tel.: +39-0984-493011

Received: 15 April 2019; Accepted: 16 May 2019; Published: 18 May 2019

Abstract: Selective vectorization of Cisplatin (CisPt) to Glioblastoma U87 cells was exploited by the fabrication of a hybrid nanocarrier composed of magnetic γ-Fe_2O_3 nanoparticles and nanographene oxide (NGO). The magnetic component, obtained by annealing magnetite Fe_3O_4 and characterized by XRD measurements, was combined with NGO sheets prepared via a modified Hummer's method. The morphological and thermogravimetric analysis proved the effective binding of γ-Fe_2O_3 nanoparticles onto NGO layers. The magnetization measured under magnetic fields up to 7 Tesla at room temperature revealed superparamagnetic-like behavior with a maximum value of M_S = 15 emu/g and coercivity $H_C \approx 0$ Oe within experimental error. The nanohybrid was found to possess high affinity towards CisPt, and a rather slow fractional release profile of 80% after 250 h. Negligible toxicity was observed for empty nanoparticles, while the retainment of CisPt anticancer activity upon loading into the carrier was observed, together with the possibility to spatially control the drug delivery at a target site.

Keywords: magnetic targeting; graphene oxide; maghemite; glioblastoma; cisplatin

1. Introduction

Malignant glioma is one of the most aggressive brain tumors, and the major cause of death from central nervous system cancers (median survival times less than 15 months from diagnosis) [1–5]. Glioma treatment is still one of the most difficult challenges for oncologists [6], and current therapies involve surgical intervention to achieve tumor debulking followed by adjuvant radio- and chemo-therapy [7]. Chemotherapy approaches are of paramount importance in the case of the most devastating and lethal grade IV glioma (Glioblastoma Multiforme, GBM), because the extensive tumor infiltration into the surrounding brain parenchyma makes surgery un-effective [8]. However, the therapeutic efficiency of chemotherapy is remains unsatisfactory for two main reasons: (i) the rare brain penetration of the anticancer agents systemically administered through the blood brain barrier (BBB) [9], and (ii) the poor glioma targeting of employed chemotherapeutics [10]. The latter issue is the main obstacle in the clinical treatment of Glioma with *cis*-diamminedichloroplatinum(II) (CisPt) [11], one of the most effective anticancer agents. CisPt suffers from a nonselective distribution between normal and tumor tissues, with the insurgence of severe adverse side effects, including acute nephrotoxicity, myelosuppression, and chronic neurotoxicity in adults [12–14], and lifelong health issues when the therapy was given in children [15,16]. Therefore, it is patently clear that, for an effective Glioma treatment, there is an urgent need for powerful and targeted CisPt delivery systems in order to promote preferential accumulation in cancer cells and thereby reduce the side effects [17]. Taking advantage of the peculiar features of tumor tissues such as the leaky neovasculature and the lack of functional lymphatic drainage, a wide range of nanoparticle drug carriers have been explored for this purpose [18].

Among others, graphene nanomaterials, mainly in the form of nanographene oxide (NGO), possess superior physicochemical, thermal, optical, mechanical, and biological properties [19–21]. NGO is widely explored for drug delivery applications by virtue of the large surface area (four times higher than that of any other nanomaterials) and the high stability of its water dispersion due to the richness of oxygen containing functional groups (e.g., carboxyl, epoxide, and hydroxyl groups) [22–24]. The suitability of NGO for the preparation of CisPt delivery vehicles with high loading efficiency is related to the presence of either the sp^2-aromatic structure or the abundant oxidized sp^3-portion on the edge, top, and bottom surfaces of each sheet [25–27], allowing the drug interaction through diverse mechanisms, including π-π stacking and hydrogen bonding [28–35].

More interestingly, functionalized NGO was found to highly accumulate in U87 human glioblastoma subcutaneous tumor xenografts [36,37], confirming that such nanocarriers can be considered a valuable tool for delivering CisPt to brain cancers. The efficiency of NGO delivery vehicles can be maximized by the incorporation of magnetic materials allowing the nanocarrier to be selectively driven into tumor tissues by the application of an external magnetic field [38]. In particular, magnetic nanoparticles based on iron oxide (maghemite γ-Fe_2O_3 or magnetite Fe_3O_4) were widely used for this purpose due to their biocompatibility and superparamagnetic properties [39,40]. The resulting NGO hybrid nanodevices were proposed as effective tools for glioblastoma treatment using Doxorubicin [41] and Irinotecan [42] as cytotoxic agents. Although possessing favorable properties for magnetic drug vectorization, the different chemical stabilities of Fe_3O_4 and γ-Fe_2O_3 may affect the toxicity of the delivery vehicle [43]. The lower chemical stability of Fe_3O_4 resulted in the release of Fe^{2+} ions from the nanoparticle cores, which can catalyze the formation of reactive oxygen species (ROS) damaging cell membrane and organelles, with the insurgence of adverse long-term side effects [44]. On the other hand, γ-Fe_2O_3 was found to be a better material owing to either the magnetic features or the high chemical stability [45].

In the present study we explored the possibility to employ NGO–Iron oxide nanohybrids (γ-Fe_2O_3@NGO) as a CisPt carrier for glioblastoma treatment by intercalating γ-Fe_2O_3 nanoparticles into NGO sheets. After characterizing the physical, chemical, and morphological properties, CisPt was loaded onto the nanocarrier for several drug-to-carrier ratios and their cytotoxicity was tested on human U87 cell lines.

2. Results and Discussion

2.1. Properties of γ-Fe_2O_3@NGO Nanohybrid

As previously reported, the size of NGO is a parameter that strongly affects the drug delivery effectiveness of NGO-based systems in vitro and in vivo [46,47]. Specifically, low-sized NGOs (lateral dimension ≈100 nm) have been reported to have the best performance [46].

The average size of our graphite oxide (GO) particles, as assessed by scanning electron microscopy (SEM), revealed an average size (lateral width) of 350–400 nm. These particles were therefore subsequently sonicated until NGO with lateral width of 80–100 nm and a thickness of 6.3 nm was attained (10 NGO sheets, assuming an interlayer distance of 0.7 nm) [48] (Figure 1a–c).

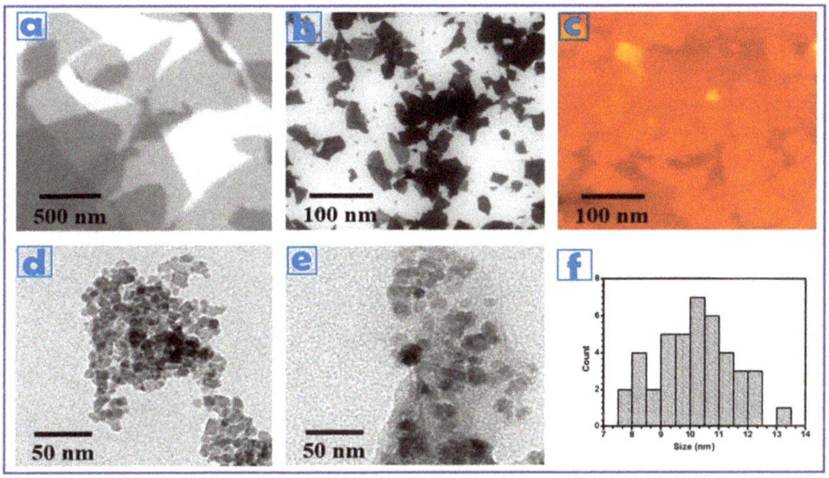

Figure 1. SEM images of (**a**) GO; and (**b**) NGO showing an average lateral width of 350–400 and 80–100 nm, respectively. (**c**) AFM image of NGO. TEM images of (**d**) γ-Fe_2O_3; and (**e**) γ-Fe_2O_3@NGO nanoparticles. (**f**) Size distribution of γ-Fe_2O_3 nanoparticles (approximately 10 nm).

The obtained NGO 100 nm were employed for the preparation of the magnetic hybrid device (γ-Fe_2O_3@NGO) as sketched in Figure 2.

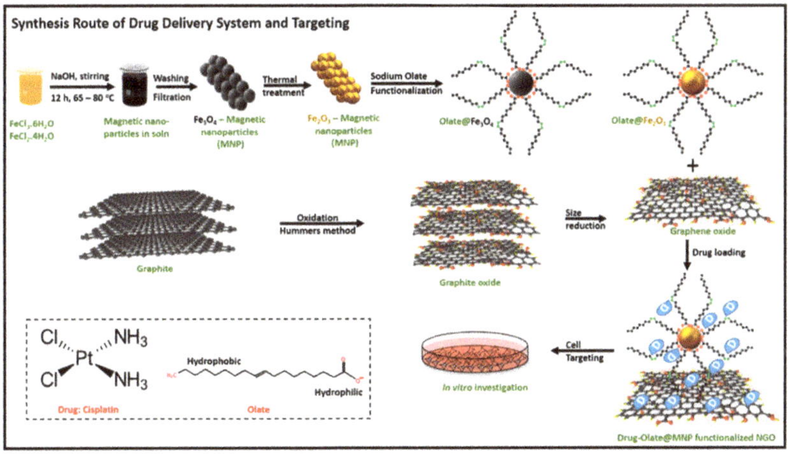

Figure 2. Schematic representation of the preparation of γ-Fe_2O_3@NGO.

Maghemite (γ-Fe_2O_3) nanoparticles were chosen to provide magnetic properties to the nanohybrids because of their high chemical stability, biocompatibility, and large magnetic moment at room temperature in its bulk form [40]. Superparamagnetism is crucial for application in biomedicine, because, despite the strong response to an external magnetic field, the absence of residual magnetic properties upon removal of the external field prevents nanoparticles from aggregation in biological environment [49–52]. γ-Fe_2O_3 nanoparticles (average size of 10 nm, see Figure 1d,f) were synthesized by annealing of magnetite Fe_3O_4 prepared by a chemical co-precipitation technique of $FeCl_3$ and $FeCl_2$ solutions [53,54], and then coated with oleic acid/sodium oleate to enhance their dispersion in water media and thus the biocompatibility features [55]. Since previously reported data proved the presence of transport systems importing fatty acids into the brain with high affinity and efficiency, it is reasonable to hypothesize that this coating strategy could be appropriate for targeting the blood brain barrier [56].

Despite the evidence of Fe_3O_4 to γ-Fe_2O_3 oxidation from the change of color of the sample (from black to reddish-brown color, see Figure 3), we investigated this phase change by XRD measurements. Figure 3 showed the XRD patterns of both compounds, and the *d*-spacing values emulated well the data deduced from the Joint Committee on Powder Diffraction Standards (JCPDS) cards 19-629 (Fe_3O_4) and 39-1346 (γ-Fe_2O_3).

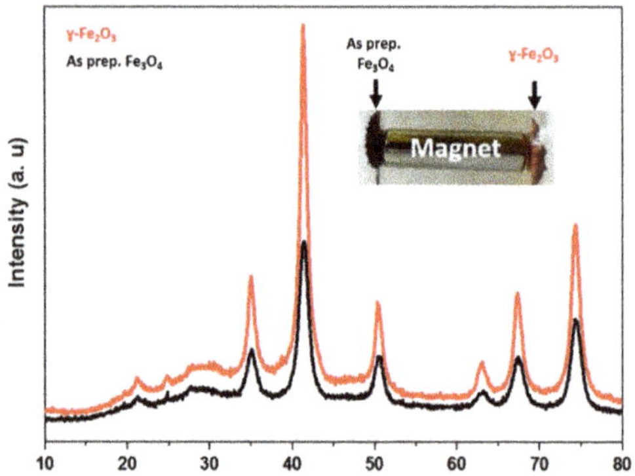

Figure 3. XRD patterns for Fe_3O_4 and γ-Fe_2O_3.

The result indicated no major differences between the two patterns, in each set of XRD patterns, the crystalline structure of magnetite and/or maghemite with indexes (hkl) ascribed to (220), (311), (400), (422), (511), and (440) were observable at the diffraction angels 2θ = 35.1°, 41.4.6°, 50.4°, 63.1°, 67.4° and 74.3° crystal planes, respectively. This result indicated that the thermal treatment of as prepared Fe_3O_4 produced γ-Fe_2O_3 (maghemite) crystal form [57].

The magnetization vs. field M(H) curves for the annealed γ-Fe_2O_3 nanoparticles showed nearly closed hysteresis loops, with zero coercivity (Figure 4).

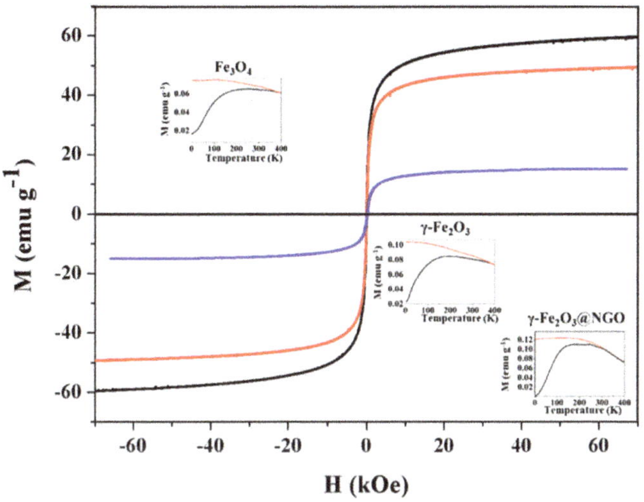

Figure 4. Hysteresis loops M(H) for Fe_3O_4 (black) and γ-Fe_2O_3 (red) and γ-Fe_2O_3@NGO (blue) nanoparticles. The insets show the Zero-field cooled (black) and field-cooled (orange) magnetization curves for Fe_3O_4, γ-Fe_2O_3, and γ-Fe_2O_3@NGO, taken with H_{FC} = 100 Oe.

The magnetization did not fully saturate within our experimentally available fields (H = 70 kOe), attaining a value of MS = 59.36 emu/g and MS = 49.25 emu/g at H = 70 kOe for Fe_3O_4 and γ-Fe_2O_3, respectively. After assembling γ -Fe_2O_3 into NGO the Ms value was 15.02 emu/g, consistent with a ≈30.5% wt. of magnetic material into NGO matrix, confirming the dispersion on magnetic nanoparticle into the hybrid platform. The coercivity values at room temperature were HC ≈ 0 for all samples. The zero field cooling (ZFC) and field cooling (FC) curves at H_{FC} = 100 Oe of Fe_3O_4, γ-Fe_2O_3 and γ-Fe_2O_3@NGO samples reflected similar features, i.e., a broad maximum in the ZFC curves originated from the distribution of blocking temperatures due to the distribution of particle sizes (see inset of Figure 4). The maxima were centered around T ≈ 194, 245, and 242 for Fe_3O_4, γ-Fe_2O_3, and γ-Fe_2O_3@NGO, respectively. These broad maxima are consistent with the blocking of the smallest nanoparticles at these temperatures, while the presence of irreversible behavior up to the highest temperature (400 K) suggests that a fraction of the largest particles are still blocked above room temperature.

The thermogravimetric analysis (TGA) curves of NGO and γ-Fe_2O_3@NGO were depicted in Figure 5.

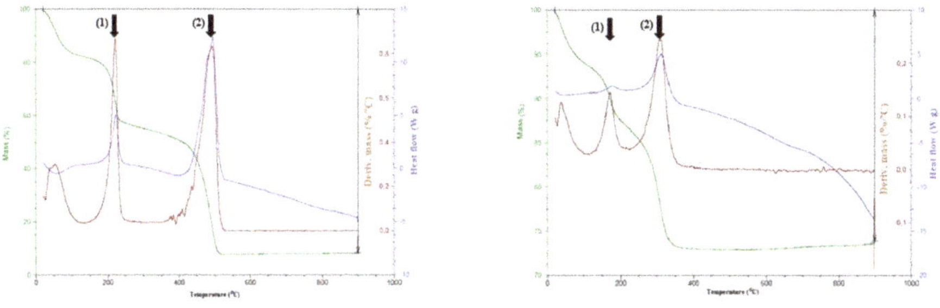

(**a**) (**b**)

Figure 5. TGA curves for NGO (**a**) and γ-Fe_2O_3@NGO (**b**).

For the NGO sample (Figure 5a), the mass loss in the range 150–250 °C with the maximum in the derivative %M/°C graph at 215 °C (arrow (1)) was ascribed to the decomposition of decorated oxygen functionalities on the basal graphene structure, while between 400 and 525 °C (maximum at 490, see arrow (2)), a high weight loss occurs due to the discard of more thermally stable oxygen groups. On the other hand, for γ-Fe_2O_3@NGO (Figure 5b), these mass losses were found to shift to lower temperatures (maximum in the derivative %M/°C graph at 170 °C and 305 °C, respectively) as a consequence of the effective binding of γ-Fe_2O_3 nanoparticles onto NGO layers.

2.2. Evaluation of Carrier Performances

Before testing the efficiency of γ-Fe_2O_3@NGO nanohybrid as CisPt carrier, we evaluated the toxicity of the empty nanoparticles (γ-Fe_2O_3, NGO, and γ-Fe_2O_3@NGO) on human glioblastoma U87 cell lines at a concentration range of 0–25 μg mL^{-1}. This range of concentration was selected because of the absence of any sign of aggregation as per Dynamic light-scattering (DLS) measurements. The viability values (>96% for all samples and concentrations, see Figure 6) proved the high biocompatibility of all nanoparticle systems, confirming their suitability as drug carrier [58].

The ultimate aim of the study is to check the suitability of γ-Fe_2O_3@NGO to selectively vectorize the cytotoxic drug to the tumor site under magnetic actuation. Indeed a key requirement for this nanocarrier is the ability to retain the drug until it reaches the target site. γ-Fe_2O_3@NGO was found to possess high affinity for CisPt (Drug Loading Efficiency of 0.37 mg mg^{-1}) and the release profiles were recorded after loading the drug by a soaking procedure (drug to carrier ratio of 10% by weight).

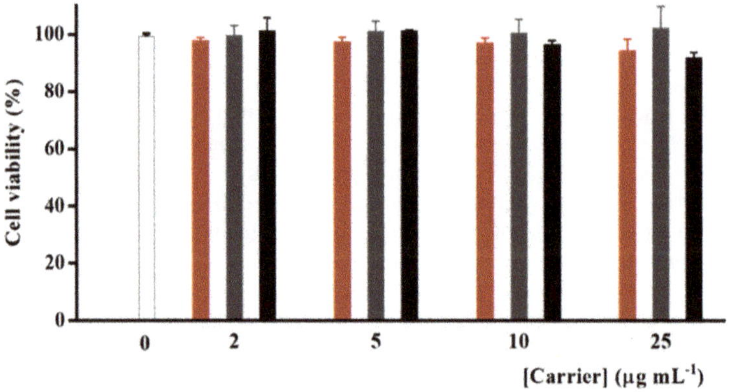

Figure 6. U87 viability after treatment with empty γ-Fe_2O_3 (**red**) and NGO (**grey**) and γ-Fe_2O_3@NGO (**black**).

The cumulative amount of drug released (M_t/M_0) was compared with those recorded when uncombined γ-Fe_2O_3 or NGO were employed as carrier (Figure 7).

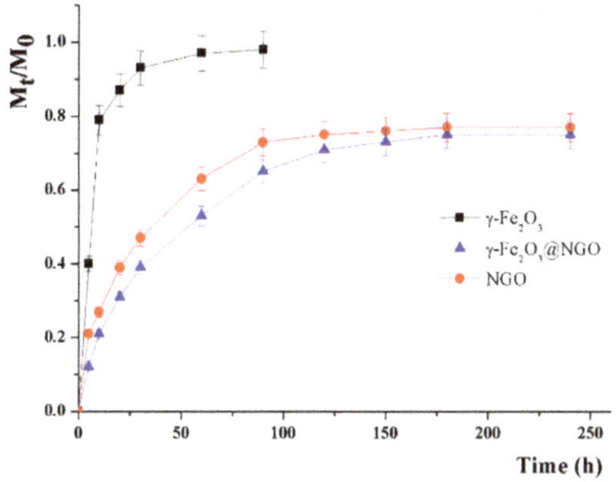

Figure 7. CisPt release profiles from γ-Fe_2O_3@NGO, γ-Fe_2O_3, and NGO.

For a more exhaustive analysis of the CisPt release profiles, a mathematical model considering the partition between the carrier and the surrounding environments and the underlying mechanism of the drug release was applied according to the literature [59]. In this model, a key parameter (α) was adopted to describe the physicochemical affinity of the drug between the carrier and solvent phases according to Equation (1):

$$\alpha = \frac{F_{max}}{1 - F_{max}} \tag{1}$$

where F_{max} represents the maximum value of relative release (M_t/M_0).

The overall drug release can be modeled according to reversible first- or second-order kinetics of Equations (2) and (3).

$$\frac{M_t}{M_0} = F_{max}\left(1 - e^{-\left(\frac{k_R}{F_{max}}\right)t}\right) \tag{2}$$

$$\frac{M_t}{M_0} = \frac{F_{max}\left(e^{2\left(\frac{k_R}{\alpha}\right)t} - 1\right)}{1 - 2F_{max} + e^{2\left(\frac{k_R}{\alpha}\right)t}} \tag{3}$$

with k_R being the release rate constant.

The time required for reaching 50% of F_{max} ($t_{1/2}$) can be obtained by applying the following Equations (4) and (5), respectively:

$$t^1_{1/2} = \frac{F_{max}}{k_R} ln2 \tag{4}$$

$$t^2_{1/2} = \frac{\alpha}{2kR} \ln(3 - 2F_{max}) \tag{5}$$

Both models are suitable for describing the CisPt release (see R^2 in Table 1), with the presence of NGO making the release better described by reversible second-order kinetics. In the absence of NGO, a fast CisPt release was recorded (M_t/M_0 of 0.90 after 20 h), with high α value indicating a low affinity of the drug towards the carrier phase (γ-Fe_2O_3). On other hand, the strong interaction between CisPt and NGO [60–62] resulted in a more extended release over time ($F_{max} < 0.8$ even after 250 h), with the same affinity (3.54) recorded for either NGO or γ-Fe_2O_3@NGO. The presence of γ-Fe_2O_3 in γ-Fe_2O_3@NGO was found to slow the release, with reduced kinetic constant (k_R) and $t_{1/2}$ values moving from 19.01 (NGO) to 29.38 (γ-Fe_2O_3@NGO) h. This could be ascribed to the hindrance to the drug diffusion from the NGO to the solvent phase by the oleate coating of γ-Fe_2O_3 nanoparticles [55].

Table 1. R^2 values and kinetic parameters for CisPt release according to the applied mathematical model.

Mathematical Model	Parameter	γ-Fe_2O_3	NGO	γ-Fe_2O_3@NGO
$\frac{M_t}{M_0} = F_{max}\left(1 - e^{-(k_R/M_{max})t}\right)$	R^2	0.9818	0.9822	0.9909
	Fmax	0.98	0.76	0.74
	α	49	3.17	2.85
	k_R (10^{-2})	12.71	2.76	1.85
	$t^1_{1/2}$ (h)	5.35	18.81	27.00
$\frac{M_t}{M_0} = \frac{F_{max}\left(e^{2(\frac{k_R}{\alpha})t} - 1\right)}{1 - 2F_{max} + e^{2(\frac{k_R}{\alpha})t}}$	R^2	0.9340	0.9908	0.9960
	Fmax	0.97	0.78	0.78
	α	32.33	3.54	3.54
	k_R (10^{-2})	18.28	3.42	2.25
	$t^2_{1/2}$ (h)	5.15	19.01	29.38

CisPt loaded γ-Fe_2O_3@NGO were employed in different drug-to-carrier ratios (concentration ranges of 0–25 μg mL^{-1} and 0–10 μM for carrier and drug, respectively, see Figure 8). From the data in Figure 8, it is clear that the lowest toxic concentrations of CisPt (10 μM) is unchanged after loading on the different carriers, with γ-Fe_2O_3@NGO being the most effective vehicle for killing cells.

To investigate the possibility of obtaining a selective vectorization of the drug, a proof of concept experiment was designed by incubating U87 cells with 10 μM CisPt loaded γ-Fe_2O_3@NGO for 24 h kept under the effect of a magnetic field generated by a permanent Nd-Fe-B magnet. As a result of the magnetic carrier driven spatial concentrations of the drug, a selective cell death at the region close to the magnet was reached, even at low drug concentration (10 μM), with no relevant toxicity detected on the region where the magnetic forces were negligible (Figure 9).

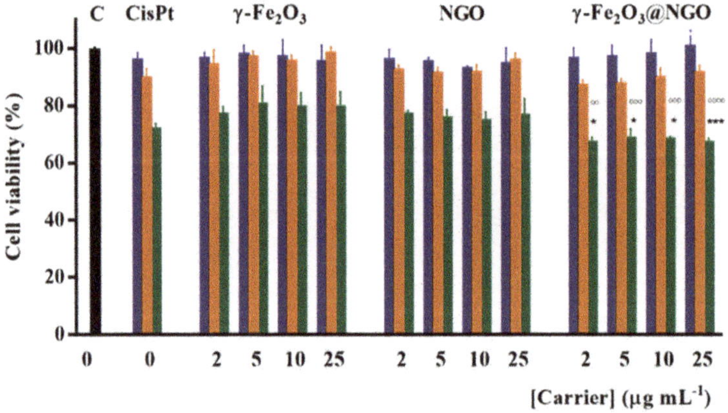

Figure 8. U87 viability after 72 h incubation with CisPt concentrations 2.5 (**blue**); 5.0 (**orange**); and 10.0 (**green**) μM in the free form and after loading on γ-Fe_2O_3; NGO; γ-Fe_2O_3@NGO. Carrier concentrations were 2.0; 5.0; 10.0; and 25.0 μg mL^{-1}. An overall p-value less than 0.05 was accepted as significant. For individual comparisons of γ-Fe_2O_3@NGO (10 μM CisPt) vs. γ-Fe_2O_3 or NGO at the same concentrations, adjusted p-values are indicate as * $p < 0.05$ vs. NGO; *** $p < 0.001$ vs. NGO; °°° $p < 0.001$ vs. γ-Fe_2O_3; °°°° $p < 0.0001$ vs. γ-Fe_2O_3. Error bars represent standard error of the mean (n = 3 independent experiments).

Overall, the obtained results are of great interest for application in cancer therapy for two main outcomes: (i) an effective magnetic vectorization of CisPt to cancer cells can be reached, since a very low amount of CisPt was released in the first 20 h ($M_t/M_0 < 0.30$) and thus negligible side toxicity can be hypothesized, and (ii) the CisPt loaded into γ-Fe_2O_3@NGO is biologically active in reducing the viability of cancerous with an efficiency comparable with that of the free drug.

Future experiments will be performed for evaluating the therapeutic performance of the designed magnetic nanohybrid, by determining the pharmacokinetics profiles with or without a magnetic field, the anticancer activity in appropriate in vivo models, and the possibility to use the system for theranostics applications.

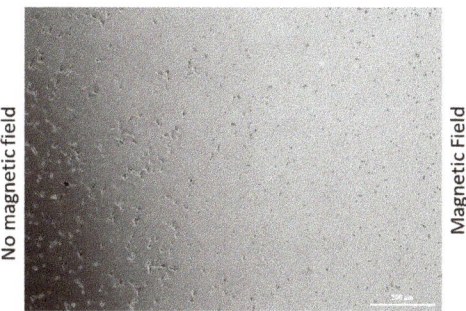

Figure 9. Optical microscope image U87 cells incubated with 10 μM CisPt loaded γ-Fe_2O_3@NGO under the effect of a permanent magnet.

3. Materials and Methods

3.1. Synthesis of Graphite Oxide

Graphite oxide particles were prepared from graphite powder (natural, -200 mesh, 99.9995% purity, Alfa Aesar) by using a modified Hummers method [63]. Graphite powder (1.0 g) was sonicated in water for 5 min, filtrated, washed with water and dried in an oven at 40 °C for 12 h. The dried graphite was transferred to a beaker and mixed with concentrated H_2SO_4 (98%, 23 mL). The mixture was left overnight under stirring at room temperature. Thereafter, 3.0 g $KMnO_4$, as an oxidizing agent, was added gradually while keeping the reaction mixture below 10 °C, in order to decorate the surfaces of graphite by various oxygen groups (hydroxy, epoxy, carboxylic, etc.). After complete addition of $KMnO_4$, the reaction mixture was stirred for 30 min at 35 °C and 45 min at 50 °C for enhancing the degree of oxidation. 46.0 mL of distilled water was added while maintaining the temperature between 98–105 °C for 30 min 10 mL of 30% H_2O_2 was added in order to terminate the reaction. The mixture of GO was washed several times with 5% HCl and water during the suction filtration. The filtrated graphite oxide was dried in an oven at 40 °C for 5 h.

3.2. Synthesis of Nanographene Oxide

NGO particles were prepared as reported previously [46]. The resultant material of graphite oxide was cracked in distilled water with different power percent and sonication time using a horn-tipped ultrasonic probe. The material was separated to different sizes by repeated centrifuge and filtration. SEM images were obtained using a FEI, NOVA NanoSEM200 (FEI, Hillsboro, OR, USA) with an acceleration voltage of 15 kV. AFM images of well-defined NGO sizes were acquired using Digital Instruments Veeco, NanoScope IIIa, operating in the tapping mode. The images were analyzed using WSxM software designed by Nanotech Electronica (Madrid, Spain). The distribution used during this study was approximately 100 nm in lateral size and 6 nm in thickness.

3.3. Synthesis of Maghemite Nanoparticles

Maghemite γ-Fe_2O_3 nanoparticles were synthesized in a three-step procedure as follows: first, the magnetite Fe_3O_4 nanoparticles were prepared by co-precipitation method in basic medium [53]. The synthesis of Fe_3O_4 nanoparticles is shown in Equation (6):

$$2FeCl_3 + FeCl_2 + 8NaOH \rightarrow Fe_3O_4\ (s) + 4H_2O + 8NaCl \quad (6)$$

Briefly, 2.25 g of $FeCl_3{\cdot}6H_2O$ and 0.825 g of $FeCl_2{\cdot}4H_2O$ were mixed in an alkaline solution (NaOH, 1.7 g). The mixture stirred at 65–80 °C for 12 h. The resultant material was filtrated and washed many times by distilled water and ethanol.

Subsequently, magnetite Fe_3O_4 nanoparticles were employed as starting material for the synthesis of maghemite γ-Fe_2O_3. An initial amount of 1.0 g of Fe_3O_4 was placed in furnace and heated up to 450 °C in the presence of Argon and $H_{2(g)}$ for 12 h [54,57]. Thereafter, the reaction was quenched down to room temperature. The resulting material was collected, washed several times in deionized water and ethanol, dried in an oven at 65 °C for 3 h. A second annealing was applied at the same conditions in order to identify the structure of Fe_2O_3 whether it was maghemite or hematite form.

In the final step, 0.5 g of γ-Fe_2O_3 were heated to 60 °C for 15 min separately. Consequently, an excess of sodium oleate (20% wt/vol) was added under vigorous stirring for 15 min. Oleate functionalized nanoparticles were collected by magnetic decantation to remove the non-magnetic materials. The product was washed with water and acetone several times, filtrated and dried in an oven at 40 °C for 2 h.

The relevant X-ray diffraction patterns were performed by using Pert Pro MPD PW3040/60 X-ray diffractometer with Co K_α radiation (λ = 0.179278 nm) at ambient temperature.

3.4. Synthesis of γ-Fe_2O_3@NGO Nanohybrid

An amount of 0.5 g of NGO -100 nm particles was sonicated for 15 min in order to homogenize it in distilled water. The solution was heated up to 60 °C for 15 min directly; an excess of γ-$F_{e2}O_3$ system was added and stirred for 15 min. The final material was separated by magnetic decantation, washed with water and acetone, filtrated and dried in an oven at 40 °C for 2 h. TEM images were recorded on HRTEM/Tecnai F30 [300 kV] (FEI, Hillsboro, OR, USA). TGA was performed on a STA 409 PC/PG-Luxx analyzer (Netzsch, Selb, Germany). Measurements were conducted in a nitrogen atmosphere (flow of 10 mL min^{-1}), with an initial sample weight of ~10 mg in the temperature range 50–900 °C at a heating rate of 10 °C min^{-1}.

Drug loading efficiency (DLE) of γ-Fe_2O_3@NGO for CisPt was estimated by mixing drug and carrier in a 1:1 ratio (by weight) and determining the amount of unloaded CisPt by UV-Vis on a Jasco V-530 UV/Vis spectrometer (Jasco Europe s.r.l., Milan, Italy) at 301 nm [64]. DLE was calculated according to the following Equation (7):

$$DLE\left(mg\ mg^{-1}\right) = \frac{W_D}{W_C} \quad (7)$$

where W_D and W_C are the amount of loaded drug and carrier, respectively. In our condition, to ensure the same amount of drug being loaded on the three carriers (γ-Fe_2O_3@NGO, γ-Fe_2O_3, or NGO) the CisPt loading procedure was performed by mixing, in separate experiments, variable amounts of CisPt solution with the carriers and drying the products under vacuum at RT.

3.5. Magnetic Characterization

Magnetization curves were measured as function of temperature M(T) in the 4 K $\leq$ T $\leq$ 400 K temperature rage, in a SQUID magnetometer (MPMS 5000 from Quantum Design). The Zero-field-cooling (ZFC) and Field-cooling (FC) curves were measured under a field-cooling field H_{FC} = 100 Oe Hysteresis loops M(H) were taken at 4 K and 300 K within the −70 kOe $\leq$ H $\leq$ +70 kOe field range. For all these measurements, the colloids were conditioned in cylindrical sample holders and diamagnetic signal were extracted from the total magnetization.

3.6. In Vitro Cisplatin Release

Release experiments were performed by dialysis methods using 5.0 mL phosphate buffer saline (10^{-3} M, pH 7.4) was releasing media and dialysis tubing cellulose membranes of 25 mm average flat width and 12,000 MW cutoff (Fisher Scientific, Waltham, MA, USA). 5.0 mg nanoparticles (γ-Fe_2O_3@NGO, γ-Fe_2O_3, and NGO) loaded with CisPt were inserted into the dialysis tubes and subject to dialysis. At predetermined time intervals, the amount of CisPt in the releasing media was determined by UV-Vis on a Jasco V-530 UV/Vis spectrometer (Jasco Europe s.r.l., Milan, Italy) at 301 nm [64]. The cumulative amount of drug released (*F*) was calculated using the following Equation (8):

$$F = \frac{M_t}{M_0} \tag{8}$$

where M_t and M_0 are the amounts of drug in solution at time t and loaded into the carrier, respectively. Sink conditions were maintained through the experiment: the maximal theoretical concentration of dissolved CisPt was 0.33 mM, with its solubility being 3.3 mM in these conditions [65].

3.7. Cell Growth Inhibition Assays

Human Glioblastoma cells (U87) were grown as a monolayer in a humidified atmosphere at 37 °C and in 5% CO_2 in the presence of Dulbecco's Modified Eagle Medium (DMEM) supplemented with 10% Fetal bovine serum (FBS), 1% L-glutamine, and 1% penicillin–streptomycin. Treatment effects on U87 cell growth were measured on the basis of the metabolic activity of cells using Alamar Blue assays [66]. Briefly, cells were plated in clear transparent 96-well plates at an optimized cell density of 2.5×10^3 cells per well 48 h prior to treatment. Cells were then treated with either CisPt loaded or unloaded carriers (γ-Fe_2O_3@NGO, γ-Fe_2O_3, NGO) and effects on cell growth assessed 72 h later. Treatments involved the combination of CisPt and carrier concentrations of 2.5; 5.0; 10.0 μM and 2.0; 5.0; 10.0; 25.0 μg mL^{-1}, respectively. Resazurin reduction was measured (excitation 530 nm, emission 590 nm) on a Versamax microplate reader (Molecular Devices, Sunnyvale, CA, USA).

To evaluate the magnetic vectorization ability, viability experiments were performed by treating 250 X 10^3 cells seeded in a 35 mm petri dish with 10 μM CisPt loaded on γ-Fe_2O_3@NGO for 24 h under the effect of a magnetic field generated by a permanent magnet (100 G).

All chemicals were purchased by from Merck/Sigma Aldrich, Taufkirchen, Germany.

3.8. Statistical Analysis

Three experiments were carried out in triplicate. Values were expressed as means ± standard error of the mean. For viability assay, statistical significance was assessed by one-way analysis of variance followed by post-hoc comparison test (Tukey's test). Significance was set at $p < 0.01$.

4. Conclusions

The possibility of CisPt delivery to specific target sites by remote actuation was reached by combining γ-Fe_2O_3 magnetic nanoparticles ensembled into a NGO nanoplatform. The correct assembly of the components was responsible for the efficiency of γ-Fe_2O_3@NGO as a drug delivery system. While NGO conferred high loading capabilities to the nanosystems, the magnetic nanoparticles provided the magnetic actuation capabilities for targeting and delivery of therapeutics.

The mathematical model of the CisPt release profiles suggested a sustained reversible second-order kinetics, which implies low amounts of CisPt released during the first seconds of the experiments. This type of release profile is of major importance if low toxicity levels are required for in vivo applications.

These findings, considered together with the retainment of CisPt toxicity upon loading and the possibility to increase the dose delivered at the target site by a magnetic actuation, make the nanocarrier developed here a valuable tool for applications in cancer therapy.

Author Contributions: Conceptualization, G.C., O.V., and S.H.; formal analysis, S.A.M., F.P.N., and A.A.E.-G.; Investigation, S.A.M., E.V., F.V., A.F., and M.C.; methodology, G.C., O.V., and A.A.E.-G.; Resources, S.H.; supervision, F.I., G.F.G., and S.H.; validation, G.C., O.V., A.A.E.-G., G.F.G., and S.H.; visualization, S.A.M., M.C., and A.A.E.-G.; writing—original draft, G.C.; writing—review and editing, F.I., F.P.N., A.A.E.-G., G.F.G., and S.H.

Funding: This research was funded by the DAAD Re-invitation Programme for Former Scholarship Holders, 2018 (57378442). G.F.G. acknowledges the partial financial support from the Spanish Ministerio de Ciencia, Innovación y Universidades (projectMAT2016-78201-P) and the Aragon Regional Government (DGA, Project No. E26).

Acknowledgments: MIUR Excellence Department Project funds, awarded to the Department of Pharmacy and Health and Nutritional Sciences, University of Calabria (L.232/2016) is acknowledged.

Conflicts of Interest: The authors declare no conflict of interest.

References

1. Ni, D.; Zhang, J.; Bu, W.; Xing, H.; Han, F.; Xiao, Q.; Yao, Z.; Chen, F.; He, Q.; Liu, J.; et al. Dual-targeting upconversion nanoprobes across the blood-brain barrier for magnetic resonance/fluorescence imaging of intracranial glioblastoma. *ACS Nano* **2014**, *8*, 1231–1242. [CrossRef] [PubMed]
2. Huse, J.T.; Holland, E.C. Targeting brain cancer: Advances in the molecular pathology of malignant glioma and medulloblastoma. *Nat. Rev. Cancer* **2010**, *10*, 319–331. [CrossRef] [PubMed]
3. Belhadj, Z.; Ying, M.; Cao, X.; Hu, X.; Zhan, C.; Wei, X.; Gao, J.; Wang, X.; Yan, Z.; Lu, W. Design of Y-shaped targeting material for liposome-based multifunctional glioblastoma-targeted drug delivery. *J. Control. Release* **2017**, *255*, 132–141. [CrossRef]
4. Cohen, Z.R.; Ramishetti, S.; Peshes-Yaloz, N.; Goldsmith, M.; Wohl, A.; Zibly, Z.; Peer, D. Localized RNAi therapeutics of chemoresistant grade IV glioma using hyaluronan-grafted lipid-based nanoparticles. *ACS Nano* **2015**, *9*, 1581–1591. [CrossRef]
5. Dong, H.; Jin, M.; Liu, Z.; Xiong, H.; Qiu, X.; Zhang, W.; Guo, Z. In vitro and in vivo brain-targeting chemo-photothermal therapy using graphene oxide conjugated with transferrin for Gliomas. *Lasers Med. Sci.* **2016**, *31*, 1123–1131. [CrossRef]
6. Gao, H.; Qian, J.; Cao, S.; Yang, Z.; Pang, Z.; Pan, S.; Fan, L.; Xi, Z.; Jiang, X.; Zhang, Q. Precise glioma targeting of and penetration by aptamer and peptide dual-functioned nanoparticles. *Biomaterials* **2012**, *33*, 5115–5123. [CrossRef]
7. Séhédic, D.; Cikankowitz, A.; Hindré, F.; Davodeau, F.; Garcion, E. Nanomedicine to overcome radioresistance in glioblastoma stem-like cells and surviving clones. *Trends Pharmacol. Sci.* **2015**, *36*, 236–252. [CrossRef] [PubMed]
8. Cheng, Y.; Morshed, R.A.; Auffinger, B.; Tobias, A.L.; Lesniak, M.S. Multifunctional nanoparticles for brain tumor imaging and therapy. *Adv. Drug Deliv. Rev.* **2014**, *66*, 42–57. [CrossRef] [PubMed]
9. Pardridge, W.M. Brain drug development and brain drug targeting. *Pharm. Res.* **2007**, *24*, 1729–1732. [CrossRef]
10. Chowdhury, S.M.; Surhland, C.; Sanchez, Z.; Chaudhary, P.; Suresh Kumar, M.A.; Lee, S.; Peña, L.A.; Waring, M.; Sitharaman, B.; Naidu, M. Graphene nanoribbons as a drug delivery agent for lucanthone mediated therapy of glioblastoma multiforme. *Nanomed. Nanotechnol. Biol. Med.* **2015**, *11*, 109–118. [CrossRef] [PubMed]
11. Zhang, C.; Nance, E.A.; Mastorakos, P.; Chisholm, J.; Berry, S.; Eberhart, C.; Tyler, B.; Brem, H.; Suk, J.S.; Hanes, J. Convection enhanced delivery of cisplatin-loaded brain penetrating nanoparticles cures malignant glioma in rats. *J. Control. Release* **2017**, *263*, 112–119. [CrossRef]
12. Duan, X.; He, C.; Kron, S.J.; Lin, W. Nanoparticle formulations of cisplatin for cancer therapy. *Wiley Interdiscip. Rev. Nanomed. Nanobiotechnol.* **2016**, *8*, 776–791. [CrossRef]
13. Ferroni, P.; Della-Morte, D.; Palmirotta, R.; McClendon, M.; Testa, G.; Abete, P.; Rengo, F.; Rundek, T.; Guadagni, F.; Roselli, M. Platinum-based compounds and risk for cardiovascular toxicity in the elderly: Role of the antioxidants in chemoprevention. *Rejuvenation Res.* **2011**, *14*, 293–308. [CrossRef]

14. Chovanec, M.; Abu Zaid, M.; Hanna, N.; El-Kouri, N.; Einhorn, L.H.; Albany, C. Long-term toxicity of cisplatin in germ-cell tumor survivors. *Ann. Oncol.* **2017**, *28*, 2670–2679. [CrossRef] [PubMed]
15. Hartmann, J.T.; Lipp, H.P. Toxicity of platinum compounds. *Expert Opin. Pharmacother.* **2003**, *4*, 889–901. [CrossRef] [PubMed]
16. Ruggiero, A.; Trombatore, G.; Triarico, S.; Arena, R.; Ferrara, P.; Scalzone, M.; Pierri, F.; Riccardi, R. Platinum compounds in children with cancer: Toxicity and clinical management. *Anti Cancer Drugs* **2013**, *24*, 1007–1019. [CrossRef]
17. Cheng, D.; Cao, N.; Chen, J.; Yu, X.; Shuai, X. Multifunctional nanocarrier mediated co-delivery of doxorubicin and siRNA for synergistic enhancement of glioma apoptosis in rat. *Biomaterials* **2012**, *33*, 1170–1179. [CrossRef] [PubMed]
18. Cassano, D.; Santi, M.; Cappello, V.; Luin, S.; Signore, G.; Voliani, V. Biodegradable passion fruit-like nano-architectures as carriers for cisplatin prodrug. *Part. Part. Syst. Charact.* **2016**, *33*, 818–824. [CrossRef]
19. Chung, C.; Kim, Y.K.; Shin, D.; Ryoo, S.R.; Hong, B.H.; Min, D.H. Biomedical applications of graphene and graphene oxide. *Acc. Chem. Res.* **2013**, *46*, 2211–2224. [CrossRef] [PubMed]
20. Kiew, S.F.; Kiew, L.V.; Lee, H.B.; Imae, T.; Chung, L.Y. Assessing biocompatibility of graphene oxide-based nanocarriers: A review. *J. Control. Release* **2016**, *226*, 217–228. [CrossRef] [PubMed]
21. Liu, J.; Cui, L.; Losic, D. Graphene and graphene oxide as new nanocarriers for drug delivery applications. *Acta Biomater.* **2013**, *9*, 9243–9257. [CrossRef] [PubMed]
22. Rahmanian, N.; Eskandani, M.; Barar, J.; Omidi, Y. Recent trends in targeted therapy of cancer using graphene oxide-modified multifunctional nanomedicines. *J. Drug Target.* **2017**, *25*, 202–215. [CrossRef] [PubMed]
23. Deb, A.; Andrews, N.G.; Raghavan, V. Natural polymer functionalized graphene oxide for co-delivery of anticancer drugs: In-vitro and in-vivo. *Int. J. Biol. Macromol.* **2018**, *113*, 515–525. [CrossRef]
24. Arosio, D.; Casagrande, C. Advancement in integrin facilitated drug delivery. *Adv. Drug Deliv. Rev.* **2016**, *97*, 111–143. [CrossRef] [PubMed]
25. Kuila, T.; Bose, S.; Mishra, A.K.; Khanra, P.; Kim, N.H.; Lee, J.H. Chemical functionalization of graphene and its applications. *Progress Mater. Sci.* **2012**, *57*, 1061–1105. [CrossRef]
26. Fangping, O.; Huang, B.; Li, Z.; Xiao, J.; Wang, H.; Xu, H. Chemical functionalization of graphene nanoribbons by carboxyl groups on stone-wales defects. *J. Phys. Chem. C* **2008**, *112*, 12003–12007. [CrossRef]
27. Zhu, S.; Li, J.; Chen, Y.; Chen, Z.; Chen, C.; Li, Y.; Cui, Z.; Zhang, D. Grafting of graphene oxide with stimuli-responsive polymers by using ATRP for drug release. *J. Nanopart. Res.* **2012**, *14*, s11051–s12012. [CrossRef]
28. Orecchioni, M.; Cabizza, R.; Bianco, A.; Delogu, L.G. Graphene as cancer theranostic tool: Progress and future challenges. *Theranostics* **2015**, *5*, 710–723. [CrossRef]
29. Kazemi-Beydokhti, A.; Zeinali Heris, S.; Reza Jaafari, M.; Nikoofal-Sahlabadi, S.; Tafaghodi, M.; Hatamipoor, M. Microwave functionalized single-walled carbon nanotube as nanocarrier for the delivery of anticancer drug cisplatin: In vitro and in vivo evaluation. *J. Drug Deliv. Sci. Technol.* **2014**, *24*, 572–578. [CrossRef]
30. Hilder, T.A.; Hill, J.M. Modelling the encapsulation of the anticancer drug cisplatin into carbon nanotubes. *Nanotechnology* **2007**, *18*. [CrossRef]
31. Tian, L.; Pei, X.; Zeng, Y.; He, R.; Li, Z.; Wang, J.; Wan, Q.; Li, X. Functionalized nanoscale graphene oxide for high efficient drug delivery of cisplatin. *J. Nanopart. Res.* **2014**, *16*. [CrossRef]
32. Wei, Y.; Zhou, F.; Zhang, D.; Chen, Q.; Xing, D. A graphene oxide based smart drug delivery system for tumor mitochondria-targeting photodynamic therapy. *Nanoscale* **2016**, *8*, 3530–3538. [CrossRef]
33. Tran, A.V.; Shim, K.; Vo Thi, T.T.; Kook, J.K.; An, S.S.A.; Lee, S.W. Targeted and controlled drug delivery by multifunctional mesoporous silica nanoparticles with internal fluorescent conjugates and external polydopamine and graphene oxide layers. *Acta Biomater.* **2018**, *74*, 397–413. [CrossRef] [PubMed]
34. Vittorio, O.; Le Grand, M.; Makharza, S.A.; Curcio, M.; Tucci, P.; Iemma, F.; Nicoletta, F.P.; Hampel, S.; Cirillo, G. Doxorubicin synergism and resistance reversal in human neuroblastoma BE(2)C cell lines: An in vitro study with dextran-catechin nanohybrids. *Eur. J. Pharm. Biopharm.* **2018**, *122*, 176–185. [CrossRef]
35. Lerra, L.; Farfalla, A.; Sanz, B.; Cirillo, G.; Vittorio, O.; Voli, F.; Grand, M.L.; Curcio, M.; Nicoletta, F.P.; Dubrovska, A.; et al. Graphene oxide functional nanohybrids with magnetic nanoparticles for improved vectorization of doxorubicin to neuroblastoma cells. *Pharmaceutics* **2019**, *11*. [CrossRef] [PubMed]

36. Yang, K.; Zhang, S.; Zhang, G.; Sun, X.; Lee, S.T.; Liu, Z. Graphene in mice: Ultrahigh in vivo tumor uptake and efficient photothermal therapy. *Nano Lett.* **2010**, *10*, 3318–3323. [CrossRef]
37. Moore, T.L.; Podilakrishna, R.; Rao, A.; Alexis, F. Systemic administration of polymer-coated nano-graphene to deliver drugs to glioblastoma. *Part. Part. Syst. Charact.* **2014**, *31*, 886–894. [CrossRef]
38. Richard, S.; Saric, A.; Boucher, M.; Slomianny, C.; Geffroy, F.; Mériaux, S.; Lalatonne, Y.; Petit, P.X.; Motte, L. Antioxidative theranostic iron oxide nanoparticles toward brain tumors imaging and ROS production. *ACS Chem. Biol.* **2016**, *11*, 2812–2819. [CrossRef]
39. Caetano, B.L.; Guibert, C.; Fini, R.; Fresnais, J.; Pulcinelli, S.H.; Ménager, C.; Santilli, C.V. Magnetic hyperthermia-induced drug release from ureasil-PEO-γ-F_e2O_3 nanocomposites. *RSC Adv.* **2016**, *6*, 63291–63295. [CrossRef]
40. Lee, N.; Yoo, D.; Ling, D.; Cho, M.H.; Hyeon, T.; Cheon, J. Iron oxide based nanoparticles for multimodal imaging and magnetoresponsive therapy. *Chem. Rev.* **2015**, *115*, 10637–10689. [CrossRef]
41. Song, M.M.; Xu, H.L.; Liang, J.X.; Xiang, H.H.; Liu, R.; Shen, Y.X. Lactoferrin modified graphene oxide iron oxide nanocomposite for glioma-targeted drug delivery. *Mater. Sci. Eng. C* **2017**, *77*, 904–911. [CrossRef] [PubMed]
42. Huang, Y.S.; Lu, Y.J.; Chen, J.P. Magnetic graphene oxide as a carrier for targeted delivery of chemotherapy drugs in cancer therapy. *J. Magn. Magn. Mater.* **2017**, *427*, 34–40. [CrossRef]
43. Roca, A.G.; Gutiérrez, L.; Gavilán, H.; Fortes Brollo, M.E.; Veintemillas-Verdaguer, S.; Morales, M.D.P. Design strategies for shape-controlled magnetic iron oxide nanoparticles. *Adv. Drug Deliv. Rev.* **2018**. [CrossRef] [PubMed]
44. Pham, B.T.T.; Colvin, E.K.; Pham, N.T.H.; Kim, B.J.; Fuller, E.S.; Moon, E.A.; Barbey, R.; Yuen, S.; Rickman, B.H.; Bryce, N.S.; et al. Biodistribution and clearance of stable superparamagnetic maghemite iron oxide nanoparticles in mice following intraperitoneal administration. *Int. J. Mol. Sci.* **2018**, *19*. [CrossRef]
45. Kumar, N.; Kulkarni, K.; Behera, L.; Verma, V. Preparation and characterization of maghemite nanoparticles from mild steel for magnetically guided drug therapy. *J. Mater. Sci. Mater. Med.* **2017**, *28*. [CrossRef]
46. Makharza, S.; Cirillo, G.; Bachmatiuk, A.; Vittorio, O.; Mendes, R.G.; Oswald, S.; Hampel, S.; Ruemmeli, M.H. Size-dependent nanographene oxide as a platform for efficient carboplatin release. *J. Mater. Chem. B* **2013**, *1*, 6107–6114. [CrossRef]
47. Rosli, N.F.; Fojtů, M.; Fisher, A.C.; Pumera, M. Graphene oxide nanoplatelets potentiate anticancer effect of cisplatin in human lung cancer cells. *Langmuir* **2019**, *35*, 3176–3182. [CrossRef]
48. Makharza, S.; Vittorio, O.; Cirillo, G.; Oswald, S.; Hinde, E.; Kavallaris, M.; Buechner, B.; Mertig, M.; Hampel, S. Graphene oxide—Gelatin nanohybrids as functional tools for enhanced carboplatin activity in neuroblastoma cells. *Pharm. Res.* **2015**, *32*, 2132–2143. [CrossRef] [PubMed]
49. Arruebo, M.; Fernández-Pacheco, R.; Ibarra, M.R.; Santamaría, J. Magnetic nanoparticles for drug delivery. *Nano Today* **2007**, *2*, 22–32. [CrossRef]
50. Mahmoudi, M.; Sant, S.; Wang, B.; Laurent, S.; Sen, T. Superparamagnetic iron oxide nanoparticles (SPIONs): Development, surface modification and applications in chemotherapy. *Adv. Drug Deliv. Rev.* **2011**, *63*, 24–46. [CrossRef] [PubMed]
51. Mojica Pisciotti, M.L.; Lima, E., Jr.; Vasquez Mansilla, M.; Tognoli, V.E.; Troiani, H.E.; Pasa, A.A.; Creczynski-Pasa, T.B.; Silva, A.H.; Gurman, P.; Colombo, L.; et al. In vitro and in vivo experiments with iron oxide nanoparticles functionalized with DEXTRAN or polyethylene glycol for medical applications: Magnetic targeting. *J. Biomed. Mater. Res. Part B Appl. Biomater.* **2014**, *102*, 860–868. [CrossRef] [PubMed]
52. Calatayud, M.P.; Riggio, C.; Raffa, V.; Sanz, B.; Torres, T.E.; Ibarra, M.R.; Hoskins, C.; Cuschieri, A.; Wang, L.; Pinkernelle, J.; et al. Neuronal cells loaded with PEI-coated Fe_3O_4 nanoparticles for magnetically guided nerve regeneration. *J. Mater. Chem. B* **2013**, *1*, 3607–3616. [CrossRef]
53. Szalai, A.J.; Manivannan, N.; Kaptay, G. Super-paramagnetic magnetite nanoparticles obtained by different synthesis and separation methods stabilized by biocompatible coatings. *Colloids Surf. A Physicochem. Eng. Asp.* **2019**, *568*, 113–122. [CrossRef]
54. Cuenca, J.A.; Bugler, K.; Taylor, S.; Morgan, D.; Williams, P.; Bauer, J.; Porch, A. Study of the magnetite to maghemite transition using microwave permittivity and permeability measurements. *J. Phys. Condens. Matter.* **2016**, *28*. [CrossRef]
55. Mei, Z.; Dhanale, A.; Gangaharan, A.; Sardar, D.K.; Tang, L. Water dispersion of magnetic nanoparticles with selective Biofunctionality for enhanced plasmonic biosensing. *Talanta* **2016**, *151*, 23–29. [CrossRef]

56. Mitchell, R.W.; Edmundson, C.L.; Miller, D.W.; Hatch, G.M. On the mechanism of oleate transport across human brain microvessel endothelial cells. *J. Neurochem.* **2009**, *110*, 1049–1057. [CrossRef] [PubMed]
57. Múzquiz-Ramos, E.M.; Guerrero-Chávez, V.; Macías-Martínez, B.I.; López-Badillo, C.M.; García-Cerda, L.A. Synthesis and characterization of maghemite nanoparticles for hyperthermia applications. *Ceram. Int.* **2014**, *41*, 397–402. [CrossRef]
58. Ryan, S.M.; Brayden, D.J. Progress in the delivery of nanoparticle constructs: Towards clinical translation. *Curr. Opin. Pharmacol.* **2014**, *18*, 120–128. [CrossRef] [PubMed]
59. Reis, A.V.; Guilherme, M.R.; Rubira, A.F.; Muniz, E.C. Mathematical model for the prediction of the overall profile of in vitro solute release from polymer networks. *J. Colloid Interface Sci.* **2007**, *310*, 128–135. [CrossRef] [PubMed]
60. Liu, P.; Wang, S.; Liu, X.; Ding, J.; Zhou, W. Platinated graphene oxide: A nanoplatform for efficient gene-chemo combination cancer therapy. *Eur. J. Pharm. Sci.* **2018**, *121*, 319–329. [CrossRef]
61. Cheng, S.J.; Chiu, H.Y.; Kumar, P.V.; Hsieh, K.Y.; Yang, J.W.; Lin, Y.R.; Shen, Y.C.; Chen, G.Y. Simultaneous drug delivery and cellular imaging using graphene oxide. *Biomater. Sci.* **2018**, *6*, 813–819. [CrossRef] [PubMed]
62. Lin, K.C.; Lin, M.W.; Hsu, M.N.; Yu-Chen, G.; Chao, Y.C.; Tuan, H.Y.; Chiang, C.S.; Hu, Y.C. Graphene oxide sensitizes cancer cells to chemotherapeutics by inducing early autophagy events, promoting nuclear trafficking and necrosis. *Theranostics* **2018**, *8*, 2477–2487. [CrossRef] [PubMed]
63. Makharza, S.; Cirillo, G.; Bachmatiuk, A.; Ibrahim, I.; Ioannides, N.; Trzebicka, B.; Hampel, S.; Ruemmeli, M.H. Graphene oxide-based drug delivery vehicles: Functionalization, characterization, and cytotoxicity evaluation. *J. Nanopart. Res.* **2013**, *15*. [CrossRef]
64. Czarnobaj, K.; Łukasiak, J. In vitro release of cisplatin from sol-gel processed porous silica xerogels. *Drug Deliv. J. Deliv. Target. Ther. Agents* **2004**, *11*, 341–344. [CrossRef]
65. Hall, M.D.; Telma, K.A.; Chang, K.-E.; Lee, T.D.; Madigan, J.P.; Lloyd, J.R.; Goldlust, I.S.; Hoeschele, J.D.; Gottesman, M.M. Say No to DMSO: Dimethylsulfoxide Inactivates Cisplatin, Carboplatin, and Other Platinum Complexes. *Cancer Res.* **2014**, *74*, 3913. [CrossRef] [PubMed]
66. Parmar, A.; Pascali, G.; Voli, F.; Lerra, L.; Yee, E.; Ahmed-Cox, A.; Kimpton, K.; Cirillo, G.; Arthur, A.; Zahra, D.; et al. In vivo [64Cu]$CuCl_2$ PET imaging reveals activity of dextran-Catechin on tumor copper homeostasis. *Theranostics* **2018**, *8*, 5645–5659. [CrossRef] [PubMed]

pharmaceuticals

MDPI

Article

Characterisation of an Isogenic Model of Cisplatin Resistance in Oesophageal Adenocarcinoma Cells

Amy M. Buckley [1], Becky AS. Bibby [2], Margaret R. Dunne [1], Susan A. Kennedy [1], Maria B. Davern [1], Breandán N. Kennedy [3], Stephen G. Maher [1,†] and Jacintha O'Sullivan [1,*,†]

1 Department of Surgery, Trinity Translational Medicine Institute, St. James's Hospital, Trinity College Dublin, Dublin 8, Ireland; bucklea6@tcd.ie (A.M.B.); margaret.a.dunne@gmail.com (M.R.D.); KENNES21@tcd.ie (S.A.K.); DAVERNMA@tcd.ie (M.B.D.); MAHERST@tcd.ie (S.G.M.)

2 Translational Radiobiology Group, Division of Cancer Sciences, University of Manchester, Manchester Academic Health Science Centre, Christie Hospital, Manchester M20 4BX, UK; becky.bibby@manchester.ac.uk

3 UCD Conway Institute & UCD School of Biomolecular and Biomedical Science, University College Dublin, Dublin 4, Ireland; brendan.kennedy@ucd.ie

* Correspondence: osullij4@tcd.ie

† These authors contributed equally to this work.

Received: 19 December 2018; Accepted: 15 February 2019; Published: 20 February 2019

Abstract: Cisplatin (cis-diamminedichloroplatinum) is widely used for the treatment of solid malignancies; however, the development of chemoresistance hinders the success of this chemotherapeutic in the clinic. This study provides novel insights into the molecular and phenotypic changes in an isogenic oesophageal adenocarcinoma (OAC) model of acquired cisplatin resistance. Key differences that could be targeted to overcome cisplatin resistance are highlighted. We characterise the differences in treatment sensitivity, gene expression, inflammatory protein secretions, and metabolic rate in an isogenic cell culture model of acquired cisplatin resistance in OAC. Cisplatin-resistant cells (OE33 Cis R) were significantly more sensitive to other cytotoxic modalities, such as 2 Gy radiation ($p = 0.0055$) and 5-fluorouracil (5-FU) ($p = 0.0032$) treatment than parental cisplatin-sensitive cells (OE33 Cis P). Gene expression profiling identified differences at the gene level between cisplatin-sensitive and cisplatin-resistant cells, uncovering 692 genes that were significantly altered between OE33 Cis R cells and OE33 Cis P cells. OAC is an inflammatory-driven cancer, and inflammatory secretome profiling identified 18 proteins secreted at significantly altered levels in OE33 Cis R cells compared to OE33 Cis P cells. IL-7 was the only cytokine to be secreted at a significantly higher levels from OE33 Cis R cells compared to OE33 Cis P cells. Additionally, we profiled the metabolic phenotype of OE33 Cis P and OE33 Cis R cells under normoxic and hypoxic conditions. The oxygen consumption rate, as a measure of oxidative phosphorylation, is significantly higher in OE33 Cis R cells under normoxic conditions. In contrast, under hypoxic conditions of 0.5% O_2, the oxygen consumption rate is significantly lower in OE33 Cis R cells than OE33 Cis P cells. This study provides novel insights into the molecular and phenotypic changes in an isogenic OAC model of acquired cisplatin resistance, and highlights therapeutic targets to overcome cisplatin resistance in OAC.

Keywords: oesophageal cancer; treatment resistance; cisplatin; metabolism; inflammation; radiation

1. Introduction

Oesophageal cancer is the sixth most common cause of cancer-related mortality globally, and unfortunately, the five-year survival rates remain low at <20% [1,2]. Oesophageal cancer consists of two different histological subtypes: oesophageal squamous cell carcinoma (OSCC) and oesophageal adenocarcinoma (OAC) [1]. In recent years, the epidemiology of oesophageal cancer dramatically shifted, wherein OAC is now the most prevalent subtype in the Western world [3]. The increasing OAC incidence in Western countries has paralleled the increasing rates of obesity, which is a known risk factor for OAC [4].

The current standard treatment of care for oesophageal cancer focusses on neoadjuvant treatment with chemotherapy alone (neoCT) or in combination with radiation, and neoadjuvant chemoradiation (neoCRT) for locally advanced tumours prior to surgery [5]. Despite the improvements demonstrated with neoadjuvant treatment versus surgery alone, only ~30% of patients achieve a complete pathological response to neoadjuvant treatment, which is a proxy for improved overall survival [6]. Surgery offers the best chance of locoregional control, and neoadjuvant treatment aims to reduce tumour burden prior to surgery to improve post-operative outcome. Thus, it is critical to improve response rates to neoadjuvant therapy to increase patient survival [5,7,8]. Treatment resistance is a major cause of treatment failure, and it is crucial to understand the molecular mechanisms and markers governing the treatment resistance phenotype.

Cisplatin is a platinum-based chemotherapy that is used to treat a wide number of solid cancers [9]. Cisplatin is administered as part of a neoadjuvant chemotherapy regimen, and is referred to as MAGIC for the treatment of OAC [10]. The MAGIC chemotherapy protocol consists of the administration of epirubicin, cisplatin, and 5-fluorouracil pre-operatively and post-operatively [11,12]. One mechanism by which cisplatin exerts its anti-cancer effect is through the generation of DNA lesions, resulting in the activation of the DNA damage response and the subsequent induction of mitochondrial-mediated apoptosis [9]. Initial responses to cisplatin are often quite promising; however, chemoresistance to cisplatin frequently develops, leading to treatment failure, and a poor response to neoadjuvant treatment is associated with poor outcome. Thus, it is critical to understand the molecular mechanisms governing resistance to cisplatin in OAC. Our first findings investigate cross-resistance and sensitivity to other cytotoxic treatments, including radiation and 5-fluorouracil (5-FU).

OAC is an inflammatory-driven upper gastrointestinal malignancy, and previous studies have reported on the role of inflammation as a negative regulator of response to radiation treatment in OAC [4,13]. Inflammation is linked with cisplatin resistance, and Cui et al. demonstrated that interleukin-7 (IL-7) upregulation was associated with cisplatin resistance in glioma cells [14]. Targeting IL-7 improved cisplatin sensitivity [14]. In the present study, we identify changes in the inflammatory secretome in an isogenic OAC model of cisplatin resistance to increase our understanding of inflammation in cisplatin resistance. Inflammation is also tightly linked to metabolism, as inflammatory cells rely on metabolites generated from the metabolic cycle to maintain their function [15]. Tumours rely on metabolism to fuel their growth, and altered energy metabolism is an emerging hallmark of cancer [16]. Metabolic alterations correlate with treatment resistance in OAC, wherein increased oxygen consumption is linked with a radioresistant phenotype in an isogenic model of OAC radioresistance [17,18]. Furthermore, in a lung cancer model, cisplatin-resistant cells have significantly elevated oxygen consumption rates compared to parental cisplatin-sensitive cells [19]. This paradigm has not yet been explored in a cisplatin-resistant model of OAC.

In this study, we examined the key differences in chemosensitivity, radiosensitivity, gene expression, inflammatory secretions, and metabolism between matched OAC cisplatin-sensitive (OE33 Cis P) cells and OAC cisplatin-resistant (OE33 Cis R) cells. Cisplatin-resistant cells are more sensitive to radiation and 5-FU treatment than cisplatin-sensitive cells. Cisplatin resistance was associated with a number of significant changes in gene expression, where KEGG pathway analysis identified four pathways upregulated in chemoresistant OE33 Cis R cells, including pathways in cancer, tumour growth factor (TGF)-beta signalling, Wnt signalling, and steroid biosynthesis. Eighteen proteins were secreted at significantly altered levels in OE33 Cis R cells compared to OE33 Cis P, with IL-7 secretion at a significantly higher level from chemoresistant OE33 Cis R cells compared with OE33 Cis P cells. Metabolic profiling revealed that the oxygen consumption rate, as a measure of oxidative phosphorylation, was significantly higher in OE33 Cis R cells under normoxic conditions ($p = 0.0040$).

In contrast, under hypoxic conditions, the oxygen consumption rate was significantly lower in OE33 Cis R cells than in OE33 Cis P cells ($p = 0.0078$). This study highlights molecular and phenotypical changes in an isogenic OAC model of acquired cisplatin resistance, and highlights key differences that could be therapeutically targeted to overcome cisplatin resistance in OAC.

2. Results

2.1. OE33 Cis R Cells Are More Sensitive to Radiation and 5-Fluorouracil (5-FU) Treatment

The relative cisplatin sensitivity of the parental cell line, OE33 Cis P, and the age and passage-matched cisplatin resistant subclone, OE33 Cis R, was evaluated by clonogenic assay. The treatment of cisplatin-sensitive OAC cells with the IC_{50} of cisplatin was previously determined in CCK8 assay (Figure 1); 1.3 μM of cisplatin significantly reduced the surviving fraction of OE33 Cis P cells to 0.303 compared to untreated OE33 Cis P cells, $p = 0.0108$ (Figure 2A). However, 1.3 μM of cisplatin did not significantly alter the surviving fraction of OE33 Cis R cells (0.944 ± 0.042 compared to untreated OE33 Cis R cells), which in itself was significantly higher than the surviving fraction of the OE33 Cis P cells treated with 1.3 μM of cisplatin, $p = 0.0011$ (Figure 2A). A ~two-fold higher concentration, 2.8 μM of cisplatin, significantly reduced the surviving fraction of OE33 Cis R cells to 0.604 ± 0.045, which was a reduction of ~39%, $p = 0.0043$ (Figure 2A). Notably, OE33 Cis P cells were not clonogenically viable with 2.8 μM of cisplatin. To investigate whether OE33 cells with acquired cisplatin resistance had altered sensitivity to other treatments, we investigated the response to both clinically relevant doses of radiation and 5-FU. The basal cell survival and radiosensitivity of cisplatin-sensitive OE33 Cis P cells and cisplatin-resistant OE33 Cis R OAC cells were assessed by clonogenic assay. Basal cell survival was assessed in OE33 Cis P and OE33 Cis R to determine if in the absence of any irradiation, there was a difference in surviving fraction. No significant difference was observed between the two cell lines under basal conditions, indicating that there is no longer-term proliferation differences between these cell lines, which might correlate with the altered radiosensitivity phenotypes (Figure 2B). To assess whether acquired cisplatin resistance conferred altered radiosensitivity, OE33 Cis P and OE33 Cis R cells were either mock-irradiated or treated with a single dose of 2 Gy X-ray radiation. Interestingly, OE33 Cis R cells were significantly more radiosensitive than OE33 Cis P cells, $p = 0.0055$ (Figure 2C). Similarly, OE33 Cis R cells were significantly more sensitive to 5-FU compared to the OE33 Cis P cells following 72 h of 5-FU treatment, $p = 0.0032$ (Figure 2D). In summary, OE33 Cis R cells were more radiosensitive and 5-FU chemosensitive when compared to the parental OE33 Cis P cells.

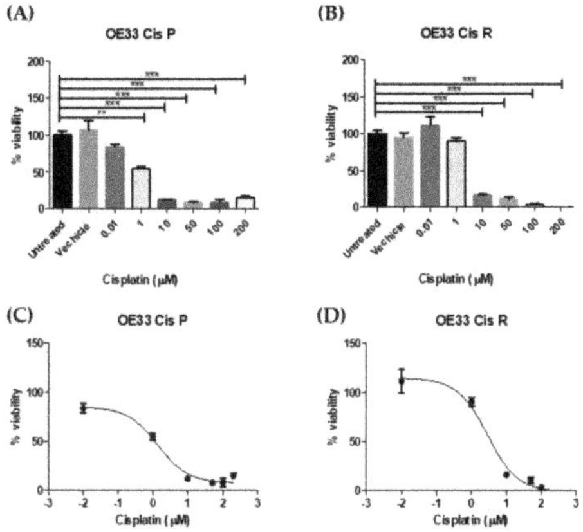

Figure 1. Oesophageal adenocarcinoma (OAC) cisplatin-sensitive (OE33 Cis P) cells were significantly more sensitive to cisplatin-induced cell death than OAC cisplatin-resistant (OE33 Cis R) cells. The toxicity to a range of increasing concentrations of cisplatin in (**A**) OE33 Cis P and (**B**) OE33 Cis R cells following 48 h of treatment was determined using a CCK-8 assay. The 48-h IC_{50} for (**C**) OE33 Cis P cells and (D) OE33 Cis R cells was 1.3 μM and 2.8 μM, respectively (n = 3). ** $p < 0.01$, *** $p < 0.001$ by an unpaired two-tailed *t*-test.

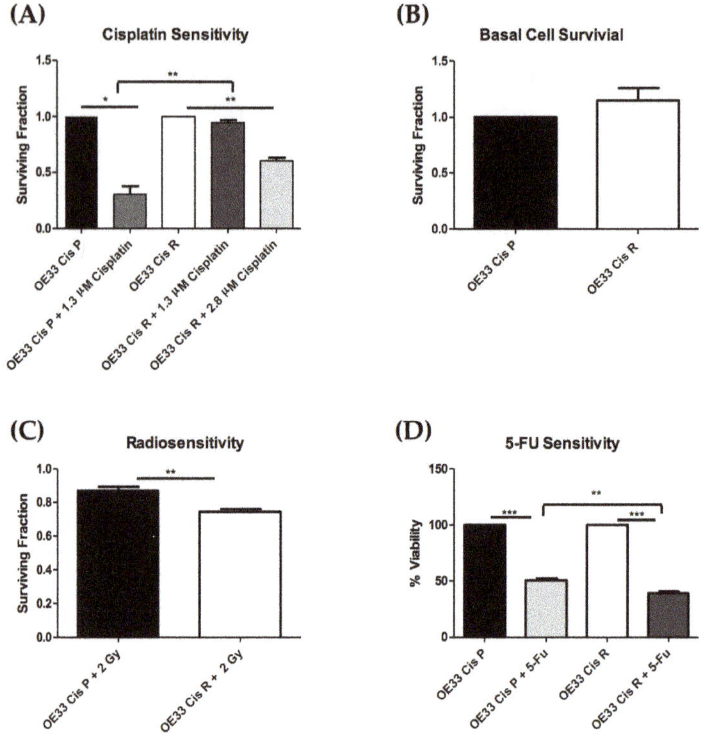

Figure 2. Cisplatin-resistant (OE33 Cis R) oesophageal adenocarcinoma cells are more radiosensitive than cisplatin-sensitive (OE33 Cis P) oesophageal adenocarcinoma (OAC) cells. (**A**) The sensitivity of cisplatin-sensitive (OE33 Cis P) and cisplatin-resistant (OE33 Cis R) OAC cells to cisplatin was assessed by clonogenic assay (n = 3). (**B**) There is no difference in the basal cell surviving fraction of cisplatin-sensitive and cisplatin-resistant OAC cells cultured in RPMI media, (n = 3). (**C**) Surviving fraction of Cis P and Cis R OAC cells following treatment of one 2 Gy fraction of irradiation, (n = 3). (**D**) The viability of the OE33 Cis R cells was significantly decreased compared to the OE33 Cis P when treated with 12 µM of 5-fluorouracil (5-FU) (n = 4). An unpaired *t*-test was used to compare between different cell lines, and a paired *t*-test was used to compare between the same cell line. Data presented as ±SEM * $p < 0.05$, ** $p < 0.01$, *** $p < 0.0001$.

2.2. Gene Expression Is Significantly Altered in OE33 Cis R Cells

OE33 Cis R cells have increased ALDH1 activity, which is a marker of stemness, compared to OE33 Cis P cells [20]. Thus, we investigated whether acquired cisplatin resistance was associated with significant changes in gene expression by whole genome digital gene expression analysis. Of the ~25,000 genes detected, 692 genes were significantly altered, 278 were upregulated, and 414 were downregulated between OE33 Cis P and OE33 Cis R cell lines. Applying a threshold of ±twofold change expression, 42 genes were upregulated (Figure 3A), and 104 genes were downregulated (Figure 3B) in the OE33 Cis R cell line compared to the OE33 Cis P cell line. Kyoto Encyclopedia of Genes and Genomes (KEGG) pathway analysis identified four pathways that were significantly upregulated in OE33 Cis R cells based on the gene expression findings, including: pathways in cancer, TGF-beta signalling, Wnt signalling, and steroid biosynthesis (Table 1A). Furthermore, eight KEGG pathways were downregulated in OE33 Cis R cells, including the MAPK signalling pathway, complement and coagulation cascades, RIG-I-like receptor signalling, sulfur metabolism, NOD-like receptor signalling, cell adhesion molecules, B cell receptor signalling, and Notch signalling (Table 1B).

In summary, OE33 Cis R cells with acquired cisplatin resistance have a significantly altered gene expression profile compared to matched cisplatin sensitive OE33 Cis P cells.

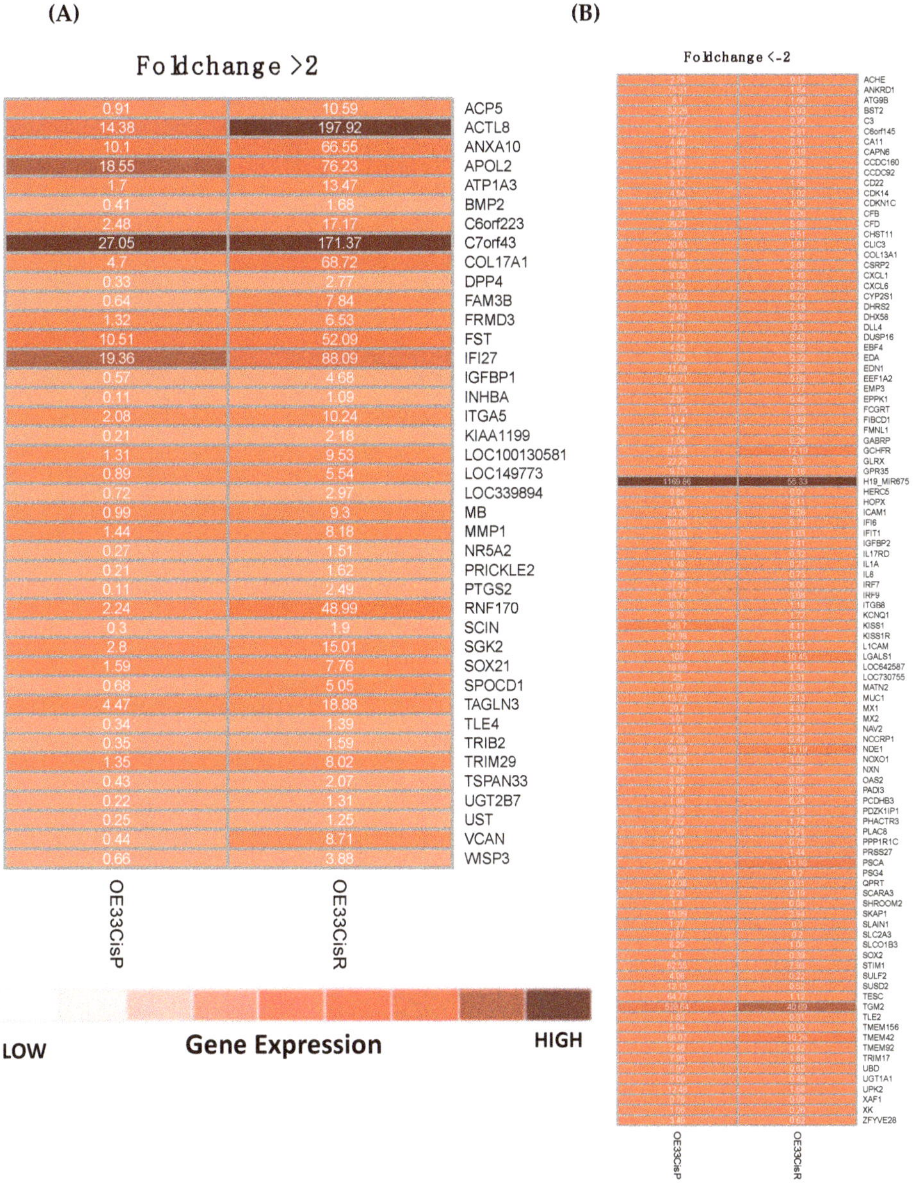

Figure 3. OE33 Cis R cells have a significantly altered gene expression profile compared to OE33 Cis P cells. Heatmaps were generated from gene expression data after applying a fold change filter ±two. (**A**) Heatmap showing 42 genes that were significantly upregulated in OE33 Cis R cells with a fold change of greater than two. (**B**) Heatmap showing 104 genes which were significantly downregulated in OE33 Cis R cells with a fold change of less than minus two. Gene expression values shown as Fragments Per Kilobase of transcript per Million mapped reads (FKPM).

Table 1. Kyoto Encyclopaedia of Genes and Genomes (KEGG) pathway analysis identifies significant pathway differences in OE33 Cis P versus OE33 Cis R cells. (**A**) KEGG pathway analysis of gene expression data identified four pathways that were significantly upregulated in OE33 Cis R cells compared to OE33 Cis P cells. (**B**) KEGG pathway analysis of gene expression data identified eight pathways that were significantly downregulated in OE33 Cis R cells compared to OE33 Cis P cells.

(**A**)

KEGG Pathway Term	Number of Identified Genes Involved	*p* Value	Gene Names
hsa05200:Pathways in cancer	13	5.29×10^{-3}	BMP4, PPARD, BMP2, BCR, PTGS2, EPAS1, PIK3CB, FOXO1, KITLG, MLH1, MMP1, RAC2, WNT9A
hsa04350:TGF-beta signalling pathway	6	1.21×10^{-2}	BMP4, INHBA, BMP2, ID2, ID1, FST
hsa00100:Steroid biosynthesis	3	2.92×10^{-2}	CYP27B1, LIPA, DHCR24
hsa04310:Wnt signalling pathway	6	9.19×10^{-2}	SENP2, PPARD, RAC2, PRICKLE2, FRAT2, WNT9A

(**B**)

KEGG Pathway Term	Number of Identified Genes Involved	*p* Value	Gene Names
hsa04010:MAPK signaling pathway	17	2.61×10^{-4}	FGFR3, PDGFA, RELB, CACNG6, CACNG4, NR4A1, STK3, JMJD7-PLA2G4B, RASGRP3, DUSP14, JMJD7, DUSP16, RRAS, HSPB1, TRAF6, GADD45B, PLA2G4B, IL1A, DUSP6
hsa04610:Complement and coagulation cascades	7	4.23×10^{-3}	PLAT, C3, CFB, SERPINA1, CFD, F2R, PLAUR
hsa04622:RIG-I-like receptor signaling pathway	6	2.09×10^{-2}	IFIH1, ISG15, IL8, IRF7, TRAF6, DHX58
hsa00920:Sulfur metabolism	3	2.84×10^{-2}	CHST11, CHST13, SULT2B1
hsa04621:NOD-like receptor signaling pathway	5	4.95×10^{-2}	CXCL1, IL8, IL18, TRAF6, BIRC3
hsa04514:Cell adhesion molecules (CAMs)	7	7.50×10^{-2}	ICAM1, CLDN9, CLDN3, ITGB8, PVRL2, CD22, L1CAM
hsa04662:B cell receptor signaling pathway	5	8.68×10^{-2}	RASGRP3, CD22, PIK3AP1, MALT1, VAV1
hsa04330:Notch signaling pathway	4	8.75×10^{-2}	HES5, DTX2, DLL4, RBPJ

2.3. Acquisition of Cisplatin Resistance Results in an Alerted Inflammatory Secretome

OAC is an inflammatory-driven upper gastrointestinal cancer, and previous studies have reported inflammation as a negative regulator of response to radiation treatment in OAC [13,21]. However, a link between inflammation and cisplatin resistance in OAC has not yet been investigated. To determine if cisplatin-resistant OE33 Cis R cells have an altered inflammatory secretome to cisplatin-sensitive OE33 Cis P OAC cells, a 47-analyte multiplex enzyme linked immunosorbent assay (ELISA) was conducted. Twenty-three proteins of 47 analytes were detected in either one or both cell lines. IL-7 was secreted at significantly higher levels from OE33 Cis R cells, $p = 0.0191$ (Figure 4A). Seventeen proteins were secreted at significantly lower levels from OE33 Cis R cells compared OE33 Cis P cells, including C-reactive protein (CRP), IL-12p70, IL-10, TNFα, macrophage-derived chemokine (MDC), intracellular adhesion molecule 1 (ICAM-1), IL-6, IL-1β, IL-13, serum amyloid A (SAA), TARC, IL-4, IL-8, IL-1RA, IL-1α, IL-2, and IP-10, as shown in Figure 4 ($p < 0.05$). There was no significant difference in the secreted levels of five of the 23 proteins detected; MCP-1, VEGF-A, VCAM, GM-CSF, and IL-15 between the cell lines (Supplemental Figure S1). OE33 Cis R cells have an altered inflammatory secretome compared to cisplatin-sensitive OE33 Cis P cells, where OE33 Cis R cells have reduced levels of a number of inflammatory chemokines and cytokines and vascular injury proteins except for IL-7, which is secreted at significantly higher levels from OE33 Cis R OAC cells.

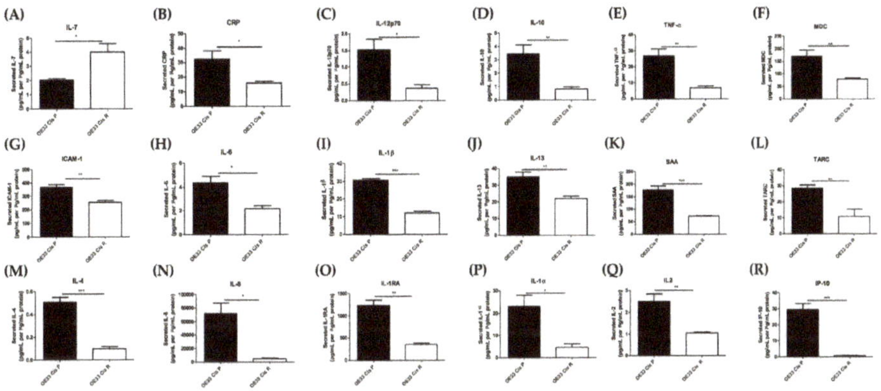

Figure 4. Inflammatory protein secretions are significantly different in cisplatin-sensitive (OE33 Cis P) versus cisplatin-resistant (OE33 Cis R) OAC cells. The secreted levels of 47 proteins in Cis P and Cis R cells was evaluated by multiplex ELISA; 23 proteins were detected in supernatant of Cis P and Cis R cells; 18 proteins were significantly different between the two cell lines, and interleukin-7 was significantly higher in Cis R cells compared to Cis P cells. Secreted levels of (**A**) Interleukin-7 (IL-7) (**B**) C-reactive protein (CRP) (**C**) Interleukin 12p70 (IL-12p70) (**D**) Interleukin 10 (IL-10) (**E**) Tumour necrosis factor α (TNF-α) (**F**) Macrophage-derived chemokine (MDC) (**G**) Intracellular adhesion molecule 1 (ICAM-1) (**H**) Interleukin 6 (IL-6) (**I**) Interleukin 1β (IL-1β) (**J**) Interleukin 13 (IL-13) (**K**) Serum amyloid A (SAA) (**L**) Thymus and activation regulated chemokine (TARC) (**M**) Interleukin 4 (IL-4) (**N**) Interleukin 8 (IL-8) (**O**) Interleukin 1 receptor antagonist (IL-1RA) (**P**) Interleukin 1α (IL-1α) (**Q**) Interleukin 2 (IL-2) (**R**) Interferon gamma-induced protein 10 (IP-10) in OE33 Cis P and OE33 Cis R cells, all secretions normalised to protein content. (n = 4). Unpaired *t*-test. * $p < 0.05$, ** $p < 0.01$, *** $p < 0.001$. Date expressed as ±SEM.

We also compared our findings from our gene expression study (Figure 3) to our inflammatory secretome data described in this section to determine if there was any overlap between the two datasets. In both our gene expression data (Figure 3B) and inflammatory secretome dataset (Figure 4G, 4N, 4P) ICAM-1, IL-8, and IL-1α were both expressed and secreted at significantly lower levels from OE33 Cis R cells compared to OE33 Cis P cells (Table 2).

Table 2. Differences in gene expression and protein secretion values of ICAM-1, IL-8, and IL-1α in OE33 Cis P and OE33 Cis R cells. This table shows the mean values of data that were used to calculate the significant differences in gene expression and protein secretions previously illustrated in Figures 3B and 4G, 4N, 4P. Fragments Per Kilobase of transcript per Million mapped reads (FKPM).

Protein	OE33 Cis P Mean Gene Expression (FPKM)	OE33 Cis R Mean Gene Expression (FPKM)	OE33 Cis P Mean Protein Secretion (pg/mL per µg/mL Protein)	OE33 Cis R Mean Protein Secretion (pg/mL per µg/mL Protein)
ICAM-1	25.26	6.08	365.64	254.39
IL-8	7.68	0.73	71822.10	4611.60
IL-1α	1.49	0.27	23.10	4.56

2.4. OE33 Cis R Cells Have an Altered Metabolic Phenotype Compared to the Parental OE33 Cis P Cells

Altered mitochondrial function is linked with treatment resistance in OAC; thus, we wanted to investigate the association between cisplatin resistance and metabolism in our model of OAC-acquired cisplatin resistance [17]. To investigate whether cisplatin-resistant OE33 Cis R cells have altered energy metabolism, we measured the two major energy pathway—oxidative phosphorylation and glycolysis—using the Seahorse XFe24 analyser under normoxic and hypoxic conditions. OE33 Cis R cells have a significantly higher ($p = 0.0040$) oxygen consumption rate (OCR), which is a measure of oxidative phosphorylation compared to OE33 Cis P cells, under normoxia. However, the oxygen consumption rate of OE33 Cis R cells was significantly lower than OE33 Cis P cells under low oxygen conditions (0.5% O_2), $p = 0.0078$, (Figure 5A). There was no significant difference in the extracellular acidification rate (ECAR), which is a measure of glycolysis, between the two cell lines under normoxic or hypoxic conditions (Figure 5B). To further investigate changes in cellular energetics both OE33 Cis P and OE33 Cis R cells were treated with oligomycin (a mitochondrial complex V inhibitor and antimycin A (a mitochondrial complex III inhibitor), which inhibit specific processes in the electron transport chain. Oligomycin and antimycin produced a similar level of OCR inhibition in both OE33 Cis P and OE33 Cis R cells, and there was no significant difference in the rate of ATP production or proton leak between cisplatin-sensitive and cisplatin-resistant cells under normoxic or hypoxic conditions (Figure 5C,D). Furthermore, treatment of OE33 Cis P and OE33 Cis R cells with the uncoupling agent carbonyl cyanide-*p*-trifluoromethoxyphenylhydrazone (FCCP) showed no significant difference in maximal respiration rate between the cell lines (Figure 5E). In addition, the rate of non-mitochondrial respiration was not significantly altered between the two cell lines (Figure 5F). In summary, OE33 Cis R cells have an alerted metabolic phenotype whereby they have a significantly elevated OCR compared to parental OE33 Cis P cells under normoxic conditions, and OE33 Cis R cells have significantly lower OCR under hypoxic conditions.

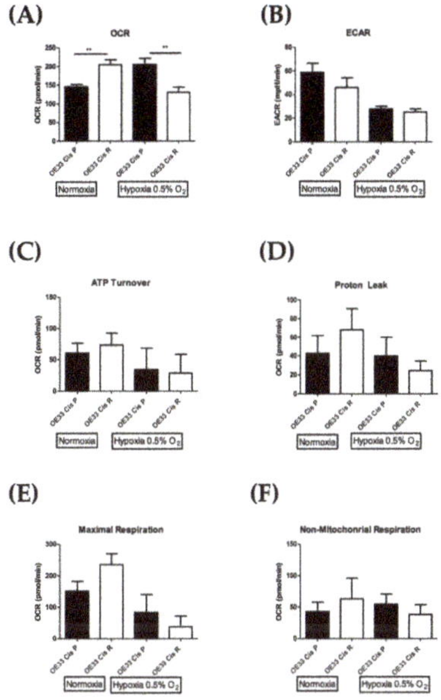

Figure 5. Cisplatin-resistant (OE33 Cis R) oesophageal adenocarcinoma cells have an altered metabolic phenotype compared to cisplatin-sensitive (OE33 Cis P) cells under normoxic and hypoxic conditions (0.5% O_2). (**A**) The oxygen consumption rate (OCR), which is a measure of oxidative phosphorylation, was evaluated in OE33 Cis P and OE33 Cis R OAC cells using the Seahorse Biosciences XFe24 extracellular flux analyser cultured under normoxic and hypoxic conditions (0.5% O_2). OE33 Cis R cells have a significantly higher OCR when compared to OE33 Cis P; cisplatin-sensitive cells, under normoxic conditions (n = 5), unpaired *t*-test, ** $p < 0.01$. (**B**) The extracellular acidification rate (ECAR), which is a measure glycolysis, was evaluated in OE33 Cis P and OE33 Cis R cells using the Seahorse Biosciences XFe24 extracellular flux analyser cultured under normoxic and hypoxic conditions (0.5% O_2), (n = 5), unpaired *t*-test. (**C**) Difference in the rate of ATP production in OE33 Cis P and OE33 Cis R cells cultured under normoxic and hypoxic conditions (0.5% O_2), (n = 5), unpaired *t*-test. (**D**) Difference in the rate of proton leak in OE33 Cis P and OE33 Cis R cells cultured under normoxic and hypoxic conditions (0.5% O_2), (n = 5), unpaired *t*-test. (**E**) Difference in maximal respiration rate in OE33 Cis P and OE33 Cis R cells cultured under normoxic and hypoxic conditions (0.5% O_2), (n = 5), unpaired *t*-test. (**F**) Difference in non-mitochondrial respiration in OE33 Cis P and OE33 Cis R cells cultured under normoxic and hypoxic conditions (0.5% O_2), (n = 5), unpaired *t*-test. Data presented as ±SEM.

3. Discussion

Cisplatin is a widely use chemotherapeutic drug for the treatment of solid cancers, including OAC; however, the development of chemoresistance to cisplatin hinders the success of this agent [9]. Previous studies in cisplatin-resistant cancer cell lines of various tissue origin report multiple mechanisms responsible for enhanced resistance, and that the cisplatin-resistant phenotype is the result of multiple microRNA, gene, and protein expression changes [22–24]. Molecular mechanisms commonly associated with cisplatin resistance include alterations in DNA repair, drug influx/efflux, drug detoxification, cell cycle dysregulation, and evasion of apoptosis [25]. In this study, we sought to characterise the key differences linked to resistance in an isogenic model of OAC cisplatin resistance, including relative chemosensitivity and radiosensitivity, whole gene expression, inflammatory protein secretions, and metabolic phenotype.

Chemoresistant OE33 Cis R cells have a significant acquired resistance to cisplatin compared to cisplatin-sensitive OE33 Cis P cells. Interestingly, cisplatin-resistant OE33 Cis R cells are more radiosensitive than matched OE33 Cis P cells. Cisplatin is often administered in combination with radiation for the treatment of numerous solid cancers, including oesophageal, head, neck, and cervical cancer [26–29]. Cisplatin has been widely shown to enhance radiosensitivity, which is potentially through the non-homologous end joining (NHEJ) DNA repair pathway [30,31]. As cisplatin is often given in combination with radiation to improve response, it was surprising that OE33 Cis R cells are more radiosensitive than OE33 Cis P cells. OE33 Cis R cells can overcome cytotoxic insult from cisplatin to a greater degree than OE33 Cis P cells, but cannot overcome radiation-induced DNA damage as efficiently as they could before the acquisition of cisplatin resistance. Whilst it was unexpected that OE33 Cis R cells are more radiosensitive, as DNA is the common target of both cisplatin and radiation, the mechanisms of action in yielding lethal events, delivery methods, and repair systems as a result of both treatments are very different. Cisplatin has to cross the plasma membrane and traffic to the nucleus; this is a process during which it can be affected in several ways, such as influx via CTR1, efflux via ABC transporters, detoxification by glutathione, trapping in lysosomes, altered trafficking between the plasma membrane and the nucleus, as well as DNA repair proficiency [32,33]. Radiation, on the other hand, largely influences DNA damage through water radiolysis (70%), and has direct effects on DNA bases (30%), but is also subject to energy transfer, glutathione scavenging, oxygen fixation, and DNA repair proficiency [34]. Radiation is responsible for the induction of double-strand breaks in DNA, whereas cisplatin treatment results in the formation of DNA adducts as a result of covalent bonds [31]. Additionally, cisplatin largely employs homologous recombination and nucleotide excision repair as its major pathways of repair, while radiation employs non-homologous end joining, base excision repair, single-strand break repair and, to a much lesser extent, homologous recombination. Thus, the DNA repair mechanics that were employed by cancer cells following either radiation or cisplatin treatment are quite different, and the significance of DNA repair in potentially driving this phenotype requires further mechanistic investigation in the future. Furthermore, OE33 Cis R cells were found to be more sensitive to 5-FU treatment compared to OE33 Cis P cells. A previous study established cisplatin-resistant and 5-FU-resistant OAC OE19 cell lines [35]. Interestingly, miRNA expression profiling in the OE19 cisplatin-resistant cell line and the OE19 5-FU-resistant cell line identified a large number of miRNA that were significantly differentially expressed in comparison to the relatively chemosensitive controls [23,31]. In the OE19 cisplatin-resistant cells 18 miRNAs were significantly dysregulated compared to controls (13 downregulated, five upregulated), of which 11 were validated including: miR-455-3p, miR-200b-3p, let-7e-5p, miR-181b-5p, miR-125a-5p, miR-181a-5p, miR-200b-5p, miR-31-5p, miR-200a-3p, miR-638, and miR-191-5p. Interestingly, the miRNA expression profile of the cisplatin-resistant cell line differed from the miRNA expression profile of the 5-FU-resistant cell line [23,31]. The differential miRNA expression profiles may be associated with the different mechanisms by which cisplatin and 5-FU induce cytotoxic damage.

The gene expression data that were presented in this study provide indications as to the potential mechanisms associated with enhanced resistance to cisplatin in the OE33 Cis R cells compared to the OE33 Cis P cells. Cell membrane transporter genes *ATP1A3*, *ABCA12*, *TMEM199*, and *TMEM22* were upregulated in the OE33 Cis R, and *TMEM156* and *TMEM42* were downregulated. The existing literature is limited with regards to these genes; however, they are members of cell membrane transporter families, some of which are associated with transport and the cellular accumulation of cisplatin, such as ATP7A/B and TMEM205 [25]. Upregulated Wnt signalling and the EMT pathway are also associated with cisplatin resistance [36,37]. The upregulation of the *PRICKLE2* gene may contribute to an increase in Wnt signalling in the OE33 Cis R cell line [38]. The *CDKN1C* gene produces the cyclin-dependent kinase inhibitor p57, which functions as a tumour suppressor in multiple cancer types [39]. Furthermore, the overexpression of p57 has been shown to enhance cisplatin sensitivity in-vitro via intrinsic mitochondrial apoptosis [40]. The downregulation of the *CDKN1C* gene in the OE33 Cis R cell line may contribute to the evasion of apoptosis and cellular resistance to cisplatin. Interestingly, TGF-β signalling, which was identified by KEGG pathway analysis to be upregulated in OE33 Cis R cells, has previously been linked to cisplatin resistance in nasopharyngeal and head and neck cancer; it would be of interest in the future to further understand the role Of TGF-β signalling in cisplatin resistance in OAC [41,42].

KEGG pathway analysis also revealed that the complement pathway was downregulated in cisplatin-resistant cells; this was an interesting finding, as levels of complement C3a and C4a of the classically activated pathway have previously been shown to be predictive of response to neoadjuvant chemoradiation therapy in OAC [13]. Considering this, we sought to investigate the larger inflammatory secretome of OAC cisplatin-resistant OE33 Cis R cells compared to that of cisplatin-sensitive OE33 Cis P cells. OAC is an inflammatory-driven cancer; thus, it is vital to understand the potential contributions of inflammatory secretions to cisplatin resistance. OE33 Cis R cells have a significantly altered inflammatory profile; only one protein, IL-7, was secreted at higher levels from OE33 Cis R cells. Whereas, 17 proteins (CRP, IL-12p70, IL-10, TNFα, MDC, ICAM-1, IL-6, IL-1β, IL-13, SAA, TARC, IL-4, IL-8, IL-1RA, IL-1α, IL-2, and IP-10) were secreted at significantly lower levels from in OE33 Cis R cells compared OE33 Cis P cells. Three of the proteins detected—ICAM-1, IL-1α and IL-8—were also found to be altered at the gene level, where they were both expressed and secreted at significantly lower levels from OE33 Cis R cells compared with OE33 Cis P cells. In a human glioma cancer model, the expression of IL-7 was positively correlated with the IC_{50} of cisplatin in both cell lines and glioma patient samples, and the overexpression of IL-7 further increased cisplatin resistance in glioma cancer cells [14]. This study supports our findings and further highlights IL-7 as a potential mediator of cisplatin resistance in OAC. IL-7 may be a useful therapeutic target for enhancing cisplatin sensitivity in OAC, and this warrants further investigation in the future.

Interleukin-1 alpha (IL-1α) is a potent inflammatory cytokine that plays a pivotal role in the inflammatory response [43]. IL-1α was both expressed and secreted at significantly lower levels from OE33 Cis R cells when compared to OE33 Cis P cells. Interestingly, IL-1α has previously been shown to play a key role in cisplatin sensitivity in human ovarian cancer cells, whereby IL-1α was shown to enhance sensitivity to cisplatin [44]. IL-1α given in combination with cisplatin was shown to enhance the anti-proliferative effect of cisplatin, increase cisplatin uptake, and increase DNA-platination in human ovarian OVCAR-3 cells [44]. Given that we have shown IL-1α to be expressed and secreted at a lower level in cisplatin resistant cells, it would be of interest to evaluate the potential chemosensitising effect of combining IL-1α with cisplatin in OE33 Cis R cells.

Similarly, intracellular adhesion molecule-1 (ICAM-1) was found to be both expressed and secreted at significantly lower levels from OE33 Cis R cells compared to cisplatin-sensitive OE33 Cis P cells. The role of ICAM-1 in carcinogenesis and drug resistance is often dependent on the cancer and cell type. ICAM-1 has previously been shown to have anti-cancer activity in numerous studies through its recruitment of immune cells to the tumour [45–47]. Furthermore, cisplatin treatment has been shown to induce ICAM-1 expression in cancer cells; thus, it is not surprising that ICAM-1 is found at lower levels in the cisplatin-resistant cells compared to the OAC cisplatin-sensitive cells [48]. On the other hand, in an oesophageal SCC cancer study, ICAM-1 was reported to enhance cisplatin resistance and tumourigenicity in-vivo. However, it is important to note that this study was carried out in immunodeficient mice [49]. Thus, the potential of targeting ICAM-1 to alter cisplatin sensitivity in OAC needs further exploration, as it has direct effects on numerous cell types, including both cancer and endothelial cells, and is reliant on interactions with the tumour microenvironment.

Inflammation and metabolism are tightly interlinked biological processes whereby inflammatory cells rely on metabolites generated from the metabolic cycle to maintain their function. Given the significant differences in inflammatory protein secretions from OE33 Cis R cells compared to OE33 Cis P cells, we sought to investigate the metabolic profile of our model of acquired cisplatin resistance. Cisplatin-resistant OE33 Cis R cells have an altered metabolic phenotype compared to matched OE33 Cis P cisplatin-sensitive cells. OE33 Cis R cells have an ~40% higher rate of oxygen consumption rate than OAC cisplatin-sensitive cells. Interestingly, a previous study by Lynam-Lennon et al. demonstrated that increased oxygen consumption rate was linked with a radioresistant phenotype in OAC [17]. However, to date, the role of oxidative phosphorylation in cisplatin resistance in OAC has been underexplored. In a human ovarian cancer model of cisplatin resistance, SKOV3/DPP cisplatin-resistant cells had a significantly higher oxygen consumption rate when compared to SKOV3 cisplatin-sensitive cells [50]. The treatment of ovarian cisplatin-resistant cells with a Bcl-2 inhibitor was found to reduce the oxygen consumption rate and enhance cisplatin sensitivity [50]. Additionally, a study by Catanzaro et al. demonstrated that the inhibition of glucose-6-phosphate dehydrogenase could sensitise cisplatin-resistant ovarian cancer cells to cytotoxic death, further highlighting the role of the oxidative phosphorylation pathway in cisplatin resistance [51]. An elevated oxygen consumption rate has also been linked to chemoresistance with other chemotherapies, such as 5-FU. A study by Denise et al. demonstrated that 5-FU-resistant colorectal cancer cells have a significantly higher oxygen consumption rate compared to parental 5-FU sensitive cells. Furthermore, an increased oxygen consumption rate has also been linked to chemoresistance in docetaxel-resistant prostate cancer cells, where treatment with metformin to inhibit oxygen consumption was found to increase chemosensitivity [52]. Thus, it would be of interest to target oxidative phosphorylation in OAC OE33 Cis R cells as a potential mechanism to enhance cisplatin sensitivity. Metabolism is also tightly influenced by environmental conditions, whereby low oxygen conditions can result in the upregulation of hypoxia-inducible glucose transporters [53]. Thus, we investigated the metabolic rate of OE33 Cis P and Cis R cells under hypoxic conditions. The metabolic profile of OE33 Cis R cells is significantly altered under moderate hypoxic conditions (0.5% O_2), where OE33 Cis R cells have a significantly lower oxygen consumption rate than parental OE33 Cis P cells. This result highlights the flexible nature of OE33 Cis R cells, whereby they are able to adapt to environmental conditions and reduce oxygen consumption rate in low oxygen conditions. Hypoxia plays a critical role in cisplatin resistance, and hypoxic tumours often display a high level of resistance to cisplatin [54,55]. Studies in lung cancer have reported that hypoxia can promote the activation of autophagy, resulting in chemoresistance [55]. In addition, cisplatin-resistant lung cancer cells display a hypoxia-induced upregulation of p53, resulting in the activation of p21 transcription, which results in the arrest of the cell cycle at the G0–G1 phase, ultimately reducing the effect of cisplatin [54]. As dynamic regions of hypoxia are found in most solid tumours, including OAC, it is critical to understand how OE33 Cis R cells adapt to their tumour microenvironment to determine the best method to target this cell population. The reduced OCR that is seen in OE33 Cis R under hypoxic conditions is something that needs to be further evaluated in future studies.

This study has investigated a number of key differences in an isogenic model of OAC cisplatin resistance. Importantly, OE33 Cis R cells have a significantly altered gene expression and inflammatory secretome profile compared to cisplatin-sensitive cells. In addition, cisplatin-resistant cells have an altered metabolic profile under normal and low oxygen conditions. The molecular differences identified in this study, including the increased sensitivity to radiation and 5-FU of cisplatin-resistant cells, provides novel insight into cisplatin resistance in OAC, and has identified molecular processes that could be targeted in the future as a means to overcome cisplatin resistance and improve therapeutic outcomes for OAC.

4. Materials and Methods

4.1. Generation of the OE33 Cis P and OE33 Cis R Cell Lines

The human OE33 oesophageal adenocarcinoma cell line was obtained from the European collection of cell cultures. The isogenic model of cisplatin-resistant OAC; Cis P (cisplatin-sensitive) and Cis R (cisplatin-resistant) cells was generated as previously described [20]. Briefly, the original OE33 cells were split to generate two passage-matched flasks of OE33 cells. One flask was mock treated, and the other was treated with a metronomic dosing of cisplatin. Both lines were developed side-by-side and treated identically, differing only in being treated with vehicle or cisplatin until cisplatin-resistant cells were developed.

4.2. *Preparation of Chemotherapeutic Drugs*

Stock solutions of cis-diamminedichloroplatinum (cisplatin) and 5-flurouracil (5-FU) were prepared in phosphate-buffered saline (PBS) and dimethyl sulfoxide (DMSO), respectively. Solutions were sterile filtered and then aliquoted and stored at −20 °C. Prior to use, the solution was incubated at 37 °C and mixed thoroughly.

4.3. *Determining IC_{50} of Cisplatin for OE33 Cis P and OE33 Cis R Cells at Using Cell Counting kit-8 (CCK8) Assay*

OE33 Cis P and OE33 Cis R cells were seeded at 5×10^3 cells/200 µL in complete Roswell Park Memorial Institute (RPMI) 1640 medium supplemented with 10% fetal calf serum (Lonza, Basal, Switzerland) and 1% penicillin-streptomycin (Lonza, Basal, Switzerland) in a 96-well flat-bottomed plate and incubated at 37 °C, 5% CO_2 overnight. Media was replaced with 180 µL of fresh complete RPMI and cells were treated with 20 µL of cisplatin at a range of increasing concentrations (0, 0.01, 1, 10, 50, 100, 200 µM). Cells were incubated for 48 h at 37 °C, 5% CO_2/95% air. 10 µL of cell counting kit-8 (CCK8) assay solution (Sigma-Aldrich, Missouri, USA) was added to each well after 48 h. Cells were incubated at 37 °C, 5% CO_2 for 1.5 to 2 h until appropriate colour development was observed. The absorbance was measured at 450 nm using a VersaMax microplate reader (Molecular Devices, Sunnyvale, CA, USA).

4.4. *Clonogenic Assay*

OE33 Cis P and OE33 Cis R cells were trypsinised, counted, and seeded at the optimised densities of 1–2.5 × 10^3 in 1.5 mL of complete RPMI, in triplicate in six-well plates and allowed to adhere overnight. For chemosensitivity assays, cells were allowed to adhere for 24 h following which time they were treated with vehicle control or cisplatin. OE33 Cis P cells were treated with 1.3 µM of cisplatin, and OE33 Cis R cells were treated with either 1.3 µM or 2.8 µM of cisplatin. For radiosensitivity assays, cell were seeded and allowed to adhere for 48 h following which time OE33 Cis P and OE33 Cis R cells were either irradiated with 2 Gy (dose rate 1.73 Gy/min 195 KV 15 mA) or mock irradiated. Colonies were allowed to grow for 7 to 14 days, at which point they were fixed and stained with crystal violet (0.5%/ 25% *v*/*v* methanol) and allowed to air dry. Colonies consisting of 50 cells or more were counted using a colony counter (GelCount, Oxford Optronix, Oxford, UK). Plating efficiency (PE), which is the fraction of colonies formed by untreated cells, was calculated using the formula: PE = No. colonies/No. cells seeded. The surviving fraction (SF), which was the number of colonies formed following treatment, and was expressed in terms of PE, was calculated using the formula: SF = No. colonies/(No. cells seeded × PE).

4.5. *Irradiation*

Irradiation was performed using a XStrahl X-ray generator, (RS225), at a dose rate of 1.75 Gray per min.

4.6. *RNA Extraction from Cell Lines*

For total RNA extraction and purification, including miRNA, the RNeasy Mini Kit was used as per the manufacturer's instructions (Qiagen, UK). Sterile RNase and DNase-free filter tips were used throughout all of the RNA experiments (TipOne Starlab, UK). Cell pellets (<5 × 10^4 cells) were resuspended in 350 µl of RLT lysis buffer and pellets >five × 104 cells were resuspended in 600 µL of RLT lysis buffer. One volume of 70% ethanol was added to the lysate and mixed well by pipetting. RNeasy mini columns were inserted into the top of two-mL collection tubes. Up to 700 µL of the lysate was added to the columns, which were then centrifuged at 8000× *g* for 15 seconds at room temperature (RT). A 700-µL volume of RW1 buffer was added to the column, and centrifuged 8000× *g* for 15 seconds at RT. The flow through was discarded, and 500 µL of RPE buffer was added to the column and centrifuged at 8000× *g* for 15 s at RT. The flow through was discarded, and 500 μL of buffer RPE was added to the column and centrifuged at 8000× *g* for 2 min at RT. The flow through was subsequently discarded, and the column was transferred to a new 1.5-mL collection tube. A 30 to 50-μL volume of RNase-free water was pipetted directly onto the column membrane and centrifuged for 1 min at 8000× *g* to elute the RNA from the silica membrane of the column. The concentration and purity of the eluted RNA was measured on the NanoDrop ND-1000 (Thermo Scientific, Delaware, USA). Then, RNA extracts were stored at −20 °C in the short term (<one month) or −80 °C in the long term (>one month).

4.7. Digital Gene Expression Sequencing

The gene expression sequencing was outsourced to LC Sciences (Texas, USA). Briefly, six μg total RNA from three biological replicates was prepared in 50-μL of DEPC (diethylpyrocarbonate) water, five μL of 3M of NaOAc, pH 5.2 and 150 μL of absolute ethanol to give a final volume of 205 μL. Samples were stored at −80 °C prior to shipping on dry ice. High-throughput sequencing was performed using Illumina sequencing by synthesis technology. LC Sciences provided analysed gene expression data and KEGG (Kyoto Encyclopaedia of Genes and Genomes) analysis. Gene expression abundance was normalised and evaluated in FPKM (Fragments Per Kilobase of transcript per Million reads) using the Cuffdiff module of Cufflinks_v2.2.1. The q-value was representative of a false discovery rate (FDR) adjusted *p*-value < 0.05. The fold change in gene expression was calculated from the equation: log2 (OE33 Cis R FPKM/OE33 Cis P PMK). Pathway analysis was performed with EASE (Expression Analysis Systematic Explorer). The KEGG pathway *p*-value is based on the EASE score: a modified Fisher exact *p*-value that measures if the probability of the (count/list total) is more than random chance compared to the background list (pop hits/pop total), where 'count' is the number of significant genes in a pathway, 'list total' is the number of genes in the submitted list associated with the category (e.g., KEGG pathway), 'pop hits' is the number of genes in the background list associated with the term, and 'pop total' is the number of genes in the background list associated with the category. Fold enrichment was calculated as (count/list total)/(pop hits/pop total). The lower the *p*-value, the more enrichment of the term. Gene expression changes were considered significant if the *p* value was <0.05. Heatmaps were generated using the 'pheatmap' package for the R project for statistical computing (version 3.5.1) [56,57].

4.8. Multiplex Enzyme Linked Immunosorbent Assay (ELISA)

Supernatant from OE33 Cis P and OE33 Cis R cells were defrosted on ice. The secretion of cytokines and angiogenic growth factors was analysed by ELISA as per the manufacturer's instructions. To assess angiogenic, vascular injury, inflammatory cytokine and chemokine secretions, a 47 multiplex kit spread across seven plates was used (Meso Scale Diagnostics, USA). The multiplex kit was used to quantify the secretions of CRP, Eotaxin, Eotaxin-3, GM-CSF, ICAM-1, IFN-γ, IL-10, IL-12/IL-23p40, IL-12p70, IL-13, IL-15, IL-16, IL-17A, IL-17A/F, IL-17B, IL-17C, IL-17D, IL-1RA, IL-1α, IL-1β, IL-2, IL-21, IL-22, IL-23, IL-27, IL-3, IL-31, IL-4, IL-5, IL-6, IL-7, IL-8, IL-8 (HA), IL-9, IP-10, MCP-1, MCP-4, MDC, MIP-1α, MIP-1β, MIP-3α, SAA, TARC, TNF-α, TNF-β, TSLP, VCAM-1, VEGF-A from OE33 Cis P and OE33 Cis R cell supernatants from cells that had been seeded at 250,000 cells per well for 48 h. Secretion data for all of the factors was normalised appropriately to cell lysate protein content using the BCA assay (Pierce).

4.9. OCR and ECAR Measurements in Cis P and Cis R Cells

OE33 Cis P and OE33 Cis R cells were seeded in five wells per treatment group at a density of 18,000 and 20,000 cells/well, respectively, in 24-well cell culture XFe24 microplates (Agilent Technologies, Santa Clara, CA, USA) at a volume of 100 μL and allowed to adhere at 37 °C in 5% CO_2/95% air. Five hours later, an additional 150 μL/well complete cell culture RPMI medium was added. Following 48 h of incubation, media was removed and cells were washed with unbuffered

Dulbecco's Modified Eagle's medium (DMEM) supplemented with 10 mM of glucose and 10 mM of sodium pyruvate, (pH 7.4) and incubated for one hour at 37 °C in a CO_2-free incubator. The oxygen consumption rate (OCR) and extracellular acidification rate (ECAR) were measured using a Seahorse Biosciences XFe24 Extracellular Flux Analyser (Agilent Technologies, Santa Clara, CA, USA). Three basal measurements of OCR and ECAR were taken over 24 min consisting of three repeats of mix (three min)/wait (2 min)/measurement (3 min) to establish basal respiration. Three additional measurements were obtained following the injection of three mitochondrial inhibitors including oligomycin (Sigma Aldrich, Missouri, USA), antimycin-A (Sigma Aldrich, Missouri, USA) and an uncoupling agent Carbonyl cyanide 4-(trifluoromethoxy)phenylhydrazone (FCCP) (Sigma Aldrich, Missouri, USA). ATP turnover was calculated by subtracting the OCR post oligomycin injection from baseline OCR prior to oligomycin addition. Proton leak was calculated by subtracting OCR post antimycin-A addition from OCR post oligomycin addition. Maximal respiration was calculated by subtracting OCR post antimycin addition from OCR post FCCP addition. Non-mitochondrial respiration was determined as the OCR value post antimycin-A addition. All of the measurements were normalised to cell number using the crystal violet assay, transferring the eluted stain to a 96-well plate before reading. For seahorse experiments carried out under (0.5% O_2) hypoxia, cells were seeded under normoxic conditions and allowed to adhere for 6 h at 37 °C 5% CO_2/95% air, following which time they were placed at 37 °C 0.5% O_2 5% CO_2 in the H35 Don whitley hypoxstation for 48 h, and seahorse measurements were carried out under hypoxia (0.5% O_2) in the i2 Whitley station using the same protocol for measuring rate as described for normoxic conditions.

4.10. Crystal Violet

Cells were fixed with 1% glutaraldehyde (Sigma-Aldrich, Missouri, USA) for 15 min at RT. The fixative was removed, and cells were washed with PBS and stained with 0.1% crystal violet for 30 min at RT. Plates were left to air dry and incubated with 50 µL of 1% Triton X-100 in PBS on a plate shaker for 30 min at RT. Absorbance was read at 595 nm on a VersaMax microplate reader (Molecular Devices, Sunnyvale, CA, USA).

4.11. Statistical Analysis

Statistical analysis was performed using GraphPad Prism version 5 software (GraphPad Software, CA, USA). Scientific data were expressed as mean ± standard error of the mean (SEM). SEM was calculated as the standard deviation of the original samples divided by the square root of the sample size. Specific statistical tests used are indicated in figure legends. For all of the statistical analysis, differences were considered statistically significant at $p < 0.05$.

Supplementary Materials: The following are available online at http://www.mdpi.com/1424-8247/12/1/33/s1, Figure S1: Inflammatory protein in cisplatin sensitive (OE33 Cis P) versus cisplatin resistant (OE33 Cis R) OAC cells. The secreted levels of 47 proteins in Cis P and Cis R cells was evaluated by multiplex ELISA, 23 proteins were detected in supernatant of Cis P and Cis R cells, there was no significant difference in secreted levels of (**A**) Monocyte chemoattractant protein-1 (MCP-1) (**B**) Vascular endothelial growth factor (VEGF-A) (**C**) Vascular adhesion molecule 1 (VCAM-1) (**D**) Granulocyte-macrophage colony-stimulating factor (GM-CSF) (**E**) Interleukin 15 (IL-15) in OE33 Cis P and OE33 Cis R cells, all secretions normalised to protein content. (n = 4). Unpaired *t*-test. Date expressed as ± SEM.

Author Contributions: Conceptualisation, A.M.B., B.A.S.B., S.G.M. and J.O.S.; Data curation, A.M.B. and B.A.S.B.; Formal analysis, A.M.B., B.A.S.B., S.G.M. and J.O.S.; Funding acquisition, M.R.D. and J.O.S.; Investigation, A.M.B., B.A.S.B. and M.R.D.; Methodology, A.M.B., B.A.S.B. and M.R.D.; Software, S.A.K.; Supervision, B.N.K., S.G.M. and J.O.S.; Visualisation, S.A.K.; Writing—original draft, A.M.B.; Writing—review & editing, A.M.B., M.R.D., S.A.K., B.N.K., S.G.M. and J.O.S.

Funding: Funding for this work was provided by the Irish Cancer Society (Grant: CRS15BUC) and Health Research Board (Grant: HRB ILP-POR-2017-055).

Conflicts of Interest: The authors declare no conflicts of interest.

Abbreviations

5-FU	Fluorouracil
Cis	Cisplatin
ECAR	Extracellular Acidification Rate
ELISA	Enzyme Linked Immunosorbent assay
DMEM	Dulbecco's Modified Eagle's medium
IL-1α	Interleukin 1 alpha
IL-7	Interleukin 7
IL-8	Interleukin 8
ICAM-1	Intracellular Adhesion Molecule 1
KEGG	Kyoto Encyclopedia of Genes and Genomes
MiRNA	Micro ribonucleic acid
NeoCRT	Neoadjuvant Chemoradiation Therapy
NHEJ	Non Homologous end joining
OAC	Oesophageal Adenocarcinoma
OCR	Oxidative Phosphorylation
PE	Plating Efficiency
RMPI	Roswell Park Memorial Institute medium
SCC	Squamous Cell Carcinoma
SF	Surviving Fraction
TGF-β	Transforming Growth Factor Beta
VEGF	Vascular Endothelial Growth Factor

References

1. Arnold, M.; Soerjomataram, I.; Ferlay, J.; Forman, D. Global incidence of oesophageal cancer by histological subtype in 2012. *Gut* **2015**, *64*, 381–387. [CrossRef] [PubMed]
2. Ferlay, J.; Soerjomataram, I.; Dikshit, R.; Eser, S.; Mathers, C.; Rebelo, M.; Parkin, D.M.; Forman, D.; Bray, F. Cancer incidence and mortality worldwide: Sources, methods and major patterns in GLOBOCAN 2012. *Int. J. Cancer* **2015**, *136*, E359–E386. [CrossRef] [PubMed]
3. Abbas, G.; Krasna, M. Overview of esophageal cancer. *Ann. Cardiothorac. Surg.* **2017**, *6*, 131–136. [CrossRef] [PubMed]
4. Picardo, S.L.; Maher, S.G.; O'Sullivan, J.N.; Reynolds, J.V. Barrett's to oesophageal cancer sequence: A model of inflammatory-driven upper gastrointestinal cancer. *Digest. Surg.* **2012**, *29*, 251–260. [CrossRef] [PubMed]
5. Cools-Lartigue, J.; Spicer, J.; Ferri, L.E. Current status of management of malignant disease: Current management of esophageal cancer. *J. Gastrointest. Surg. Off. J. Soc. Surg. Aliment. Tract.* **2015**, *19*, 964–972. [CrossRef] [PubMed]
6. Donohoe, C.L.; Reynolds, J.V. Neoadjuvant treatment of locally advanced esophageal and junctional cancer: The evidence-base, current key questions and clinical trials. *J. Thorac. Dis.* **2017**, *9*, S697–S704. [CrossRef] [PubMed]
7. Walsh, T.N.; Noonan, N.; Hollywood, D.; Kelly, A.; Keeling, N.; Hennessy, T.P.J. A Comparison of Multimodal Therapy and Surgery for Esophageal Adenocarcinoma. *N. Engl. J. Med.* **1996**, *335*, 462–467. [CrossRef] [PubMed]
8. Jin, H.-L.; Zhu, H.; Ling, T.-S.; Zhang, H.-J.; Shi, R.-H. Neoadjuvant chemoradiotherapy for resectable esophageal carcinoma: A meta-analysis. *World J. Gastroenterol. WJG* **2009**, *15*, 5983–5991. [CrossRef] [PubMed]
9. Galluzzi, L.; Senovilla, L.; Vitale, I.; Michels, J.; Martins, I.; Kepp, O.; Castedo, M.; Kroemer, G. Molecular mechanisms of cisplatin resistance. *Oncogene* **2012**, *31*, 1869–1883. [CrossRef] [PubMed]
10. Reynolds, J.V.; Preston, S.R.; O'Neill, B.; Baeksgaard, L.; Griffin, S.M.; Mariette, C.; Cuffe, S.; Cunningham, M.; Crosby, T.; Parker, I.; et al. ICORG 10-14: NEOadjuvant trial in Adenocarcinoma of the oEsophagus and oesophagoGastric junction International Study (Neo-AEGIS). *BMC Cancer* **2017**, *17*, 401. [CrossRef]
11. Cunningham, D.; Allum, W.H.; Stenning, S.P.; Thompson, J.N.; Van de Velde, C.J.H.; Nicolson, M.; Scarffe, J.H.; Lofts, F.J.; Falk, S.J.; Iveson, T.J.; et al. Perioperative Chemotherapy versus Surgery Alone for Resectable Gastroesophageal Cancer. *N. Engl. J. Med.* **2006**, *355*, 11–20. [CrossRef]

12. Van Hagen, P.; Hulshof, M.C.C.M.; van Lanschot, J.J.B.; Steyerberg, E.W.; Henegouwen, M.I.V.B.; Wijnhoven, B.P.L.; Richel, D.J.; Nieuwenhuijzen, G.A.P.; Hospers, G.A.P.; Bonenkamp, J.J.; et al. Preoperative Chemoradiotherapy for Esophageal or Junctional Cancer. *N. Engl. J. Med.* **2012**, *366*, 2074–2084. [CrossRef] [PubMed]
13. Maher, S.G.; McDowell, D.T.; Collins, B.C.; Muldoon, C.; Gallagher, W.M.; Reynolds, J.V. Serum proteomic profiling reveals that pretreatment complement protein levels are predictive of esophageal cancer patient response to neoadjuvant chemoradiation. *Ann. Surg.* **2011**, *254*, 809–816. [CrossRef] [PubMed]
14. Cui, L.; Fu, J.; Pang, J.C.-S.; Qiu, Z.-K.; Liu, X.-M.; Chen, F.-R.; Shi, H.-L.; Ng, H.-K.; Chen, Z.-P. Overexpression of IL-7 enhances cisplatin resistance in glioma. *Cancer Biol. Therapy* **2012**, *13*, 496–503. [CrossRef] [PubMed]
15. Andrejeva, G.; Rathmell, J.C. Similarities and Distinctions of Cancer and Immune Metabolism in Inflammation and Tumors. *Cell Metabol.* **2017**, *26*, 49–70. [CrossRef] [PubMed]
16. Hanahan, D.; Weinberg, R.A. Hallmarks of cancer: The next generation. *Cell* **2011**, *144*, 646–674. [CrossRef] [PubMed]
17. Lynam-Lennon, N.; Maher, S.G.; Maguire, A.; Phelan, J.; Muldoon, C.; Reynolds, J.V.; O'Sullivan, J. Altered Mitochondrial Function and Energy Metabolism Is Associated with a Radioresistant Phenotype in Oesophageal Adenocarcinoma. *PLoS ONE* **2014**, *9*, e100738. [CrossRef] [PubMed]
18. Lynam-Lennon, N.; Reynolds, J.V.; Pidgeon, G.P.; Lysaght, J.; Marignol, L.; Maher, S.G. Alterations in DNA repair efficiency are involved in the radioresistance of esophageal adenocarcinoma. *Radiat. Res.* **2010**, *174*, 703–711. [CrossRef]
19. Wangpaichitr, M.; Theodoropoulos, G.; Wu, C.; You, M.; Feun, L.; Kuo, M.T.; Savaraj, N. The Relationship of Thioredoxin-1 and Cisplatin Resistance: Its Impact on ROS and Oxidative Metabolism in Lung Cancer Cells. *Mol. Cancer Ther.* **2012**. [CrossRef]
20. Lynam-Lennon, N.; Heavey, S.; Sommerville, G.; Bibby, B.A.S.; Ffrench, B.; Quinn, J.; Gasch, C.; O'Leary, J.J.; Gallagher, M.F.; Reynolds, J.V.; et al. MicroRNA-17 is downregulated in esophageal adenocarcinoma cancer stem-like cells and promotes a radioresistant phenotype. *Oncotarget* **2017**, *8*, 11400–11413. [CrossRef]
21. Buckley, A.M.; Lynam-Lennon, N.; Kennedy, S.A.; Dunne, M.R.; Aird, J.J.; Foley, E.K.; Clarke, N.; Ravi, N.; O'Toole, D.; Reynolds, J.V.; et al. Leukaemia inhibitory factor is associated with treatment resistance in oesophageal adenocarcinoma. *Oncotarget* **2018**, *9*, 33634–33647. [CrossRef] [PubMed]
22. Stordal, B.; Davey, M. Understanding cisplatin resistance using cellular models. *IUBMB Life* **2007**, *59*, 696–699. [CrossRef] [PubMed]
23. Hummel, R.; Sie, C.; Watson, D.I.; Wang, T.; Ansar, A.; Michael, M.Z.; Van der Hoek, M.; Haier, J.; Hussey, D.J. MicroRNA signatures in chemotherapy resistant esophageal cancer cell lines. *World J. Gastroenterol. WJG* **2014**, *20*, 14904–14912. [CrossRef] [PubMed]
24. Xie, X.-Q.; Zhao, Q.-H.; Wang, H.; Gu, K.-S. Dysregulation of mRNA profile in cisplatin-resistant gastric cancer cell line SGC7901. *World J. Gastroenterol.* **2017**, *23*, 1189–1202. [CrossRef]
25. Shen, D.W.; Pouliot, L.M.; Hall, M.D.; Gottesman, M.M. Cisplatin resistance: A cellular self-defense mechanism resulting from multiple epigenetic and genetic changes. *Pharmacol. Rev.* **2012**, *64*, 706–721. [CrossRef] [PubMed]
26. Adelstein, D.J.; Li, Y.; Adams, G.L.; Wagner, H., Jr.; Kish, J.A.; Ensley, J.F.; Schuller, D.E.; Forastiere, A.A. An Intergroup Phase III Comparison of Standard Radiation Therapy and Two Schedules of Concurrent Chemoradiotherapy in Patients With Unresectable Squamous Cell Head and Neck Cancer. *J. Clin. Oncol.* **2003**, *21*, 92–98. [CrossRef]
27. Keys, H.M.; Bundy, B.N.; Stehman, F.B.; Muderspach, L.I.; Chafe, W.E.; Suggs, C.L.; Walker, J.L.; Gersell, D. Cisplatin, Radiation, and Adjuvant Hysterectomy Compared with Radiation and Adjuvant Hysterectomy for Bulky Stage IB Cervical Carcinoma. *N. Engl. J. Med.* **1999**, *340*, 1154–1161. [CrossRef]
28. Tu, L.; Sun, L.; Xu, Y.; Wang, Y.; Zhou, L.; Liu, Y.; Zhu, J.; Peng, F.; Wei, Y.; Gong, Y. Paclitaxel and cisplatin combined with intensity-modulated radiotherapy for upper esophageal carcinoma. *Radiat. Oncol.* **2013**, *8*, 75. [CrossRef]
29. Ilson, D.H.; Minsky, B.; Kelsen, D. Irinotecan, cisplatin, and radiation in esophageal cancer. *Oncology* **2002**, *16*, 11–15.
30. Myint, W.K.; Ng, C.; Raaphorst, G.P. Examining the non-homologous repair process following cisplatin and radiation treatments. *Int. J. Radiat. Biol.* **2002**, *78*, 417–424. [CrossRef]

31. Boeckman, H.J.; Trego, K.S.; Henkels, K.M.; Turchi, J.J. Cisplatin sensitizes cancer cells to ionizing radiation via inhibition of non-homologous end joining. *Mol. Cancer Res. MCR* **2005**, *3*, 277–285. [CrossRef] [PubMed]
32. Eljack, N.D.; Ma, H.Y.; Drucker, J.; Shen, C.; Hambley, T.W.; New, E.J.; Friedrich, T.; Clarke, R.J. Mechanisms of cell uptake and toxicity of the anticancer drug cisplatin. *Metall. Integr. Biomet. Sci.* **2014**, *6*, 2126–2133. [CrossRef] [PubMed]
33. Kilari, D.; Guancial, E.; Kim, E.S. Role of copper transporters in platinum resistance. *World J. Clin. Oncol.* **2016**, *7*, 106–113. [CrossRef]
34. Baskar, R.; Dai, J.; Wenlong, N.; Yeo, R.; Yeoh, K.-W. Biological response of cancer cells to radiation treatment. *Front. Mol. Biosci.* **2014**, *1*, 24. [CrossRef] [PubMed]
35. Hummel, R.; Watson, D.I.; Smith, C.; Kist, J.; Michael, M.Z.; Haier, J.; Hussey, D.J. Mir-148a improves response to chemotherapy in sensitive and resistant oesophageal adenocarcinoma and squamous cell carcinoma cells. *J. Gastrointest. Surg. Off. J. Soc. Surg. Aliment. Tract.* **2011**, *15*, 429–438. [CrossRef] [PubMed]
36. Singh, A.; Settleman, J. EMT, cancer stem cells and drug resistance: An emerging axis of evil in the war on cancer. *Oncogene* **2010**, *29*, 4741–4751. [CrossRef]
37. Piskareva, O.; Harvey, H.; Nolan, J.; Conlon, R.; Alcock, L.; Buckley, P.; Dowling, P.; O'Sullivan, F.; Bray, I.; Stallings, R.L. The development of cisplatin resistance in neuroblastoma is accompanied by epithelial to mesenchymal transition in vitro. *Cancer Lett.* **2015**, *364*, 142–155. [CrossRef] [PubMed]
38. Katoh, M. Networking of WNT, FGF, Notch, BMP, and Hedgehog signaling pathways during carcinogenesis. *Stem Cell Rev.* **2007**, *3*, 30–38. [CrossRef] [PubMed]
39. Matsuoka, S.; Edwards, M.C.; Bai, C.; Parker, S.; Zhang, P.; Baldini, A.; Harper, J.W.; Elledge, S.J. p57KIP2, a structurally distinct member of the p21CIP1 Cdk inhibitor family, is a candidate tumor suppressor gene. *Genes Dev.* **1995**, *9*, 650–662. [CrossRef]
40. Vlachos, P.; Nyman, U.; Hajji, N.; Joseph, B. The cell cycle inhibitor p57(Kip2) promotes cell death via the mitochondrial apoptotic pathway. *Cell Death Differ.* **2007**, *14*, 1497–1507. [CrossRef]
41. Oshimori, N.; Oristian, D.; Fuchs, E. TGF-β Promotes Heterogeneity and Drug Resistance in Squamous Cell Carcinoma. *Cell* **2015**, *160*, 963–976. [CrossRef] [PubMed]
42. Bissey, P.-A.; Law, J.H.; Bruce, J.P.; Shi, W.; Renoult, A.; Chua, M.L.K.; Yip, K.W.; Liu, F.-F. Dysregulation of the MiR-449b target TGFBI alters the TGFβ pathway to induce cisplatin resistance in nasopharyngeal carcinoma. *Oncogenesis* **2018**, *7*, 40. [CrossRef]
43. Di Paolo, N.C.; Shayakhmetov, D.M. Interleukin 1α and the inflammatory process. *Nat. Immunol.* **2016**, *17*, 906. [CrossRef]
44. Benchekroun, M.N.; Parker, R.; Dabholkar, M.; Reed, E.; Sinha, B.K. Effects of interleukin-1 alpha on DNA repair in human ovarian carcinoma (NIH:OVCAR-3) cells: Implications in the mechanism of sensitization of cis-diamminedichloroplatinum(II). *Mol. Pharmacol.* **1995**, *47*, 1255–1260. [PubMed]
45. Webb, D.S.; Mostowski, H.S.; Gerrard, T.L. Cytokine-induced enhancement of ICAM-1 expression results in increased vulnerability of tumor cells to monocyte-mediated lysis. *J. Immunol.* **1991**, *146*, 3682–3686.
46. Jonjic, N.; Alberti, S.; Bernasconi, S.; Peri, G.; Jilek, P.; Anichini, A.; Parmiani, G.; Mantovani, A. Heterogeneous susceptibility of human melanoma clones to monocyte cytotoxicity: Role of ICAM-1 defined by antibody blocking and gene transfer. *Eur. J. Immunol.* **1992**, *22*, 2255–2260. [CrossRef] [PubMed]
47. Guo, P.; Huang, J.; Wang, L.; Jia, D.; Yang, J.; Dillon, D.A.; Zurakowski, D.; Mao, H.; Moses, M.A.; Auguste, D.T. ICAM-1 as a molecular target for triple negative breast cancer. *Proc. Natl. Acad. Sci. USA* **2014**, *111*, 14710–14715. [CrossRef]
48. Takizawa, K.; Kamijo, R.; Ito, D.; Hatori, M.; Sumitani, K.; Nagumo, M. Synergistic induction of ICAM-1 expression by cisplatin and 5-fluorouracil in a cancer cell line via a NF-κB independent pathway. *Br. J. Cancer* **1999**, *80*, 954. [CrossRef]
49. Tsai, S.T.; Wang, P.J.; Liou, N.J.; Lin, P.S.; Chen, C.H.; Chang, W.C. ICAM1 Is a Potential Cancer Stem Cell Marker of Esophageal Squamous Cell Carcinoma. *PLoS ONE* **2015**, *10*, e0142834. [CrossRef]
50. Xu, Y.; Gao, W.; Zhang, Y.; Wu, S.; Liu, Y.; Deng, X.; Xie, L.; Yang, J.; Yu, H.; Su, J.; et al. ABT737 reverses cisplatin resistance by targeting glucose metabolism of human ovarian cancer cells. *Int. J. Oncol.* **2018**, *53*, 1055–1068. [CrossRef]
51. Catanzaro, D.; Gaude, E.; Orso, G.; Giordano, C.; Guzzo, G.; Rasola, A.; Ragazzi, E.; Caparrotta, L.; Frezza, C.; Montopoli, M. Inhibition of glucose-6-phosphate dehydrogenase sensitizes cisplatin-resistant cells to death. *Oncotarget* **2015**, *6*, 30102–30114. [CrossRef] [PubMed]

52. Ippolito, L.; Marini, A.; Cavallini, L.; Morandi, A.; Pietrovito, L.; Pintus, G.; Giannoni, E.; Schrader, T.; Puhr, M.; Chiarugi, P.; et al. Metabolic shift toward oxidative phosphorylation in docetaxel resistant prostate cancer cells. *Oncotarget* **2016**, *7*, 61890–61904. [CrossRef]
53. Zhao, F.Q.; Keating, A.F. Functional properties and genomics of glucose transporters. *Curr. Genomics* **2007**, *8*, 113–128. [CrossRef] [PubMed]
54. Guo, Q.; Lan, F.; Yan, X.; Xiao, Z.; Wu, Y.; Zhang, Q. Hypoxia exposure induced cisplatin resistance partially via activating p53 and hypoxia inducible factor-1alpha in non-small cell lung cancer A549 cells. *Oncol. Lett.* **2018**, *16*, 801–808. [PubMed]
55. Wu, H.M.; Jiang, Z.F.; Ding, P.S.; Shao, L.J.; Liu, R.Y. Hypoxia-induced autophagy mediates cisplatin resistance in lung cancer cells. *Sci. Rep.* **2015**, *5*, 12291. [CrossRef] [PubMed]
56. Kolde, R. Pheatmap: Pretty Heatmaps. R Package Version 1.0.10. 2018. Available online: https://CRAN.R-project.org/package=pheatmap (accessed on 4 January 2019).
57. Team, R.C. *R: A Language and Environment for Statistical Computing*; R Foundation for Statistical Computing: Vienna, Austria, 2018.

pharmaceuticals

MDPI

Article

3-Vinylazetidin-2-Ones: Synthesis, Antiproliferative and Tubulin Destabilizing Activity in MCF-7 and MDA-MB-231 Breast Cancer Cells

Shu Wang [1], Azizah M. Malebari [2,†], Thomas F. Greene [1,†], Niamh M. O'Boyle [1], Darren Fayne [3], Seema M. Nathwani [3], Brendan Twamley [4], Thomas McCabe [4], Niall O. Keely [1], Daniela M. Zisterer [3] and Mary J. Meegan [1,*]

1 School of Pharmacy and Pharmaceutical Sciences, Trinity College Dublin, Trinity Biomedical Sciences Institute, 152-160 Pearse Street, Dublin 2 DO2R590, Ireland; wangsh@tcd.ie (S.W.); tgreene@tcd.ie (T.F.G.); Niamh.OBoyle@tcd.ie (N.M.O.); nkeely@tcd.ie (N.O.K.)

2 Department of Pharmaceutical Chemistry, College of Pharmacy, King Abdulaziz University, Jeddah 21589, Saudi Arabia; amelibary@kau.edu.sa

3 School of Biochemistry and Immunology, Trinity College Dublin, Trinity Biomedical Sciences Institute, 152-160 Pearse Street, Dublin 2 DO2R590, Ireland; FAYNED@tcd.ie (D.F.); seema.nathwani@outlook.com (S.M.N.); dzistrer@tcd.ie (D.M.Z.)

4 School of Chemistry, Trinity College Dublin, Dublin 2 DO2R590, Ireland; TWAMLEYB@tcd.ie (B.T.); TMCCABE@tcd.ie (T.M.)

* Correspondence: mmeegan@tcd.ie; Tel.: +353-1-896-2798; Fax: +353-1-8962793

† These authors contributed equally to this work.

Received: 1 March 2019; Accepted: 7 April 2019; Published: 11 April 2019

Abstract: Microtubule-targeted drugs are essential chemotherapeutic agents for various types of cancer. A series of 3-vinyl-β-lactams (2-azetidinones) were designed, synthesized and evaluated as potential tubulin polymerization inhibitors, and for their antiproliferative effects in breast cancer cells. These compounds showed potent activity in MCF-7 breast cancer cells with an IC_{50} value of 8 nM for compound **7s** 4-[3-Hydroxy-4-methoxyphenyl]-1-(3,4,5-trimethoxyphenyl)-3-vinylazetidin-2-one) which was comparable to the activity of Combretastatin A-4. Compound **7s** had minimal cytotoxicity against both non-tumorigenic HEK-293T cells and murine mammary epithelial cells. The compounds inhibited the polymerisation of tubulin in vitro with an 8.7-fold reduction in tubulin polymerization at 10 μM for compound **7s** and were shown to interact at the colchicine-binding site on tubulin, resulting in significant G2/M phase cell cycle arrest. Immunofluorescence staining of MCF-7 cells confirmed that β-lactam **7s** is targeting tubulin and resulted in mitotic catastrophe. A docking simulation indicated potential binding conformations for the 3-vinyl-β-lactam **7s** in the colchicine domain of tubulin. These compounds are promising candidates for development as antiproiferative microtubule-disrupting agents.

Keywords: Combretastatin A-4; β-lactam; 3-vinylazetidin-2-ones; antiproliferative activity; tubulin; antimitotic

1. Introduction

Antimitotic agents such as taxol and the vinca alkaloids vinblastine and vincristine are a major class of drugs used clinically in the treatment of many cancers [1–3]. Microtubule-destabilizing agents (e.g., vinblastine) typically bind with tubulin at the vinca alkaloid site [4], while colchicine **1** exerts its biological effects at the intrasubunit interface within a tubulin dimer [5]. Stilbene-based compounds have attracted the attention of chemists and pharmacologists due to their many biological properties such as anticancer, antioxidant and anti-inflammatory activities, and are often used in traditional medicine for a variety of therapeutic effects [6]. The combretastatins are a group of stilbenes isolated from the South African bush willow tree *Combretum caffrum* [7], and are shown to have outstanding potency in binding to the colchicine-binding site of tubulin and thus inhibiting the formation of the mitotic spindle [8]. Combretastatin A-4 **2a** and Combretastatin A-1 **2c** demonstrate exceptionally potent antiproliferative activity against a range of human cancer cell lines (Figure 1) [7]. Additionally, antivascular effects are produced by these compounds in vivo [9,10]. Although some combretastatin compounds have progressed to clinical trials[11,12], there are major problems associated with combretastatins including poor water solubility and *cis/trans* isomerization during administration or storage, which results in an extensive loss of potency. Water soluble prodrugs such as the combretastatin phosphate CA-4P, (fosbretabulin) **2b** [13,14] are currently in clinical trials for advanced anaplastic thyroid carcinoma [15], ovarian cancer [16], and in combination with Bevacizumab for patients with advanced cancer [17]. Recently, the potential combination therapy of CA-4P and vincristine in the treatment of hepatocellular carcinoma was reported to show a beneficial effect in reducing doses of drugs with narrow therapeutic windows [18]. Ombrabulin is a serine prodrug whose derivatives display the same activity as CA-4 and has completed a phase III clinical trial for the treatment of advanced stage soft tissue sarcoma [19,20]. There is ongoing interest in the clinical development of combretastatin A1 diphosphate (OXi 4503) **2d** [21]. The structurally related benzophenones phenstatin **3a**, phenstatin phosphate **3b** [22] and the lignin podophyllotoxin **4** also destabilize microtubules [23].

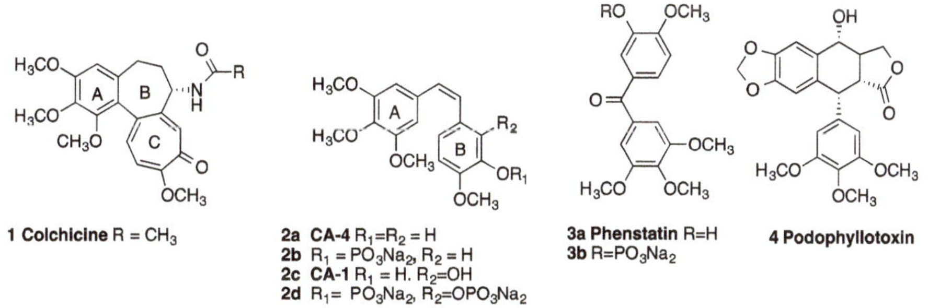

Figure 1. Colchicine (**1**), Combretastatins (**2a–2d**), phenstatins (**3a**, **3b**) and podophyllotoxin (**4**).

Many heterocyclic scaffold structures have been introduced to replace the alkene of the stilbene structure of CA-4 and to provide conformational restriction by locking the stilbene in the *cis* configuration (Rings A and B) required for biological activity [24]. Small molecule tubulin polymerization inhibitors have been reported in which the *cis* double bond of CA-4 has been replaced by various heterocycles such as furan [25], indole[26,27], imidazole [28], isoxazole [29], triazole [30], tetrazole [31], benzoxepine [32], pyrazole [33], pyridine [34], benzimidazole [35] and related heterocycles [36]. While β-lactam antibiotics have occupied a central role in the treatment of pathogenic bacteria, the antiproliferative activity of compounds containing the β-lactam (azetidin-2-one) ring has also been investigated [37–42]. The synthesis and antitumour activity of a number of chiral β-lactam bridged CA-4 analogues have been reported [37,38]. Additional impetus for research efforts on β-lactam chemistry has been provided by the use of β-lactams as synthetic intermediates in organic synthesis [43].

We have previously investigated the antiproliferative and SERM (selective estrogen receptor modulator) activity of the azetidin-2-one(β-lactam) scaffold [44] and also demonstrated the effectiveness of 1,4-diarylazetidin-2-ones in breast cancer cell lines as tubulin targeting agents. [45,46]. These compounds also demonstrated both anti-angiogenic effects in MDA-MB-231 breast adenocarcinoma cells. In addition, we established that these compounds inhibited the migration of MDA-MB-231 cells indicating a potential anti-metastatic function for these compounds [47]. To further our understanding of the antiproliferative activity of these compounds, we wished to investigate the design, synthesis and evaluation of a series of azetidin-2-ones containing a vinyl substituent at C3 of the azetidin-2-one ring, and to explore the effect of this hydrophobic substituent on the biological activity of these compounds in which the *cis* configuration (Rings A and B) is locked into the azetidin-2-one ring structure. The introduction of this vinyl substituent at C-3 also allowed us to examine further chemical transformations of the alkene, and to determine structure-activity relationships for the series. On this basis, we now aimed to investigate a new series of novel 3-vinylazetidinones compounds with an improved biochemical profile particularly in triple negative breast cancer for potential development in preclinical study of breast cancer as tubulin destabilising agents. Therefore, we focused our efforts on the preparation of a library of 1,4-diarylazetidin-2-ones which contain a vinyl substituent at C-3. The synthesis of phosphate esters and amino acid amide type prodrugs of the most potent 1,4-diarylazetidin-2-ones were examined, together with the antiproliferative and tubulin targeting effects.

2. Results and Discussion

2.1. Chemistry: Synthesis of β-lactams

There are many synthetic routes available for the construction of the β-lactam ring [43,48]. The choice of route depends on the structural features required in the final product. In the present work, the Staudinger reaction between an imine and a ketene was chosen for the formation of the β-lactam ring because of its ease of use, adaptability for use with structurally diverse imines and acid chlorides, and readily available starting materials. A series of analogues with a variety of substituents at C4 of the β-lactam ring B was synthesized from the appropriate imines. The preparation of the Schiff bases **5a–5r** was achieved by the condensation of the appropriately substituted benzaldehyde with the 3,4,5-trimethoxyaniline in ethanol in the presence of a catalytic amount of sulphuric acid, (Scheme 1). The 3,4,5-trimethoxy substituted A-Ring of CA-4 plays an important role in inhibiting tubulin polymerisation, and is confirmed in the docking of CA-4 in tubulin [49]. The substituents located at the para-position of C-4 aryl Ring B included halogens (compounds **5a–5c**), nitro (**5d**), dimethylamino (**5e**), methyl (**5g**), alkoxyl (**5h–5j**), phenoxy (**5k**), benzyloxy (**5l**), nitrile (**5q**) and thiomethyl (**5r**) together with naphthyl (compounds **5m** and **5n**). **5s** was similarly obtained by reaction of 4-methoxybenzaldehyde with 3,5-dimethoxyaniline. For the synthesis of β-lactam derivatives with a phenolic hydroxy group to mimic Ring B of CA-4, it was necessary to use the benzyl ether **5l** and *tert*-butyldimethylsilyl ether **5o**. A further series of Schiff bases (**6a–6k**) was obtained from 3,4,5-trimethoxybenzaldehyde with appropriate anilines using the same procedure as above, (Scheme 1). An example of the crystal structure of the imine **6k** is displayed in Figure 2, showing the *E* configuration of the imine N1-C2 bond (bond length 1.278(2) Å) (Table 1).

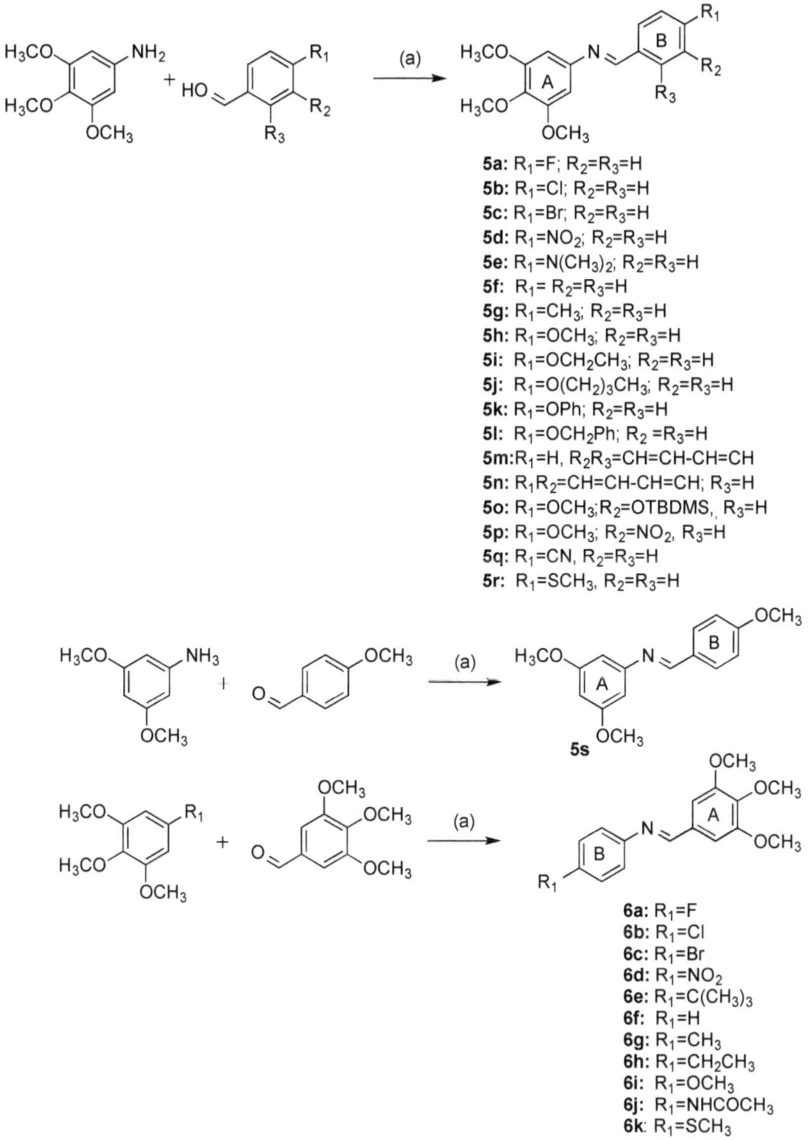

Scheme 1. Synthesis of imines **5a–5s**, **6a–6k**. Reagents and conditions: (a) EtOH, conc H_2SO_4, reflux, 4 h, (67–100%).

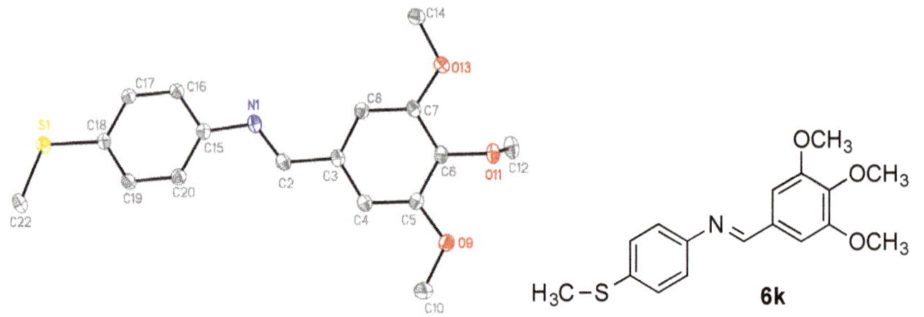

Figure 2. ORTEP representation of the X-ray crystal structure of compound **6k** with the thermal ellipsoids set at 50% probability.

Table 1. Crystal data, details of data collections and refinement **6k, 7h, 8h, 8i, 8k**.

Compound	6k	7h	8h	8i	8k
Empirical formula	$C_{17}H_{19}NO_3S$	$C_{21}H_{23}NO_5$	$C_{22}H_{25}NO_4$	$C_{21}H_{23}NO_5$	$C_{21}H_{23}NO_4S$
M (g/mol)	317.39	369.40	367.43	369.40	385.46
Crystal System	monoclinic	monoclinic	monoclinic	triclinic	triclinic
SG	$P2_1$ (No. 4)	$P2_1$ (No. 4)	$P2_1/n$ (No. 14)	$P\bar{1}$ (No. 2)	$P\bar{1}$ (No. 2)
a (Å)	7.8282(3)	20.1106(7)	7.2135(14)	10.9022(5)	8.2131(4)
b (Å)	7.7880(3)	9.1481(3)	26.440(5)	13.0315(6)	10.5047(5)
c (Å)	13.2937(6)	22.6378(8)	10.389(2)	14.9787(8)	12.5704(6)
α (°)	-	-	-	94.994(2)	107.9218(16)°
β (°)	106.4320(10)	110.6238(14)	101.41(3)	105.024(2)°	96.7759(18)°
γ (°)	-	-	-	108.284(2)°	103.3909(18)°
V (Å3)	777.36(6)	3897.9(2)	1942.3(7)	1918.37(16)	982.64(8)
T (*K*)	100(2)	100(2)	150(2)	100(2)	100(2)
Z	2	8	4	4	2
Dcalc (g/cm^3)	1.356	1.259	1.256	1.279	1.303
μ (mm^{-1})	0.220 (Mo Kα)	0.738 (Cu Kα)	0.086 (Mo Kα)	0.091 (Mo Kα)	0.191 (Mo Kα)
Total reflns	27644	59468	14461	29738	14916
Indep. reflns	4394	14180	3492	9673	4903
R(int)	0.0258	0.0602	0.0565	0.0532	0.0304
S	1.058	1.047	1.188	1.006	1.038
R_1 * [I > 2σ(I)]	0.0251	0.0364	0.0666	0.0509	0.0388
wR_2 * [all data]	0.0676	0.0945	0.1509	0.1191	0.0918
Flack	0.027(12)				
CCDC number	1820354	1820355	1820358	1820356	1820357

* $R_1 = \Sigma||F_o| - |F_c||/\Sigma|F_o|$, w$R_2 = [\Sigma w(F_o^2 - F_c^2)^2/\Sigma w(F_o^2)^2]^{1/2}$.

A series of novel β-lactams (**7a–7r**) was obtained by reaction of imines **5a–5r** with crotonyl chloride using Staudinger reaction conditions requiring the slow addition of a solution of the appropriate acid chloride to a refluxing solution of imine and TEA, (Scheme 2) [50,51]. One enantiomer is illustrated in each case and products are obtained as a racemic mixture. β-Lactam (**7s**) containing the required Ring B phenolic group of CA-4 was successfully synthesised from the silyl ether imine **5o** and crotonyl chloride to afford the silyl ether β-lactam **7o** which was deprotected in situ by treatment with tBAF to yield the phenol **7s** (Scheme 2). This series of compounds **7a–7r** differ only in the substituent pattern of aryl ring at C-4 of the β-lactam ring B.

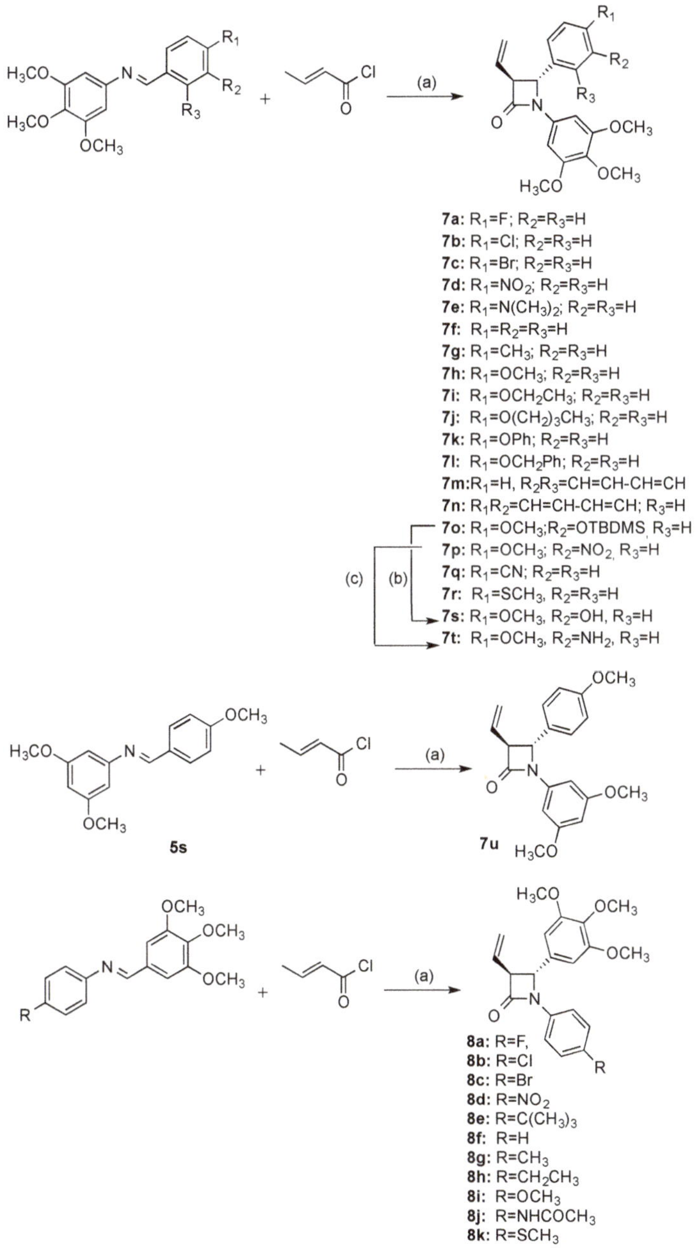

Scheme 2. Synthesis of β-lactams **7a–7u**, **8a–8k**; Reagents and conditions: (a) triethylamine, CH_2Cl_2, reflux, 5 h, (17–61%); (b) TBAF, dry THF, 0 °C, 30 min, (20%); (c) Zn dust, acetic acid, 20 °C, 7 days, (43%).

Many potentially useful CA-4 derivatives contain the amino substituent replacing the phenol on ring B and have shown interesting biochemical activity[52]. We were interested in the preparation of β-lactam CA-4 type compounds containing an amino substituent in Ring B, and the subsequent conversion to a water-soluble prodrug by conjugation with an amino acid. The nitro containing C-3-vinyl-β-lactam **7p** was successfully reduced to the amino product **7t** using zinc dust in the presence of acetic acid (Scheme 2). To investigate the effect of replacement of the 3,4,5-trimethoxy ring A of CA-4 with 3,5-dimethoxy substituted ring A, the β-lactam **7u** was prepared in a similar route from the imine **5s**. Tripodi et al. reported that 3,5-dimethoxy substituted ring A compounds demonstrated comparable activity to the β-lactam compounds containing the 3,4,5-trimethoxy ring A of CA-4 [53]. A further series of β-lactam compounds (**8a–8k**), was also prepared containing the 3,4,5-trimethoxyphenyl substituent (Ring A of the Combretastatin A-4) at C-4 position, (Scheme 2).

The products of the Staudinger reaction with imines and crotonyl chloride show IR absorptions at approximately ν 1750 cm^{-1} characteristic of the carbonyl group of the β-lactam ring. All of the β-lactams were obtained with exclusively *trans* stereochemistry, with coupling constants of 1–3 Hz for the β-lactam ring protons (e.g., for compound **7s**, H-4 is identified as a doublet δ 4.69, $J_{3,4}$ = 2.52 Hz). Coupling constants of 5–6 Hz are usually observed for β-lactams with *cis* stereochemistry [46].

Subsequent to our initial biochemical evaluation of the 3-vinyl-β-lactam CA-4 analogues, a further series of 3-substituted β-lactams was prepared from 3-unsubstituted β-lactams by aldol type reaction with a suitable electrophile [54,55]. We were particularly interested in the introduction of modified alkene substituents at C-3, due to the exceptional biochemical activity displayed by the 3-vinyl β-lactam **7s**. Lithium enolates of 3-unsubstituted β-lactams **9a** and **9b** were reacted with selected aldehydes and ketones to provide alcohol products **10a–10i**, (Scheme 3). The β-lactams **9a** and **9b** were obtained via the Reformatsky reaction of ethyl bromoacetate with imines **5h** and **5o** using microwave conditions. Treatment of **9b** with tBAF afforded the phenol **9c**. Similarly, for the preparation of compounds **10a**, **10c**, **10d**, **10f**, **10g**, **10h** the initially obtained *t*BDMS ether intermediate was subsequently deprotected in situ using *t*BAF to yield the desired phenolic product. The enolate chemistry is stereoselective, favouring *trans* stereochemistry for the products. The presence of a diastereomeric mixture for products is confirmed from the ^{1}H NMR spectra (e.g., for **10h** where H-3 and H-4 appear as two sets of doublets, δ 3.20 and δ 4.83 respectively, with J = 2.4 Hz, ratio H_3/H_4 1.14:1.00). To investigate the role of the alcohol group at C-5 in the biochemical activity of the products **10a–10h**, the alcohol **10i** was oxidised to the corresponding ketone **11** using pyridinium chlorochromate. An alternative route to **11** was identified where treatment of the 3-unsubstituted β-lactam **9b** with LDA followed by addition of acetyl chloride to gave the desired product **11** but only in low yields (11%) with the alcohol **10a** also isolated (22%), (Scheme 3).

To further investigate the role of the 3-vinyl substitution pattern in the biochemical activity of. β-lactams, a 3-ethylidene product **12** was investigated. The initial route attempted involved the chlorination of the alcohol **10i** using thionyl chloride followed by dehydrohalogentation with a suitable base such as DBU. However, a more successful method to give the 3-ethylidene β-lactams was the dehydration of the alcohol **10i** under Mitsunobu conditions and subsequent deprotection by treatment with *t*BAF to yield **12** in 63% yield overall, (Scheme 3). The Peterson olefination of 3-unsubstituted β-lactams has also been reported by Kano et al. as an alternative route to 3-ethylidene β-lactams [56], while the Mitsunobu reaction for the dehydration of alcohols has been described by Plantan et al. in the synthesis of a trinem β-lactamase inhibitor [57]. The product **12** was obtained as a mixture of *Z*/*E* isomers in a 1:1 ratio. The configuration of the separated isomers was determined by examining the chemical shifts associated with the C-6 methyl protons. The further downfield doublet signal (δ 2.05, J = 4.16 Hz) is more deshielded, and so is assigned to the *Z* isomer while the signal at δ 1.62, (J = 4.40 Hz) is assigned to the *E* isomer [51].

The introduction of a diol functionality at C-3 was now explored. The diol **13** was synthesised in 39% yield by the oxidation of the alkene **7s** with osmium tetroxide (Scheme 3). The ^{1}H NMR spectrum for **13** clearly illustrates the formation of a diastereomeric product. H-3 appears as a pair of double doublets at δ 3.16 (0.7H) and δ 3.19 (0.3H) with coupling constants of 2.42 Hz and 5.55 Hz, while H-4 appears as two separate doublets at δ 4.90 (0.3H) and δ 5.00 (0.7H), J = 2.37 Hz.

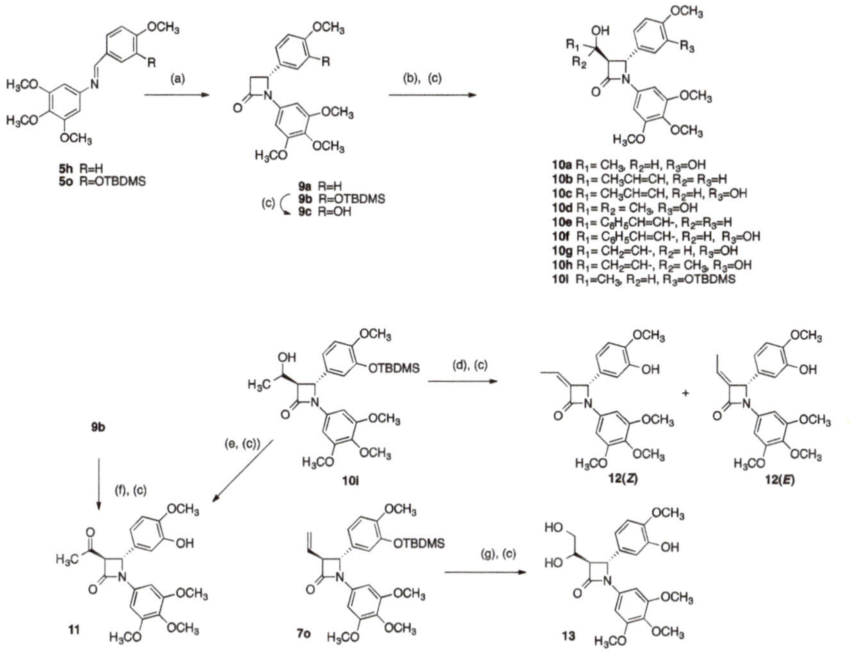

Scheme 3. Synthesis of azetidinones **10a–10i**, **11–13**. Scheme reagents and conditions: (a) Zn, $BrCH_2CO_2Et$, microwave, 100 °C, 30 min, (37–39%) (b) LDA, THF, R_1COR_2, −78 °C, 30 min, (17–38%); (c) TBAF, THF, 0 °C, 1.5 h (for compounds **10a**, **10c**, **10d**, **10f**, **10g**, **10h**, **11**, **12**, **13**), (17–52%); (d) Ph_3P, DEAD, CH_2Cl_2, 0 °C, 3 min, (52%); (e) PCC, CH_2Cl_2, 20 °C, 18 h, (7%) (f) LDA, THF, CH_3COCl, −78 °C, 30 min, (11%); (g) OsO_4, pyridine, 0 °C 1 min, then 20 °C, 22 h, (39%).

The amino acid alanine was chosen for prodrug formation of the β-lactam **7t** [58]. The protected amino acid prodrug **14** was obtained from **7t** using the coupling agent DCC with HOBt in dry DMF (Scheme 4). The FMOC protecting group was easily removed from **14** by treatment with 2N sodium hydroxide over 24 h to afford the amino acid prodrug conjugate **15** (57%). Controlled esterification of the phenolic β-lactams **7s** and **9c** with dibenzyl phosphite using diisopropylethylamine and dimethylaminopyridine afforded dibenzyl phosphate β-lactams **16a** and **16b** respectively, (Scheme 4). The dimethyl and diethylethyl phosphate esters of compound **9c**, **16c** and **16d** respectively, were also prepared (Scheme 4). The phosphate **17a** was obtained by treatment of dibenzylphosphate ester **16a** with bromotrimethylsilane. Hydrogenation of the dibenzylphosphate ester **16b** with palladium/carbon catalyst removed the dibenzyl protecting groups and also reduced the double bond at C-3 position of the β-lactam ring to afford phosphate **17c**. For the preparation of compound **17b**, where removal of the benzyl protecting groups and retention of the double bond was required, reaction of the dibenzyl phosphate ester **16b** with bromotrimethylsilane was effective.

Preliminary stability studies of the representative β-lactam **7s** were carried out at acidic, neutral and basic conditions (pH 4, 7.4 and 9) and in plasma using HPLC. The half-life ($t_{\frac{1}{2}}$) was determined to be greater than 24 h at pH 4, 7.4 and 9 and in plasma for compound **7s**. The phosphate esters **17b** and **17c** were also found to be stable over the range of pH and in plasma, with half-life ($t_{\frac{1}{2}}$) determined to be greater than 24 h. The cleavage of phosphate prodrugs **17b** and **17c** was also investigated in whole blood. They were cleaved much more rapidly in whole blood (62% and 34% remaining after 6 h respectively) than in human plasma (94% and 92% remaining after 6 h respectively). Based on this stability study the β-lactam **7s** would be suitable for further development.

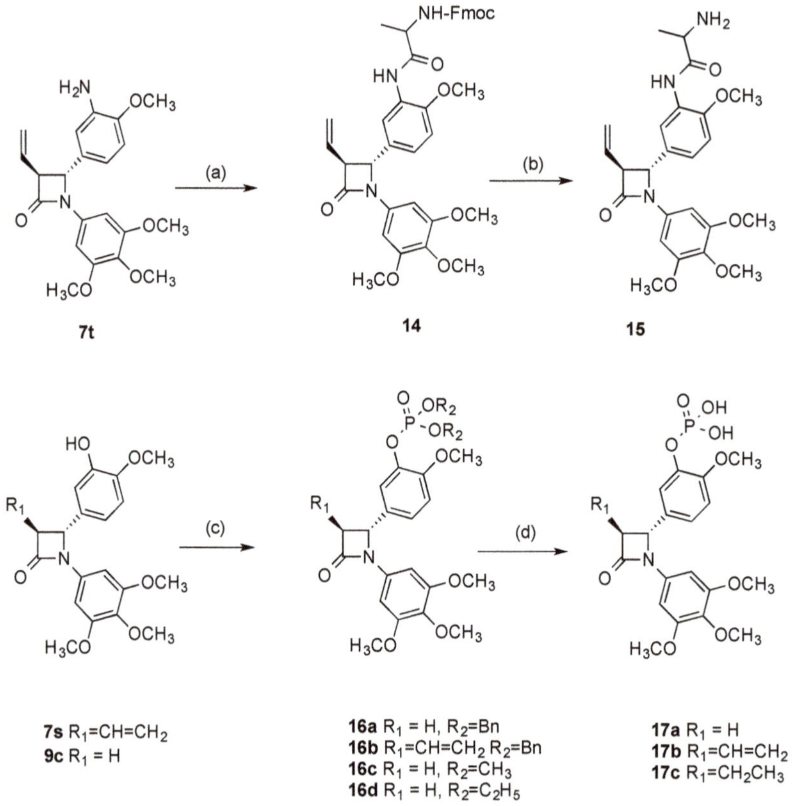

Scheme 4. Synthesis of amino acid prodrugs **15**, **17a–c**. Reagents and conditions: (a) Fmoc-L-alanine, anhydrous DMF, DCC, HOBt.H_2O, 20 °C, 24 h (58%); (b) 2N NaOH aq, CH_3OH, CH_2Cl_2, 20 °C, 24 h (57%); (c) for compounds **16a–16b**, dibenzyl phosphate, DIPEA, DMAP, CCl_4, CH_3CN, −10 °C–20 °C, 3h (60–61%); for compound **16c**, dimethyl phosphate, DIPEA, DMAP, CCl_4, CH_3CN, −10 °C–20 °C, 3h (52%); for compound **16d** diethyl phosphate, DIPEA, DMAP, CCl_4, CH_3CN, −10 °C–20 °C, 3h (79%); (d) for compounds **17a**, **17b**: bromotrimethylsilane, dry DCM, 45 min, 0 °C, (91–63%); for compound **17c**: H_2/Pd/C, ethanol-ethyl acetate, 1:1, 3 h, 20 °C, (98%).

2.2. X-Ray Structural Study

The X-ray crystal structures of compounds **7h, 8i, 8k** and **8h** are displayed in Figure 3 and confirm the structural assignment. The crystal data for the compounds are shown in Tables 1 and 2. For each compound the two aryl rings at N-1 and C-4 position are in a pseudo *cis* arrangement while the phenyl ring at C4 and the alkene group are on opposite sides of the β-lactam (*trans* configuration). The structure of the compounds **7h, 8h, 8i** and **8k** clearly demonstrated a non-coplanar configuration for rings A and B of the β-lactams, with the β-lactam ring providing a rigid scaffold. For compound **7h** even though both enantiomers are present, the compound crystallizes out in a chiral space group. The *trans* configuration of the aryl rings A and B at C-3 and C-4 is also evident. The dihedral angle H3/H4 is observed for compounds **7h, 8h, 8i** and **8k** respectively, which is consistent with the small *trans* coupling constant observed in the ^{1}H NMR spectrum of 2.00 Hz, 2.52 Hz, 2.48 Hz and 2.44 Hz respectively for these compounds. The β-lactam C=O bond lengths are 1.209(3) Å, 1.214(3) Å, 1.2077(17) Å and 1.2077(17) Å for compounds **7h, 8h, 8i** and **8k** respectively, which is consistent with data previously reported for the carbonyl bond length of monocyclic β-lactams of 1.217(3) Å [59] and 1.207(2) Å [60].

The ring A/B torsional angles for compounds **7h**, **8h**, **8i** and **8k** were observed as −59.5°, 59.7°, −73.5° and −77.0° respectively; these values are significantly greater than those observed for the corresponding rings A/B in the DAMA-colchicine **1b** [5], Combretastatin A-4 **2a** [61] and related 4-arylcoumarin [62] as 53°, 55° and 48.3° respectively (Table 2). The azetidinone N1-C4 bond length was observed at 1.372(3) Å, 1.376(3) Å, 1.367(2) Å and 1.3767(18) Å for compounds **7h**, **8h**, **8i** and **8k** respectively, which compares with 1.334(4)Å reported for the alkene C=C of combretastatin A-4 [61]. The C26-C27 alkene bond length for **7h**, **8h**, **8i** and **8k** were observed at 1.303(3) Å, 1.3174 Å, 1.308(3) Å and 1.316(2) Å respectively, while the alkene C=C bond length for *iso*-combretastatin CA-4 has been reported as 1.329(3) Å [63]. The C-N bonds lengths in the β-lactam ring are unequal with N1-C4 bond lengths of 1.487(3) Å, 1.483(3) Å, 1.4774(19) Å and 1.4801(17) Å for compounds **7h**, **8h**, **8i** and **8k** respectively, compared to 1.372(3) Å, 1.376(3) Å, 1.367(2) Å and 1.3767(18) Å for the N1/C2 bond in compounds **7h**, **8h**, **8i** and **8k** respectively, indicating some degree of amide resonance [59].

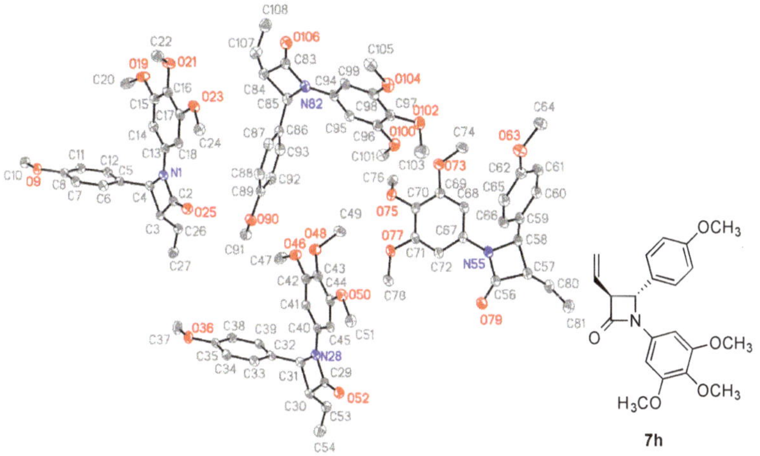

(**A**)

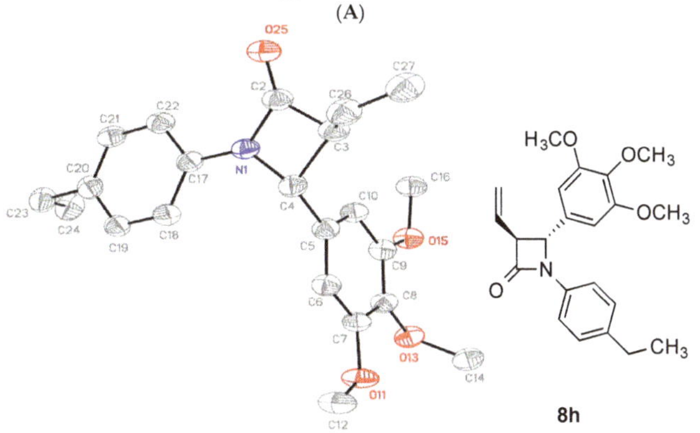

(**B**)

Figure 3. *Cont.*

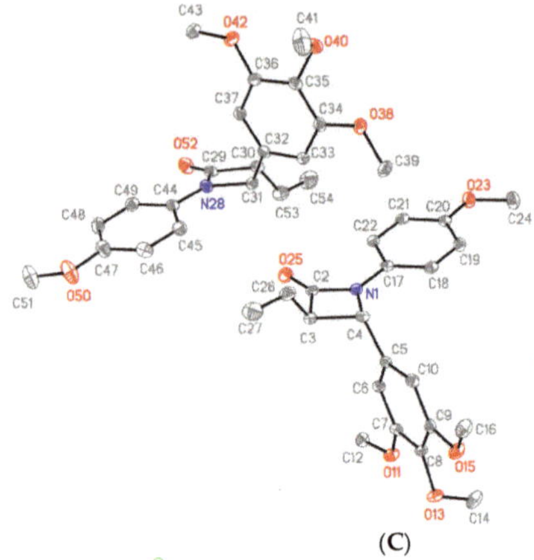

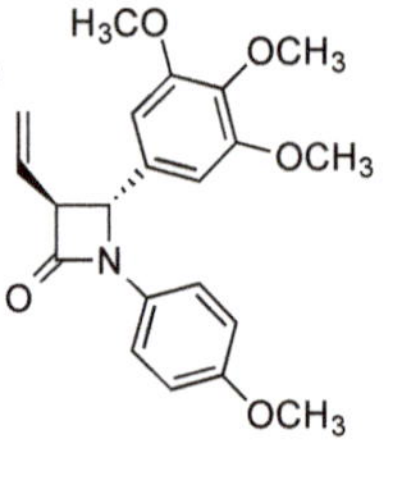

8i

(C)

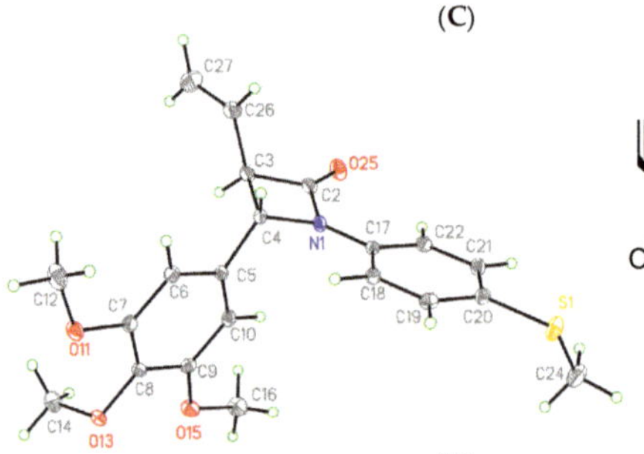

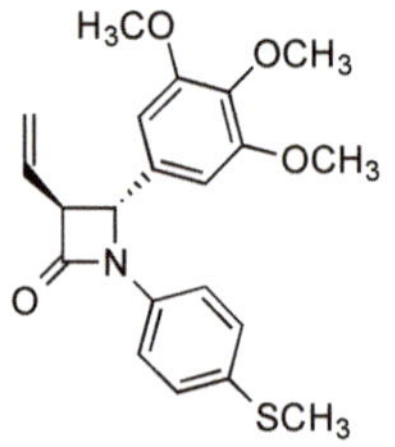

8k

(D)

Figure 3. ORTEP representation of the X-ray crystal structure of (**A**) compound **7h**, (**B**) compound **8i**, (**C**) compound **8j** and (**D**) compound 8kwith the thermal ellipsoids set at 50% probability.

Table 2. X-Ray data and torsional angles for compounds **7h**, **8h**, **8i**, **8k**.

Compound	Ring Plane Normal AB Angle(°)	Ring A to Central Torsion (°) [a]	Ring B to Central Torsion (°) [b]	RingAB Torsion (°) [c]	Ring B Vinyl Torsion (°) [d]
7h *	82.79(8)	177.0(2)	137.7(2)	−59.5(3)	124.8(2)
	75.19(8)	179.4(2)	137.1(2)	−53.8(5)	123.8(2)
	100.51(8)	177.6(2)	−136.1(2)	58.1(3)	−126.1(2)
	85.35(8)	−167.5(2)	−138.9(2)	59.7(3)	−120.9(2)
8h	93.14(7)	−171.6(3)	−130.1(2)	59.7(3)	−124.4(2)
8i §	86.28(5)	170.67(17)	150.21(14)	−73.5(2)	127.75(18)
	85.68(6)	165.62(18)	155.26(16)	−73.2(2)	127.49(16)
8k	85.60(5)	162.50(17)	156.94(13)	−77.0(2)	122.95(15)

a	b	c	d
C14-C13-N1-C2	C12-C5-C4-N1	C13-N1-C4-C5	C5-C4-C3-C26
C18-C17-N1-C2	C10-C5-C4-N1	C17-N1-C4-C5	C5-C4-C3-C26
C18-C17-N1-C2	C6-C5-C4-N1	C17-N1-C4-C5	C5-C4-C3-C26
C18-C17-N1-C2	C6-C5-C4-N1	C17-N1-C4-C5	C5-C4-C3-C26
C14-C13-N1-C2	C10-C5-C4-N1	C13-N1-C4-C5	C5-C4-C3-C26

* Four independent molecules in the asymmetric unit. § = 2 independent molecules in the asymmetric unit. Each angle given but only the first atom numbering scheme is outlined above.

2.3. Biological Results and Discussion

2.3.1. In vitro Antiproliferative Activities

The synthesized compounds were first evaluated for their antiproliferative activity against the human breast cancer cell line MCF-7 and compared with CA-4 as a reference compound (IC_{50} = 3.9 nM) [64,65]. The results are shown in Table 3 (**7a–7n**, **7p–7t**, **8a–8k**), and Table 4 (**10a–h**, **11–13**, **15** and **17a–c**). All β-lactams were evaluated as the *trans* isomer. The most potent compounds were identified as **7s** and **7t**, with IC_{50} values of 8 νM and 17 nM respectively. Compound **7s** is a direct analogue of CA-4, while **7t** is the corresponding amino compound and this type of substitution has been demonstrated to confer potency in many CA-4 analogues [52]. Compounds having the methoxy, ethoxy and thiomethyl substituents at C-4 of Ring B displayed potent antiproliferative effects, with IC_{50} values of 20 nM, 37 nM and 51 nM respectively for compounds **7h**, **7i** and **7r** respectively. The halo substituted compounds, **7b** and **7c** and 4-methyl compound **7g** were less effective with IC_{50} values of 690 nM, 445 nM and 355 nM respectively. Selectivity in antiproliferative effect was demonstrated by the 1 and 2-naphthyl compounds **7m** (IC_{50} = 1.738 μM) and **7n** (IC_{50} = 68 nM). This result compares favourably with the naphthyl CA-4 analogues reported by Medarde et al. in which the 2-naphthalene ring directly replaces the Ring B of CA-4 [66].

The IC_{50} of compound **7u** containing the 3,5-dimethoxyphenyl Ring A was determined as 170 nM in MCF-7 cells, demonstrating retention of antiproliferative potency with slightly reduced activity compared to the 3,4,5-trimethoxy ring A substituted compound **7h**. This observation could infer that the *para*-methoxy aryl group is less important for activity and the 3,5-dimethoxyaryl substituted Ring A is favourable for interaction of the molecule with the colchicine binding site of tubulin [53]. Compounds **8a–8k** containing the 3,4,5-trimethoxyphenyl substituent (Ring A of CA-4) at the C-4 position were generally observed to have poorer antiproliferative activity than the corresponding compounds **7a–7t**, containing the 3,4,5-trimethoxyphenyl substituent (Ring A of the Combretastatin A-4) at the N-1 position, (Table 3). The exceptions were compounds **8a** (4-fluoro) and **8j** (4-$NHCOCH_3$) with IC_{50} values of 1.066 μM and 4.024 μM respectively. The relative positions of the 3,4,5-trimethoxyphenyl Ring A and Ring B on the β-lactam ring at positions N-1 and C-4 have a significant effect on the antiproliferative activity of the compounds as we previously reported [45].

The effects of various structural modifications on the activity of the more potent 3-vinylazetidinones were next explored, (Table 4). The most potent compound in this series is the 3-styryl containing compound **10f**, with IC_{50} = 46 nM. The alcohol **10a** showed interesting activity (65 nM) while the introduction of an additional methyl group at C-5 to afford the alcohol **10d** resulted in reduced efficacy with IC_{50} = 544 nM. The diol **13** also proved noteworthy with IC_{50} = 69 nM. The 3-acetyl compound **11** and 3-ethylidene compound **12** resulted in similar antiproliferative effects (IC_{50} = 414 nM and 502 nM respectively). Additional compounds containing the hydroxyalkene substituent at C-3 (e.g., compounds **10b**, **10c**, **10e**, **10g**, **10h**) were found to be moderately active (IC_{50} values 288–570 nM).

The amino acid prodrug amide **15** was evaluated in MCF-7 breast cancer cells to determine if it retained any antiproliferative activity when compared with the parent compound **7t** which was extremely potent with IC_{50} = 17 nM. The IC_{50} for **15** (3.251 μM) was lower than expected; however metabolic activation in vivo may be required for the hydrolysis of the amide [67]. The phosphate esters **17a–17c** displayed impressive antiproliferative activity, with IC_{50} values of 22 nM, 27 nM and 21 nM respectively (Table 4). The IC_{50} values for the corresponding phenols **7s** and **9c** in MCF-7 cells are 8 nM and 17 nM respectively. Comparison of the 3-vinyl **17b** (IC_{50} = 27 nM) with the 3-ethyl **17c** (IC_{50} = 21 nM) indicated that introduction of the 3-vinyl or 3-ethyl substituent, together with the 3-unsubstituted **17a** (22 nM) retains potency and optimum activity. The potent activity displayed for the phosphate esters **17a–17c**, together with the predicted improvement in water solubility, indicate that these compounds are useful prodrugs for future development. Rapid in vivo dephosphorylation would be expected to occur for the β-lactam phosphates **17a–c** as observed for CA-4P [11].

Table 3. Antiproliferative activities of β-lactams **7a–7n**, **7p–7u**, **8a–8k** in human MCF-7 breast cancer cells.

Compound Number	Antiproliferative Activity IC_{50} (μM) [a]
7a	8.314 ± 1.40
7b	0.690 ± 0.11
7c	0.445 ± 0.07
7d	3.827 ± 0.53
7e	4.047 ± 0.45
7f	4.034 ± 0.42
7g	0.355 ± 0.03
7h	0.020 ± 0.0025
7i	0.037 ± 0.0033
7j	13.990 ± 1.81
7k	57.041 ± 3.72
7l	8.015 ± 0.63
7m	1.738 ± 0.17
7n	0.068 ± 0.01
7p	0.618 ± 0.10
7q	6.251 ± 5.05
7r	0.051 ± 0.001
7s	0.008 ± 0.00071
7t	0.017 ± 0.0018
7u	0.170 ± 0.07.
8a	1.066 ± 0.14
8b	29.150 ± 1.14
8c	10.400 ± 0.87
8d	59.150 ± 4.16
8e	68.840 ± 3.63
8f	50.460 ± 4.25
8g	43.130 ± 2.16
8h	36.400 ± 2.13
8i	65.120 ± 5.55
8j	4.024 ± 0.64
8k	>50
CA-4 [b]	0.0039 ± 0.00032

[a] IC_{50} values are half maximal inhibitory concentrations required to block the growth stimulation of MCF-7 cells. Values represent the mean ± SEM (error values × 10^{-6}) for at least three experiments performed in triplicate. [b] The IC_{50} value obtained for CA-4 (0.0039 μM for MCF-7) is in good agreement with the reported values [64,65].

Table 4. Antiproliferative activities of β-lactams **10a–h**, **11–13**, **15a** and **17a–c** in human MCF-7 breast cancer cells [a].

Compound Number	Antiproliferative Activity IC_{50} (nM) [a]
10a	65 ± 15
10b	292 ± 50
10c	5701 ± 246
10d	544 ± 310
10e	537 ± 80
10f	46 ± 41
10g	288 ± 76
10h	467 ± 0.253
11	414 ± 132
12	502 ± 212
13	69 ± 29
15	3251 ± 270
17a	22 ± 1.5
17b	27 ± 2
17c	21 ± 1.5
CA-4 [b]	39 ± 3.2

[a] IC_{50} values are half maximal inhibitory concentrations required to block the growth stimulation of MCF-7 cells. Values represent the mean ± SEM (error values × 10^{-6}) for at least three experiments performed in triplicate. [b] The IC_{50} value obtained for CA-4 (39 nM for MCF-7) is in good agreement with the reported values [64,65].

Triple-negative breast cancers (TNBC) are characterised by the absence of estrogen receptors (ER-), progesterone receptors (PR-) and human epidermal growth factor receptor 2 (HER2-). TNBC does not respond to hormonal therapy (such as tamoxifen or aromatase inhibitors) or therapies that target HER2 receptors, such as Herceptin. Treatment options are limited leading to poor prognosis, as indicated by low 5-year survival rates. A number of the more potent compounds were evaluated in the triple negative MDA-MB-231 cell line (Table 5). Compound **7s** was the most effective of the series with an IC_{50} value of 10 nM. Compounds **7h, 7t, 17a, 17b** and **17c** were also seen to be effective with IC_{50} values of 31 nM, 30 nM, 30 nM, 49 nM and 44 nM respectively, and compared favourably with the positive CA-4 (control IC_{50} = 43 nM) [34,63,68].

Table 5. Antiproliferative activities of selected β-lactams in human MDA-MB-231 breast cancer cells [a].

Compound Number	Antiproliferative Activity IC_{50} (nM) [a]
7b	191 ± 16
7h [b]	31.7
7i	61 ± 7
7n	77 ± 9
7s [b]	10
7t	30 ± 2
17a	30 ± 4
17b [b]	48.6
17c	44 ± 7
CA-4 [c]	43

[a] IC_{50} values are half maximal inhibitory concentrations required to block the growth stimulation of MDA-MB-231 cells. Values represent the mean ± SEM (error values × 10^{-6}) for at least three experiments performed in triplicate. [b] Antiproliferative activity against MDA-MB-231 from NCI (see Supplementary Information). [c] The IC_{50} value obtained for CA-4 in this assay is 43 nM for MDA-MB-231 in good agreement with reported values for CA-4 in MTT assay on human MDA-MB-231 breast cancer cell line [34,63,68].

Compound **7h** was also evaluated in the triple-negative Hs578T breast cancer cell line and its isogenic subclone Hs578Ts(i)8 cells to examine the activity of β-lactams as CA-4 analogues and as anti-tubulin agents for metastasis. Hs578Ts(i)8 cells are 3-fold more invasive and 2.5-fold more migratory than the parental cell line (Hs578T). In addition, Hs578Ts(i)8 cells had 30% more CD44+/CD24-/low cells that could enhance the invasive properties but with a significantly increased capacity to proliferate, migrate and produce tumours in vivo in nude mice [69]. Compound **7h** exhibited an excellent anti-proliferative activity in Hs578T cells (IC_{50} 31 nM) and interestingly retained potency in invasive Hs578Ts(i)8 cells (IC_{50} 76 nM). The values for CA4 in these cells were 8 nM and 20 nM respectively. These results could indicate the ability of β-lactams as CA-4 analogues to inhibit tumour invasion and angiogenesis which are characteristic of tumour growth and metastasis. These β-lactam compounds may provide potential development leads for this subset of aggressive breast cancers. Compound **7s** was also evaluated in the leukemia cell lines HL-60 and K562 and was found to be extremely potent with IC_{50} values of 17 nM and 26 nM respectively, comparing favourable with CA-4 [IC_{50} values of 4 nM (HL-60) and 4 nM (K562)].

The novel compounds **7h, 7s, 7t, 17b** and **17c** were selected for further investigation based on analysis of their drug-like properties (Lipinski) from a Tier-1 profiling screen, together with predictions of blood brain barrier partition, permeability, plasma protein binding, metabolic stability and human intestinal absorption properties which confirmed that these compounds are moderately lipophilic-hydrophilic drugs and are suitable candidates for further investigation (Tables S1 and S2, Supporting information).

2.3.2. Evaluation of β-Lactams in the NCI60 Cell Line Screen

A series of the more potent compounds **7h, 7s, 7t, 17b** and **17c** were evaluated in the National Cancer Institute (NCI)/Division of Cancer Treatment and Diagnosis (DCTD)/Developmental Therapeutics Program (DTP) [70], in which the activity of each compound was determined using approximately 60 different cancer cell lines of diverse tumor origins. The results are summarized in Tables S3–S5, Supplementary Information. The compounds were tested for inhibition of growth (GI_{50}) and cytotoxicity (LC_{50}) in the NCI panel of cancer cell lines and showed excellent broad-spectrum antiproliferative activity against tumor cell lines derived from leukemia, non-small-cell lung cancer, colon cancer, CNS cancer, melanoma, ovarian cancer, renal cancer, breast cancer and prostate cancer [71] using the sulforhodamine B (SRB) protein assay [72], (Tables S3–S5 Supplementary Information). The NCI results confirmed our in-house evaluations in MCF-7 cells with GI_{50} values for compounds **7h**, **7s**, **7t**, **17b** and **17c** of 30.6, <10, <10, 39.4 and 25.1 nM respectively.

Compound **7s**, the most potent compound in our panel, demonstrated a mean GI_{50} value of 23 nM across all NCI cell lines tested. The GI_{50} values for **7s** were in the sub-micromolar range for each of the cell lines investigated, except for two cell lines (melanoma cell line UACC-257 and the breast cancer cell line T-47D). For compound **7s** the GI_{50} values obtained were below 10 nM for 28 of the cell lines investigated and below 40 nM in all but eight of the panel cell lines tested. Activity was demonstrated for compound **7s** against all of the non-small cell lung (GI_{50} value 85.5 - <10 nM), colon (GI_{50} value 429 - <10 nM), CNS (GI_{50} value 40.5 - <10 nM), ovarian (GI_{50} value 45.3 - <10 nM), prostate (GI_{50} value <10 nM) and renal (GI_{50} value 40.2 - <10 nM) cancer cell lines tested. The mean GI_{50} values over the full 60 cell line panel for compounds **7h**, **7t** and **17c** of 52, 48 and 73 nM respectively (see Supplementary Information, Table S5) compares very favourably with the GI_{50} value for CA-4 of 99 nM.

LC_{50} values for compound **7s** were greater than 100 μM in all but three cell lines tested indicating minimal toxicity and the potential use of this compound for a wide range of therapeutic applications (Tables S3–S5 Supplementary Information). A similar result was obtained for compound **7h** with LC_{50} values > 100 μM in all cell lines tested.

The NCI COMPARE algorithm allows a comparison of the activities of β-lactams **7h** and **7s** with compounds of a known mechanism of antiproliferative action in the NCI Standard Agents Database. Compounds **7h** and **7s** showed high correlation to tubulin targeting agents such as maytansine, rhizoxin and the clinically important anticancer drugs vincristine and vinblastine, (see Supplementary Information, Tables S6 and S7).

2.3.3. Evaluation of Toxicity of 7s in Normal Murine Mammary Epithelial Cells

The cytotoxic effect of a selected number of 3-vinyl-β-lactams in MCF-7 cells at 10 μM concentration was initially determined in the lactate dehydrogenase (LDH) assay [73]. The 3-vinyl-β-lactams **7d**, **7h**, **7i**, **7q**, **7r** and **7u** resulted in low cytotoxicity with 7.2%, 2.4%, 8.5%, 4.5%, 4.5% and 3.5% cell death respectively while compounds **7s** and **7t** displayed increased cytotoxicity of 16.1% and 25% cell death in this assay. The 3-(1-hydroxyl-1-methylethyl) and 3-(1-hydroxy-1-phenylallyl) substituted compounds **10d** and **10f** resulted in 9.8% and 7.6% cell death respectively while cell death of 8.4% was obtained for the 3-ethylidene compound **12**. CA-4 was used as the positive control in this assay and resulted in 11.8% cell death at 10 μM concentration.

The cytotoxicity of the most potent compound **7s** on non-tumourigenic cell line HEK-293 (normal human embryonic kidney) was also investigated. We demonstrated an IC_{50} value greater than 5 μM in HEK-293T cells for **7s**. Cell viability of HEK-293T cells was significantly higher than MCF-7 cells at 10, 1 and 0.5 μM concentrations of compound **7s** (Figure 4A), demonstrating the lack of cellular toxicity of the compounds in these non-cancerous cells.

Further toxicity studies were carried out on the most potent compound β-lactam **7s** in primary cells (mouse mammary healthy epithelial cells) at two different cell concentrations (25,000 and 50,000 cells/mL), with CA4 as a positive control. The cells were harvested from mid- to late-pregnant CD-1 mice and were cultured as previously reported [74,75]. Both CA-4 [76] and **7s** were not cytotoxic at concentrations up to 10 μM in the NCI cell line panel (See Tables S8 and S9 Supplementary Information). The IC_{50} values for both compounds **7s** and CA-4 evaluated in normal murine mammary epithelial cells was greater than 10 μM which indicated a minimal toxicity for these compounds (Figure 4B). At both 25,000 cells/mL and 50,000 cells/mL and a concentration of 10 μM, CA-4 was lethal to the highest percentage of cells. The percentage of viable murine mammary epithelial cells at the IC_{50} value of each compound in MCF-7 cells (see Table 3) was calculated in order to give an estimation of the toxicity at this value. At 50,000 cells/mL, over 90% of cells were viable after 72 h for compound **7s**, (Figure 4B). At 25,000 cells/mL, the percentage of cells remaining viable after treatment with compound **7s** for 72 h was 93%, compared to 74% for CA-4. (Supplementary Information Tables S8 and S9).

These results indicate a favourable toxicity profile for **7s** in comparison to CA4. This provides further evidence, in addition to the NCI60 LC_{50} values for **7s**, that the β-lactam compound developed in this study is minimally toxic to cells that are not proliferating.

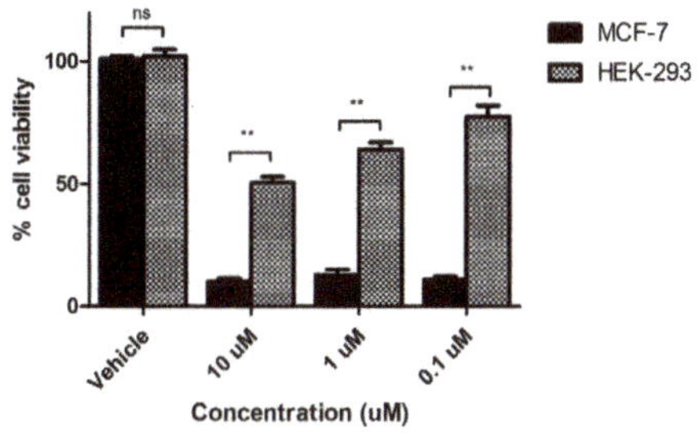

(**A**)

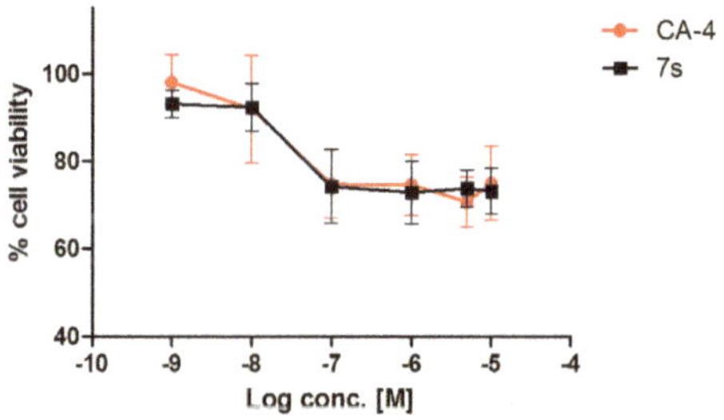

(**B**)

Figure 4. (**A**) Antiproliferative activity of β-lactam **7s** in tumorigenic MCF-7 cells and non-tumourigenic HEK-293T cells. Values represent the mean for two independent experiments. Statistical analysis was performed using a non-paired two-tailed t-test (ns, not significant; **, $p < 0.01$). (**B**) Cell viability for compound **7s** and CA-4 in murine mammary epithelial cells. Mouse mammary epithelial cells were harvested from mid- to late- pregnant CD-1 mice and cultured. The isolated mammary epithelial cells were seeded at 50,000 cells/mL. After 24 h, they were treated with 2 μL volumes of test compound which had been pre-prepared as stock solutions in ethanol to furnish the concentration range of study, 1 nM–100 μM, and re-incubated for a further 72 h. Control wells contained the equivalent volume of the vehicle ethanol (1%, *v*/*v*). The cytotoxicity was assessed using alamar blue dye.

2.3.4. Effect of β-Lactam 7s on Cell Cycle and Apoptosis

It is well recognised that tubulin destabilizing agents arrest the cell cycle in the G_2/M phase due to cytoskeleton disruption and microtubule depolymeriztion. The effects of β-lactam **7s** on cell cycle events and induction of apoptosis in MCF-7 cells were next explored. Initial analysis by flow cytometry of propidium iodide stained MCF-7 cells showed G_2M arrest at 24 h by compound **7s** [64% (10 nM) and 82% (100 nM)] (Figure 5C). A time dependent increase in the percentage of apoptotic cells (sub-G_0G_1) after 72 h (14% and 26% respectively for 10 nM and 100 nM concentration) was also evident compared to the vehicle control (6% at 72 h), (Figure 5A), with a corresponding decrease of cells in the G_0–G_1 phase of the cell cycle, (Figure 5C). The positive control CA-4 (100 nM) showed 52% of cells in G_2M arrest at 48 h, and 9.4% in the sub-G_0G_1 population.

To characterize the mode of cell death induced by **7s** in MCF-7 cells, analysis of apoptosis was performed using propidium iodide (PI), which stains DNA and enters only dead cells, and annexin-V, which binds selectively to phosphatidyl serine (Figure 6). Dual staining for annexin-V and PI facilitates discrimination between live cells (annexin-V-/PI-), early apoptotic cells (annexin-V+/PI-), late apoptotic cells (annexin-V+/PI+) and necrotic cells (annexin-V-/PI+). Each concentration induced an accumulation of annexin-V positive cells when compared to the vehicle control (5%), Figure 6.

About 13.6% of cells were found to be apoptotic (annexin-V positive) when treated with compound **7s** at 10 nM for 72 h. With an increase in concentration of **7s**, 31.9% of cells were found to be apoptotic at 100 nM. The positive control CA-4 (50 nM) resulted in 34.6% apoptotic cells. The observed effect of compound **7s** on cell cycle resulting in G_2M arrest followed by apoptosis is typical of tubulin targeting compounds. However, we have previously reported that prolonged exposure of colon cancer cells CT-26, CaCo-2 and HT-29 to our structurally related 3-aryl-β-lactams induced autophagy [77]; it is possible that autophagy may be the cell death mechanism in the present case, because of the level of apoptosis observed.

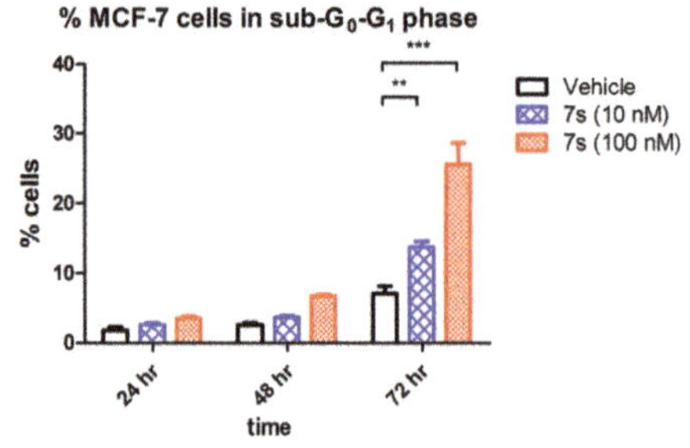

(A)

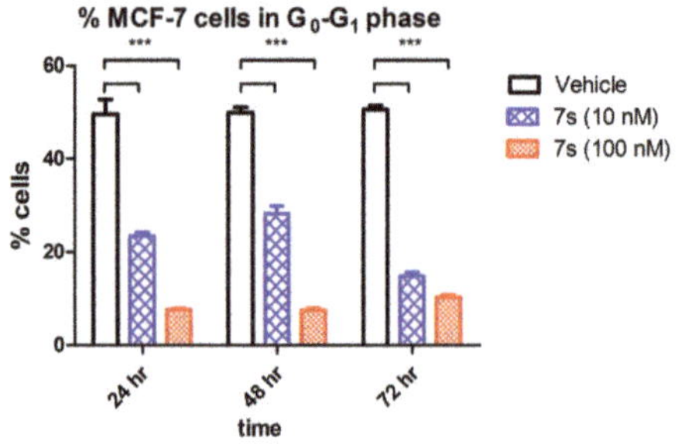

(B)

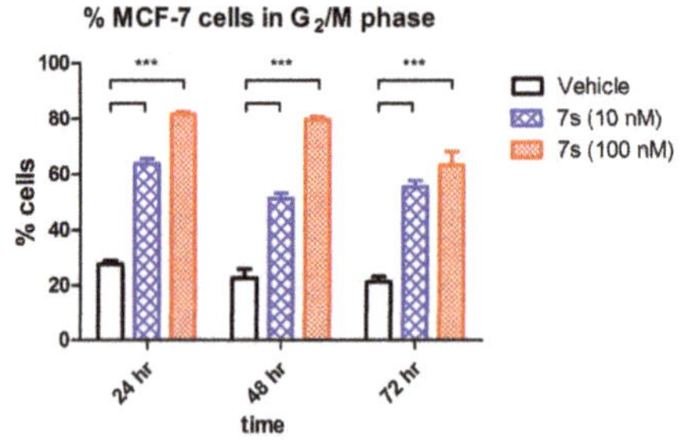

(C)

Figure 5. Effect of compound **7s** on the cell cycle and apoptosis in MCF-7 cells. Cells were treated with either vehicle [0.1% ethanol (*v*/*v*)], **7s** (10 nM and 100 nM) for 24 h, 48 h and 72 h. Cells were then fixed, stained with PI, and analyzed by flow cytometry. Cell cycle analysis was performed on histograms of gated counts per DNA area (FL2-A). The number of cells with (**A**) <2N (sub-G_1), (**B**) 2N(G_0G_1), and (**C**) 4N (G_2/M) DNA content was determined with CellQuest software. Values represent the mean ± SEM for three independent experiments. Statistical analysis was performed using two-way ANOVA (**, $p < 0.01$; ***, $p < 0.001$).

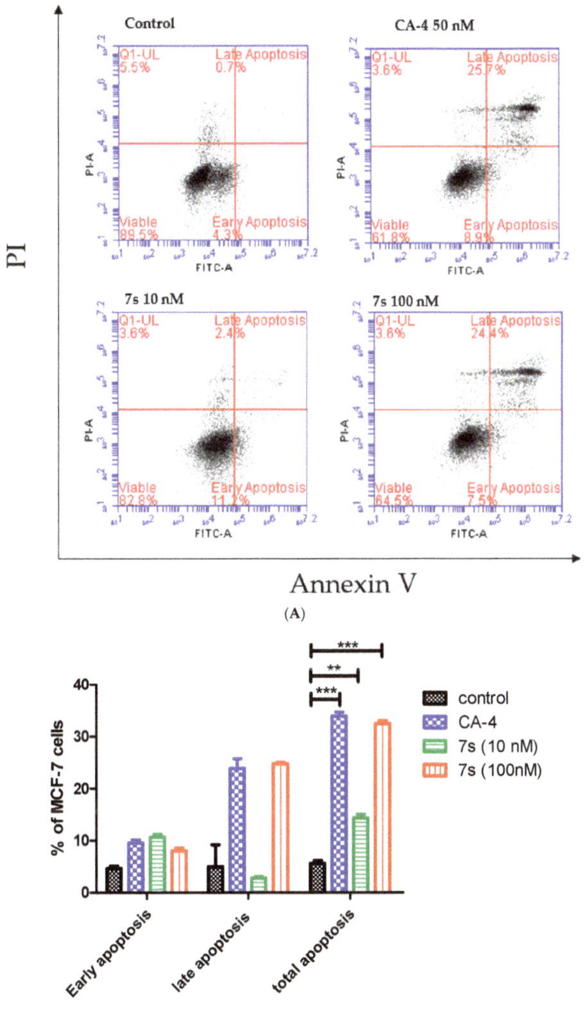

Figure 6. Compound **7s** potently induces apoptosis in MCF-7 cells (Annexin V/PI FACS). (**A**) Effect of compound 7s and CA-4 on apoptosis in MCF-7 cells analysed by flow cytometry after double staining of the cells with Annexin-V-FITC and PI. MCF-7 cells treated with 10 and 100 nM of compound 7s or 50 nM of CA-4 for 72 h and collected and processed for analysis. (**B**) Quantitative analysis of apoptosis. Values represent the mean ± SEM for three independent experiments. Statistical analysis was performed using two-way ANOVA (**, $p < 0.01$; ***, $p < 0.001$).

2.3.5. Tubulin Polymerization Studies

The effect of selected β-lactam CA-4 compounds (**7h**, **7i**, **7s**, **7t**) which demonstrated the most potent antiproliferative effects in vitro was assessed on the assembly of purified bovine tubulin. CA-4 which effectively inhibits the assembly of tubulin was used as a positive control, while paclitaxel was used to demonstrate effective tubulin polymerization. Tubulin polymerization was determined for compounds **7h**, **7i** and **7t** at 10 μM for 30 min and compound **7s** at 1, 5 and 10 μM for 60 min by measuring the increase in absorbance at 340 nm, (Figure 7A,B) [78]. The degree of light scattering by microtubules is proportional to their degree of polymerization. For the paclitaxel control the v_{max} was found to be 89.4 mOD/min. The v_{max} value provides a sensitive indication of the tubulin/ligand interactions for the tubulin polymerization. The most potent antiproliferative compound **7s** (10 μM) demonstrated a significant 8.7-fold reduction in v_{max} value while exposure to CA-4 (10 μM) brings about a 5.28-fold reduction in the v_{max} value. Compound **7s** compares very favourably to CA-4 in this respect. These effects are in good agreement with the antiproliferative data recorded for both CA-4 (IC_{50} = 4.2 nM) and **7s** (IC_{50} = 8 nM) in the MCF-7 cell line. The v_{max} value for compounds **7h, 7i** and **7t** was determined as 3.43, 3.84 and 0.92 mOD/min respectively, together with the fold-reduction in the v_{max} values of 2.45, 2.19 and 9.15 respectively for the tubulin polymerization with reference to ethanol control. These results confirm that the molecular target of these antiproliferative 3-vinyl-β-lactams is tubulin and that they are microtubule-destabilising agents.

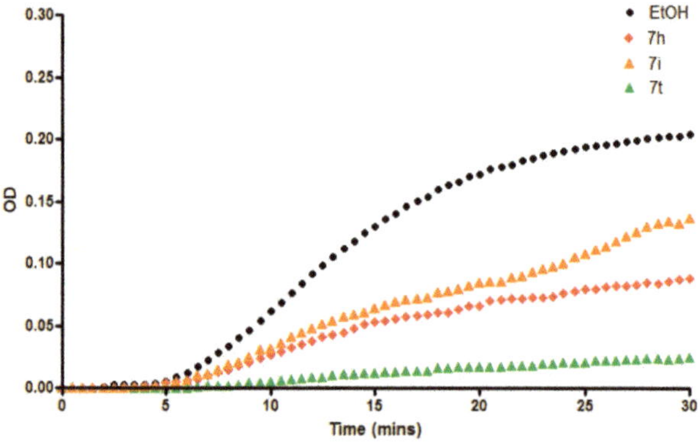

(A)

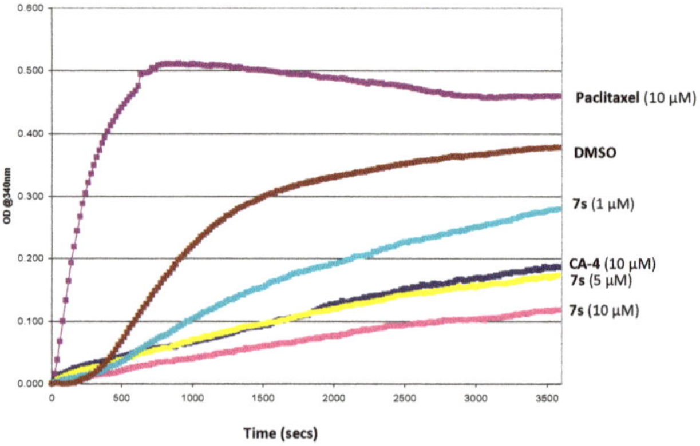

(B)

Figure 7. (**A**) Effect of compounds **7h, 7i, 7t** on tubulin polymerization in vitro. (**B**) Tubulin polymerization assay for compound **7s** at 10 μM, 5μM and 1μM. Paclitaxel (10 μM) and CA4 (10 μM) were used as references while ethanol (1% *v*/*v*) was used as a vehicle control. Purified bovine tubulin and GTP were mixed in a 96-well plate. The polymerization reaction was initated by warming the solution from 4 °C to 37 °C. The effect on tubulin assembly was monitored in a Spectramax 340PC spectrophotometer at 340 nm at 30 s intervals for 60 min at 37 °C. DMSO. Fold inhibition of tubulin polymerization was calculated using the V_{max} value for each reaction. The results represent the mean for three separate experiments.

The dose-dependent effect of **7s** on tubulin polymerization is illustrated in Figure 7. Exposure of the tubulin to 10 µM, 5 µM and 1 µM of **7s** resulted in a dose-dependent fold reduction of v_{max} of 8.70, 7.31 and 2.61 respectively while the IC_{50} value for **7s** for the inhibition of polymerization was calculated to be 1.37 µM, Figure 7. Taken together, these results demonstrate that for these novel β-lactam containing CA4 analogues, antiproliferative activity against the MCF-7 cell line and the inhibition of tubulin polymerization are closely related. It has also been shown that the most potent antiproliferative compound synthesised (**7s**) inhibits tubulin polymerization to a greater extent than CA-4.

2.3.6. Immunofluorescence Microscopy

Alterations in the microtubule network induced by β-lactam **7s** in MCF-7 cells were investigated using immunofluorescence and confocal microscopy (Figure 8). A well organised microtubular network was observed in MCF-7 control cells when stained with α-tubulin mAb (Figure 8) and in untreated cells (data not shown). Formation of microtubule bundles and pseudo asters was demonstrated for cells when exposed to paclitaxel (a microtubule-stabilising agent), Figure 8 [79]. A complete loss of microtubule formation was induced in cells exposed to CA-4 or β-lactam **7s** for 16 h. This effect is consistent with depolymerised microtubules. Following treatment with CA-4 or β-lactam **7s**, MCF-7 cells were observed to contain multiple micronuclei. Mitotic catastrophe resulting from premature or inappropriate entry of cells into mitosis is a type of programmed cell death in response to DNA damage, and is characterised by multinucleated cells [80]. CA-4 induced mitotic catastrophe has also been reported in non-small cell lung cancer cells [81,82], human endothelial cells (HUVEC) [83], human lung carcinoma cells (H460) [83] and human breast cancer cells (MCF-7) [84]. Taken together with the effects demonstrated above in Section 2.3.5 on the inhibition of polymerisation of isolated tubulin, the confocal imaging results confirm that β-lactam **7s** is targeting tubulin.

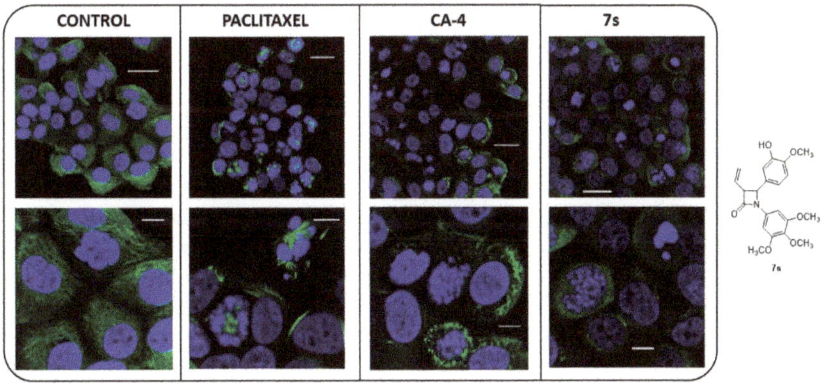

Figure 8. CA-4 and β-lactam (**7s**) depolymerise the microtubule network of MCF-7 cells. MCF-7 cells were treated with vehicle control [1% ethanol (*v*/*v*)], paclitaxel (1 µM), CA-4 (100 nM) or **7s** (*trans* isomer, 100 nM) for 16 h. Cells were fixed in 4% paraformaldehyde and stained with mouse monoclonal anti-α-tubulin-FITC antibody (clone DM1A) (green), Alexa Fluor 488 dye and counterstained with DAPI (blue). Images were captured by Leica SP8 confocal microscopy with Leica application suite X software. Representative confocal micrographs of three separate experiments are shown. Scale bar: 30 µM (top images); 10 µM (bottom images).

2.3.7. Interaction of β-Lactam 7s with Colchicine Binding Site of Tubulin

The binding of the lead compound **7s** to the colchicine binding site of tubulin was confirmed in a whole cell-based assay. *N,N′*-ethylene-bis(iodoacetamide) (EBI) is an alkylating agent that cross-links cysteine residues 239 and 354 in the colchicine-binding site of tubulin to form the β-tubulin-EBI adduct that migrates faster than β-tubulin [85,86], and is detected by Western blotting. However, when the

MCF-7 cells are pre-treated with colchicine or a colchicine-site ligand such as CA-4, the formation of the β-tubulin-EBI adduct is prevented. The MCF-7 cells were initially treated with selected β-lactam **7s** (10 μM) or CA- 4 for 2 h, then followed by addition of EBI for a further 1.5 h (Figure 9). The presence of the β-tubulin-EBI adduct was demonstrated for the control samples (no drug) at a lower position on the gel, indicating that EBI has cross-linked Cys239 and Cys354 on β-tubulin. When the cells are treated with β-lactam **7s** and CA-4, the EBI adduct formation is inhibited, indicating that **7s** is interacting with tubulin at the colchicine site of tubulin.

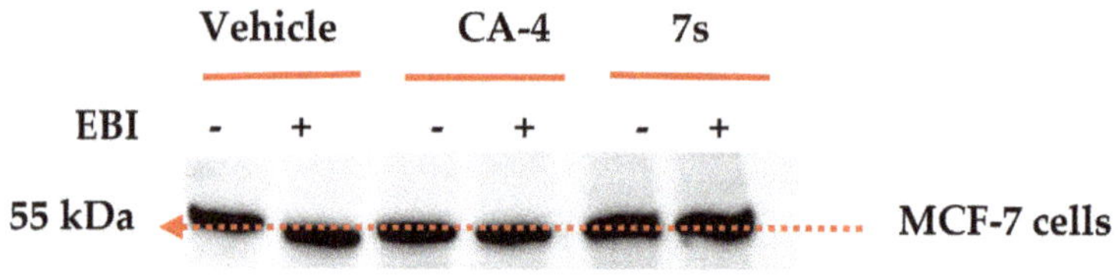

Figure 9. Colchicine binding assay: Effect of compound **7s** on the inhibition of the bisthioalkylation of Cys239 and Cys354 of β-tubulin by *N,N′*-ethylene-bis(iodoacetamide) (EBI) in MCF-7 cells. MCF-7 cells were treated with vehicle control [ethanol 0.1% (*v/v*)], **CA-4** and **7s** (10 μM) for 2 h; selected samples were then treated with EBI (100 μM) for an additional 1.5 h. Cells were harvested, lysed and analysed using sedimentation and Western blotting for β-tubulin and β-tubulin-EBI adduct.

2.4. Molecular Modelling Studies

The 3-vinyl-β-lactam compound **7s** represents the most potent compound synthesised in the study with IC_{50} value of 8 nM in MCF-7 breast cancer cells. The tubulin binding and immunofluorescence studies of 3-vinyl-β-lactam **7s** have demonstrated that the colchicine binding site of tubulin is the target for the compound. Flexible alignment of compound **7s** with CA-4 resulted in a good degree of overlap between the trimethoxyphenyl rings (Ring A) and the phenolic hydroxyl group of ring B (Figure 10A). The energy minimised structure of compound **7s** demonstrates the inter-atomic distances of the oxygens of the methoxy groups of ring A and ring B as 9.17 Å, which is similar to that calculated for CA-4 (9.27 Å).

The X-ray structure of CA-4 co-crystallised with tubulin has been determined suggesting that *cis*-CA-4 inhibits tubulin polymerization by preventing the transition from curved to straight tubulin [49]. The X-ray structure of *cis* and *trans* stereoisomers of a 3-methyl-1,4-diarylazetidinone [87] co-crystallised with tubulin was reported by Zhou et al. [37,38]. In the present study the potential interaction of our novel synthesised 3-vinyl-β-lactams with the colchicine binding site of tubulin, a series of docking calculations using MOE 2018.0101 [88] was undertaken on both the 3*S*/4*R* and 3*R*/4*S* enantiomers of the β–lactams **7s** and **7t** using the tubulin co-crystallised with DAMA-colchicine X-ray crystal structure (PDB entry 1SA0) [5]. Only results for the 3*S*/4*R* studies will be discussed as these stereoisomers were more highly ranked than the 3*R*/4*S* enantiomer and this is also supported by the crystallographic evidence [37,38]. The 3*S*/4*R* enantiomers of the hydroxyl **7s** and amino **7t** substituted analogues overlay their B-rings on the C-ring of DAMA-colchicine, collocate the trimethoxyphenyl substituents, overlap the 3-hydroxyl/amino groups on the DAMA-colchicine carbonyl oxygen atom and form HBA interactions with Lys β352 as shown in Figure 10B and 10C. The 3,4,5-trimethoxyphenyl groups of all analogues are able to make favourable van der Waals contacts within the lower subpocket delineated by Val β318 and Cys β241. The β-lactam carbonyl oxygen atom can make an HBA interaction with the backbone amine of Asp β251 for both analogues. For both compounds, the *trans* geometry at C3/C4 facilitates a more favourable interaction of rings A and B with the residues of the β-tubulin colchicine binding site. Protein-ligand interactions for **7s** are illustrated in Figure 11. The enantioselective synthesis of **7s** and **7t** are in progress which will provide the optimum configuration of these compounds to be determined for biological activity.

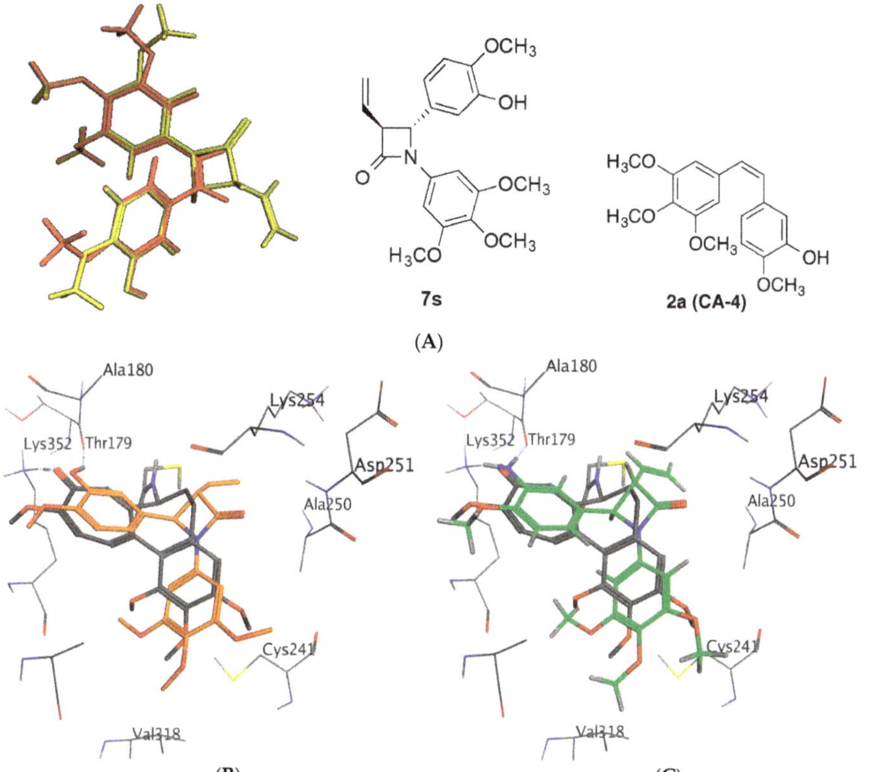

Figure 10. (**A**): Flexible alignment of **7s** (yellow) and CA-4 (**2a**)(red). (**B**,**C**): Overlay of the X-ray structure of tubulin cocrystallised with DAMA-colchicine (PDB entry 1SA0) on the best ranked docked poses of the 3S/4R enantiomers of (**B**) **7s** and (**C**) **7r**. The B-ring substituted analogues both overlap well on the C-ring of DAMA-colchicine. Ligands are rendered as tube and amino acids as line. Tubulin amino acids and DAMA-colchicine are coloured by atom type, **7s** orange and **7t** green. The atoms are coloured by element type, carbon = grey, hydrogen = white, oxygen = red, nitrogen = blue, sulphur = yellow. Key amino acid residues are labelled and multiple residues are hidden to enable a clearer view.

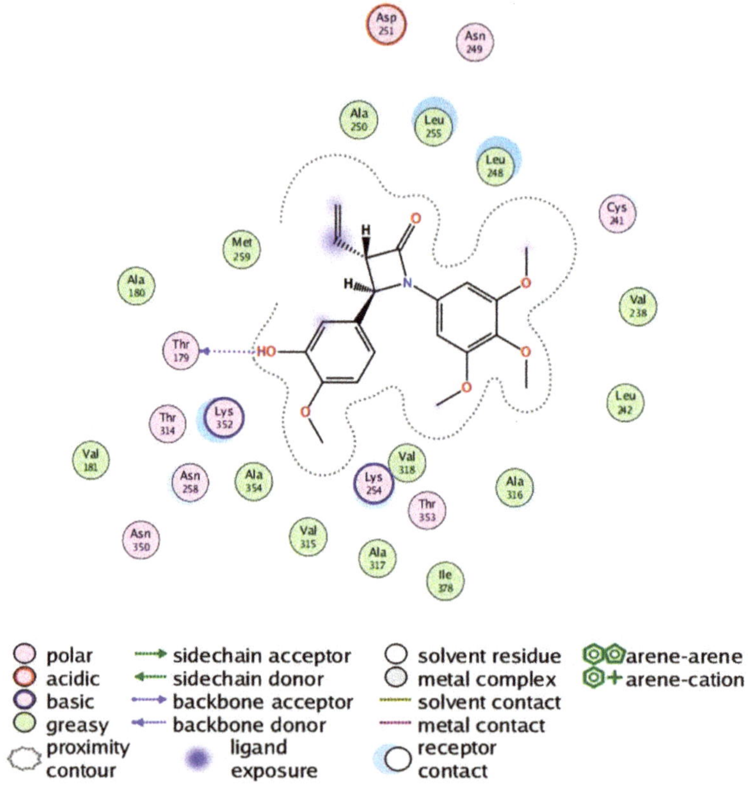

Figure 11. Protein-ligand interactions for the 3-vinyl-β-lactam compound (**7s**). 2D representation of the ligand–protein interactions of **7s** with the colchicine-binding site rendered using LigX module of MOE.

3. Conclusions

We have developed an interesting series of 3-vinylazetidinones which selectively modulate the activity of the tubulin protein, resulting in significant cytotoxicity to cancer cells and minimum cytotoxic effects to normal cells. Molecular modelling studies indicated that these compounds could interact with the colchicine binding site of tubulin, and consequently disrupt tubulin polymerization. X-Ray crystallographic studies confirmed that the torsional angle between Ring A and Ring B of the β-lactam was similar to CA-4 and was important in maintaining antiproliferative and tubulin disrupting activity. Biochemical evaluation of these compounds coupled with a molecular modeling study contributes to our understanding of the attributes of the 3-vinylazetidinones such as **7s** and **7t** that result in exceptional antiproliferative activity and dose-dependent microtubule assembly inhibition. Analysis of DNA content by flow cytometry demonstrated that the cells were arrested in the G_2/M phase; induction of apoptosis was confirmed by an increase in the sub-G_0G_1 population, which was confirmed by Annexin-V staining. Immunofluorescence staining with α-tubulin antibodies in MCF-7 cells demonstrated disorder and fragmentation of the microtubule network and disruption of mitotic spindle formation. The phosphate prodrugs **17a–c** were found to retain antitumour potency. The potent antiproliferative activity of the 3-vinylazetidinones **7s** and **7t** in breast cancer cells MCF-7 and notably in the triple negative MDA-MB-231 cell line reported in the present study compare very favourably with examples from the related series of 3-arylazetidinone compounds previously reported by our research group [45]. Vinyl substitution at C-3 of these azetidinones also results potent tubulin destabilizing effects in these derivatives of combretastatin A-4.

In summary, these novel 3-vinyl-β-lactam analogues of CA-4 which we now report show potent antiproliferative effects in preliminary in vitro investigations on MCF-7 and MDA-MB231 breast cancer cells. Further studies to establish the long-term effect of these compounds on cancer cell growth, migration and the potential vascular disrupting effects of these molecules are ongoing.

4. Experimental Section

4.1. Chemistry

All reagents were commercially available and were used without further purification unless otherwise indicated. Tetrahydrofuran (THF) was distilled immediately prior to use from Na/Benzophenone under a slight positive pressure of nitrogen, toluene was dried by distillation from sodium and stored on activated molecular sieves (4Å) and dichloromethane was dried by distillation from calcium hydride prior to use. Uncorrected melting points were measured on a Gallenkamp SMP 11 melting point apparatus. Infra-red (IR) spectra were recorded as thin film on NaCl plates, or as potassium bromide discs on a Perkin Elmer FT-IR Spectum 100 spectrometer, (PerkinElmer Inc., 940 Winter Street, Waltham, MA, USA). ^{1}H and ^{13}C nuclear magnetic resonance (NMR) spectra were recorded at 27 °C on a Brucker Avance DPX 400 spectrometer (Bruker, 40 Manning Road, Billerica, MA, USA), (400.13 MHz, ^{1}H; 100.61 MHz, ^{13}C) at 20 °C in either $CDCl_3$ (internal standard tetramethylsilane TMS) or CD_3OD by Dr. John O'Brien and Dr. Manuel Ruether in the School of Chemistry, Trinity College Dublin. For $CDCl_3$, ^{1}H-NMR spectra were assigned relative to the TMS peak at δ 0.00 ppm and ^{13}C-NMR spectra were assigned relative to the middle $CDCl_3$ triplet at δ 77.00 ppm. For CD_3OD, ^{1}H and ^{13}C-NMR spectra were assigned relative to the centre peaks of the CD_3OD multiplets at δ 3.30 and 49.00 ppm respectively. Electrospray ionisation mass spectrometry (ESI-MS) was performed in the positive ion mode on a liquid chromatography time-of-flight (TOF) mass spectrometer (Micromass LCT, Waters Ltd., Manchester, UK) equipped with electrospray ionization (ES) interface operated in the positive ion mode at the High Resolution Mass Spectrometry Laboratory by Mr. Brian Talbot in the School of Pharmacy and Pharmaceutical Sciences, Trinity College Dublin and Dr. Martin Feeney in the School of Chemistry, Trinity College Dublin. Mass measurement accuracies of < ±5 ppm were obtained. Low resolution mass spectra (LRMS) were acquired on a Hewlett-Packard 5973 MSD GC-MS system in electron impact (EI) mode, (Hewlett-Packard, 6280 America Center, San Jose, CA, USA). R_f values are quoted for thin layer chromatography on silica gel Merck F-254 plates, unless otherwise stated, (Merck, 2000 Galloping Hill Road, Kenilworth, NJ, USA). Flash column chromatography was carried out on Merck Kieselgel 60 (particle size 0.040–0.063 mm). Chromatographic separations were also carried out on Biotage SP4 instrument, (Biotage AB, Box 8, Uppsala, Sweden). All products isolated were homogenous on TLC. Analytical high-performance liquid chromatography (HPLC) to determine the purity of the final compounds was performed using a Waters 2487 Dual Wavelength Absorbance detector, a Waters 1525 binary HPLC pump, a Waters In-Line Degasser AF and a Waters 717plus Autosampler, (Waters, 34 Maple St, Milford, MA, USA). The column used was a Varian Pursuit XRs C18 reverse phase 150 × 4.6 mm chromatography column (Agilent Technologies, 5301 Stevens Creek Blvd, Santa Clara, CA, USA). Samples were detected using a wavelength of 254 nm. Imines **5a** [87], **5b** [89], **5c** [46], **5d** [46], **5e** [84], **5f** [90], **5g** [91], **5h** [45], **5i** [84], **5m** [46], **5n** [84], **5o** [45], **5p** [45], **5q** [46], **5r** [46], **5s** [53], **6a** [92], **6b** [93], **6c** [94], **6f** [45], **6g** [95], **6h** [96], **6i** [45], **6j** [97], **6k** [96] were prepared as previously reported (See Supplementary Information).

4.1.1. 3-(tert-Butyldimethylsilyloxy)-4-methoxybenzaldehyde

To a solution of 3-hydroxy-4-methoxybenzaldehyde (20 mmol) and *tert*-butyl-dimethylsilylchloride (24 mmol) in dry CH_2Cl_2 (60 mL) under a nitrogen atmosphere, 1,8-diazabicyclo[5.4.0]undec-7-ene (DBU) (32 mmol) was added dropwise via syringe. The resulting mixture was stirred at room temperature under a nitrogen atmosphere until reaction was complete on thin layer chromatography. The solution was then diluted with CH_2Cl_2 (80 mL) and washed successively with water (60 mL), 0.1M HCl (60 mL) and saturated aqueous $NaHCO_3$ (60 mL), retaining the organic layer each time, before drying over anhydrous Na_2SO_4. The solvent was removed under reduced pressure to yield the protected benzaldehyde, yield 82% [45]. IR (NaCl, film) ν_{max}: 1692 (C=O) cm^{-1}. ^1H NMR (400 MHz, $CDCl_3$): δ 0.19 (s, 6H), 1.02 (s, 9H), 3.91 (s, 3H), 6.97 (d, *J* = 8.56 Hz, 1H), 7.38 (d, *J* = 2.00 Hz, 1H), 7.48–7.51 (m, 1H), 9.84 (s, 1H). ^{13}C NMR (100 MHz, $CDCl_3$): δ -5.07, 17.97, 25.19 (OTBDMS), 55.13, 110.71, 119.63, 125.82, 129.75, 145.12, 156.16, 190.48. HRMS: found 266.1349 (M^+); $C_{14}H_{22}O_3Si$ requires 266.1338.

4.1.2. General Method I: Preparation of Imines **5a–5s**, **6a–6k**

The appropriately substituted benzaldehyde (10 mmol) and corresponding substituted aniline (10 mmol) were heated reflux in ethanol (40 mL) for 4 h with a catalytic amount of concentrated sulphuric acid. The volume of reaction was then reduced to approximately 10 mL in vacuo. The Schiff base precipitated from solution upon standing at room temperature overnight. The solid product obtained was filtered and purified by recrystallisation from ethanol.

(*E*)-1-(4-Butoxyphenyl)-*N*-(3,4,5-trimethoxyphenyl)methanimine (**5j**)

Preparation as described above from 4-butoxybenzaldehyde and 3,4,5-trimethoxyaniline. The product was obtained as pale yellow solid, yield 67%, Mp: 107–108 °C. IR (KBr) ν_{max}: 1607 (C=N) cm^{-1}. ^1H NMR (400 MHz, $CDCl_3$): δ 1.01 (t, *J* = 7.26Hz, 3H), 1.51–1.56 (m, 2H), 1.79–1.84 (m, 2H), 3.88 (s, 3H), 3.92 (s, 6H), 4.06 (t, *J* = 6.48 Hz, 2H), 6.42 (br s, 2H), 7.00 (d, *J* = 8.52 Hz, 2H), 7.87 (br s, 2H), 8.41 (s, 1H). ^{13}C NMR (100 MHz, $CDCl_3$): δ 13.87, 19.24, 31.22, 56.13, 61.04, 67.93, 98.11, 114.76, 128.57, 130.65, 136.12, 148.17, 153.56, 159.24, 162.09. HRMS: found 344.1859 (M^++H); $C_{20}H_{26}NO_4$ requires 344.1862.

(*E*)-1-(4-Phenoxyphenyl)-*N*-(3,4,5-trimethoxyphenyl)methanimine (**5k**)

Preparation as described above from 4-phenoxybenzaldehyde and 3,4,5-trimethoxyaniline. The product was obtained as pale yellow solid, yield 74%, Mp 86–88 °C. IR (KBr) ν_{max}: 1631 (C=N) cm^{-1}. ^1H NMR (400 MHz, $CDCl_3$): δ 3.88 (s, 3H), 3.92 (s, 6H), 6.51 (s, 2H), 7.08–7.10 (m, 5H), 7.39–7.41 (m, 2H), 7.89 (d, *J* = 7.52 Hz, 2H), 8.45 (s, 1H). ^{13}C NMR (100 MHz, $CDCl_3$): δ 55.68, 60.58, 97.68, 117.80, 119.34, 123.78, 124.51, 129.53, 130.10, 135.83, 147.48, 153.12, 155.57, 158.32, 160.06. HRMS: found 364.1534 (M^++H); $C_{22}H_{22}NO_4$ requires 364.1549.

(*E*)-1-(4-(Benzyloxy)phenyl)-*N*-(3,4,5-trimethoxyphenyl)methanimine (**5l**)

Preparation as described above from 4-(benzyloxy)benzaldehyde and 3,4,5-trimethoxyaniline. The product was obtained as colourless solid, yield 79%, Mp 113–115 °C. IR (KBr) ν_{max}: 1623 (C=N) cm^{-1}. ^1H NMR (400 MHz, $CDCl_3$): δ 3.88 (s, 3H), 3.92 (s, 6H), 5.17 (s, 2H), 6.51 (s, 2H), 7.09 (d, *J* = 7.84 Hz, 2H), 7.41–7.46 (m, 5H), 7.89 (d, *J* = 7.84 Hz, 2H), 8.42 (s, 1H). ^{13}C NMR (100 MHz, $CDCl_3$): δ 55.67, 60.58, 69.66, 97.65, 114.69, 127.90, 127.06, 127.75, 128.23, 128.30, 128.66, 130.16, 135.97, 147.19, 153.10, 158.63, 161.07. HRMS: found 378.1713 (M^++H); $C_{23}H_{24}NO_4$ requires 378.1705.

(*E*)-*N*-(4-Nitrophenyl)-1-(3,4,5-trimethoxyphenyl)methanimine (**6d**)

Preparation as described above from 3,4,5-trimethoxybenzaldehyde and 4-nitroaniline. The product was obtained as yellow solid, yield 72%, Mp 161–162 °C. IR (KBr) ν_{max}: 1627 (C=N) cm^{-1}. ^1H NMR (400 MHz, $CDCl_3$): δ 3.96 (s, 3H), 3.97 (s, 6H), 7.20 (s, 2H), 7.27 (d, *J* = 8.52 Hz, 2H), 8.28 (d, *J* = 9.04 Hz, 2H), 8.34 (s, 1H). ^{13}C NMR (100 MHz, $CDCl_3$): δ 55.82, 55.85, 60.62, 105.93, 120.86, 124.62, 130.12, 141.48, 144.97, 153.12, 155.56, 161.70. HRMS: found 317.1135 (M^++H); $C_{16}H_{17}N_2O_5$ requires 317.1137.

(*E*)-*N*-(4-(tert-Butyl)phenyl)-1-(3,4,5-trimethoxyphenyl)methanimine (**6e**)

Preparation as described above from 3,4,5-trimethoxybenzaldehyde and 4-(*tert*-butyl)aniline. The product was obtained as red solid, yield 100%, Mp 81–82 °C. IR (KBr) ν_{max}: 1623 (C=N) cm^{-1}. ^1H NMR (400 MHz, $CDCl_3$): δ 1.37 (s, 9H), 3.94 (s, 3H), 3.97 (s, 6H), 7.15–7.21 (m, 4H), 7.44 (d, *J* = 8.52 Hz,

2H), 8.40 (s, 1H). ^{13}C NMR (100 MHz, $CDCl_3$): δ 30.98, 34.07, 55.82, 60.55, 105.29, 120.10, 125.61, 131.31, 140.41, 148.59, 148.70, 153.05, 158.78. HRMS: found 328.1899 (M^++H); $C_{20}H_{26}NO_3$ requires 328.1913.

4.1.3. General method II: Preparation of 2-azetidinones **7a–7u**, **8a–8k**

To a stirring, refluxing solution of the imine (5 mmol) and triethylamine (6 mmol) in anhydrous dichloromethane (40 mL), a solution of crotonyl chloride (6 mmol) in anhydrous dichloromethane (10 mL) was injected dropwise through a rubber septum over 45 min under nitrogen. The reaction was heated at reflux for 5 h and stirred at room temperature overnight, continuously under nitrogen. The reaction mixture coled and washed with water (2 × 100 mL), with the organic layer being retained each time. The reaction was dried over anhydrous sodium sulfate and the solvent was then removed under reduced pressure. The crude product was purified by flash chromatography over silica gel (eluent: *n*-hexane: ethyl acetate, 4:1).

4-(4-Fluorophenyl)-1-(3,4,5-trimethoxyphenyl)-3-vinylazetidin-2-one (**7a**)

Preparation as described above from crotonyl chloride and (4-fluorobenzylidene)-3,4,5-trimethoxyphenylamine (**5a**). The product was obtained as yellow solid, yield 36%, Mp 147–149 °C. IR (KBr) ν_{max}: 1749 (C=O) cm^{-1}. ^{1}H NMR (400 MHz, $CDCl_3$): δ 3.73 (s, 6H), 3.74–3.75 (m, 1H), 3.78 (s, 3H), 4.78 (d, *J* = 2.52 Hz, 1H), 5.35–5.43 (m, 2H), 5.99–6.08 (m, 1H), 6.53 (s, 2H), 7.09–7.13 (m, 2H), 7.36–7.38 (m, 2H). ^{13}C NMR (100 MHz, $CDCl_3$): δ 55.57, 60.51, 60.51, 63.51, 94.20, 115.76, 115.97, 119.74, 127.18, 127.25, 129.81, 132.63, 133.16, 134.09, 153.10, 161.10, 164.56. HRMS: found 356.1303 (M^+-H); $C_{20}H_{19}FNO_4$ requires 356.1298.

4-(4-Chlorophenyl)-1-(3,4,5-trimethoxyphenyl)-3-vinylazetidin-2-one (**7b**)

Preparation as described above from crotonyl chloride and (4-chlorobenzylidene)-(3,4,5-trimethoxyphenyl)amine (**5b**) to afford the product as a yellow solid, yield 30%, Mp 104 °C. IR (KBr) ν_{max}: 1754 (C=O) cm^{-1}. ^{1}H NMR (400 MHz, $CDCl_3$): δ 3.70–3.71 (m, 1H), 3.72 (s, 6H), 3.77 (s, 3H), 4.77 (d, *J* = 2.48 Hz, 1H), 5.33–5.41 (m, 2H), 5.97–6.06 (m, 1H), 6.51 (s, 2H), 7.32 (d, *J* = 6.52 Hz, 2H), 7.38 (d, *J* = 8.56 Hz, 2H). ^{13}C NMR (100 MHz, $CDCl_3$): δ 56.06, 60.88, 60.95, 63.93, 94.64, 120.30, 127.28, 129.50, 130.19, 133.55, 134.54, 134.59, 135.89, 153.58, 164.89. HRMS: found 372.1017 (M^+-H); $C_{20}H_{19}{}^{35}ClNO_4$ requires 372.1003.

4-(4-Bromophenyl)-1-(3,4,5-trimethoxyphenyl)-3-vinylazetidin-2-one (**7c**)

Preparation as described above from crotonyl chloride and (4-bromobenzylidene)-3,4,5-trimethoxyphenylamine (**5c**) to afford the product as a brown oil, yield 48%. IR (NaCl) ν_{max}: 1751 (C=O) cm^{-1}. ^{1}H NMR (400 MHz, $CDCl_3$): δ 3.71–3.72 (m, 1H), 3.74 (s, 6H), 3.79 (s, 3H), 4.76 (d, *J* = 2.52 Hz, 1H), 5.35–5.43 (m, 2H), 5.99–6.08 (m, 1H), 6.53 (s, 2H), 7.27 (d, *J* = 8.52 Hz, 2H), 7.55 (d, *J* = 8.52 Hz, 2H). ^{13}C NMR (100 MHz, $CDCl_3$): δ 55.63, 60.50, 60.52, 63.43, 94.19, 119.88, 122.19, 127.08, 129.69, 132.01, 133.06, 135.95, 139.98, 153.13, 164.42. HRMS: found 418.0643 (M^++H); $C_{20}H_{21}{}^{79}BrNO_4$ requires 418.0654.

4-(4-Nitrophenyl)-1-(3,4,5-trimethoxyphenyl)-3-vinylazetidin-2-one (**7d**)

Preparation as described above from crotonyl chloride and (4-nitrobenzylidene)-3,4,5-trimethoxyphenylamine (**5d**) to afford the product as a brown solid, yield 28%, Mp 132–133 °C. IR (KBr) ν_{max}: 1754 (C=O) cm^{-1}. ^{1}H NMR (400 MHz, $CDCl_3$): δ 3.73 (s, 6H), 3.75–3.76 (m, 1H), 3.78 (s, 3H), 4.92 (d, *J* = 2.48 Hz, 1H), 5.39–5.45 (m, 2H), 6.01–6.06 (m, 1H), 6.50 (s, 2H), 7.56 (d, *J* = 9.04 Hz, 2H), 8.28 (d, *J* = 9.04 Hz, 2H). ^{13}C NMR (100 MHz, $CDCl_3$): δ 55.68, 60.03, 60.52, 63.53, 94.16, 120.46, 124.14, 126.26, 129.24, 132.75, 134.44, 144.28, 147.61, 153.27, 163.83. HRMS: found 385.1389 (M^++H); $C_{20}H_{21}N_2O_6$ requires 385.1400.

4-(4-Dimethylaminophenyl)-1-(3,4,5-trimethoxyphenyl)-3-vinylazetidin-2-one (**7e**)

Preparation as described above from crotonyl chloride and (4-(dimethylamino)benzylidene)-3,4,5-trimethoxyphenylamine (**5e**) to afford the product as a brown oil, yield 61%. IR (NaCl) ν_{max}: 1746 (C=O) cm^{-1}. ^1H NMR (400 MHz, $CDCl_3$): δ 2.98 (s, 6H), 3.73 (s, 6H), 3.77 (s, 3H), 3.78–3.92 (m, 1H), 4.70 (d, *J* = 2.00 Hz, 1H), 5.30–5.40 (m, 2H), 5.99–6.08 (m, 1H), 6.60 (s, 2H), 6.74 (d, *J* = 8.04 Hz, 2H), 7.27 (d, *J* = 9.04 Hz, 2H). ^{13}C NMR (100 MHz, $CDCl_3$): δ 40.01, 55.55, 60.49, 61.27, 63.30, 94.27, 112.20, 119.15, 126.67, 130.38, 133.58, 134.62, 137.93, 147.60, 152.95, 165.25. HRMS: found 381.1819 (M^+-H); $C_{22}H_{25}N_2O_4$ requires 381.1814.

4-Phenyl-1-(3,4,5-trimethoxyphenyl)-3-vinylazetidin-2-one (**7f**)

Preparation as described above from crotonyl chloride and benzylidene-(3,4,5-trimethoxyphenyl) amine (**5f**) to afford the product as a yellow solid, yield 29%, Mp 109–111 °C. IR (KBr) ν_{max}: 1750 (C=O) cm^{-1}. ^1H NMR (400 MHz, $CDCl_3$): δ 3.72 (s, 6H), 3.78 (s, 3H), 3.80–3.81 (m, 1H), 4.79 (d, *J* = 2.52 Hz, 1H), 5.35–5.43 (m, 2H), 6.01–6.06 (m, 1H), 6.56 (s, 2H), 7.39–7.41 (m, 5H). ^{13}C NMR (100 MHz, $CDCl_3$): δ 55.54, 60.51, 61.22, 63.35, 94.22, 119.57, 125.44, 125.53, 128.31, 128.80, 130.02, 133.34, 133.97, 136.85, 153.04, 164.75. HRMS: found 338.1383 (M^+-H); $C_{20}H_{20}NO_4$ requires 338.1392.

4-p-Tolyl-1-(3,4,5-trimethoxyphenyl)-3-vinylazetidin-2-one (**7g**)

Preparation as described above from crotonyl chloride and (4-methylbenzylidene)-(3,4,5-trimethoxyphenyl)amine (**5g**) to afford the product as a yellow solid, yield 35%, Mp 106–107 °C. IR (KBr) ν_{max}: 1746 (C=O) cm^{-1}. ^1H NMR (400 MHz, $CDCl_3$): δ 2.37 (s, 3H), 3.72 (s, 6H), 3.75 (m, 1H), 3.77 (s, 3H), 4.76 (d, *J* = 2.04 Hz, 1H), 5.32–5.41 (m, 2H), 5.99–6.08 (m, 1H), 6.56 (s, 2H), 7.21 (d, *J* = 8.00 Hz, 2H), 7.28 (d, *J* = 8.00 Hz, 2H). ^{13}C NMR (100 MHz, $CDCl_3$): δ 20.76, 55.54, 60.49, 61.07, 63.39, 94.22, 119.44, 125.48, 129.45, 130.11, 133.40, 133.78, 133.92, 138.18, 153.01, 164.87. HRMS: found 354.1706 (M^++H); $C_{21}H_{24}NO_4$ requires 354.1705.

4-(4-Methoxyphenyl)-1-(3,4,5-trimethoxyphenyl)-3-vinylazetidin-2-one (**7h**)

Preparation as described above from crotonyl chloride and (4-methoxybenzylidene)-3,4,5-trimethoxyphenylamine (**5h**) to afford the product as a brown oil, yield 34% [98]. IR (NaCl) ν_{max}: 1747 (C=O) cm^{-1}. ^1H NMR (400 MHz, $CDCl_3$): δ 3.64 (s, 6H), 3.67–3.68 (m, 1H), 3.69 (s, 3H), 3.72 (s, 3H), 4.70 (d, *J* = 2.00 Hz, 1H), 5.22–5.32 (m, 2H), 5.91–6.00 (m, 1H), 6.51 (s, 2H), 6.85 (d, *J* = 8.52 Hz, 2H), 7.26 (d, *J* = 8.52 Hz, 2H). ^{13}C NMR (100 MHz, $CDCl_3$): δ 55.37, 56.03, 60.97, 61.37, 63.92, 94.70, 114.61, 119.90, 127.31, 129.14, 130.58, 133.86, 133.93, 153.48, 159.90, 165.39. HRMS: found 370.1658 (M^++H); $C_{21}H_{24}NO_5$ requires 370.1654.

4-(4-Ethoxyphenyl)-1-(3,4,5-trimethoxyphenyl)-3-vinylazetidin-2-one (**7i**)

Preparation as described above from crotonyl chloride and (4-ethoxybenzylidene)-(3,4,5-trimethoxyphenyl)amine (**5i**) to afford a colourless solid, yield 33%, Mp 92–93 °C. [98] IR (KBr) ν_{max}: 1749 (C=O) cm^{-1}. ^1H NMR (400 MHz, $CDCl_3$): δ 1.43 (t, *J* = 6.84 Hz, 3H), 3.73 (s, 6H), 3.75–3.76 (m, 1H), 3.78 (s, 3H), 4.05 (q, *J* = 6.86 Hz, 2H), 4.73 (d, *J* = 2.48 Hz, 1H), 5.33–5.42 (m, 2H), 6.00–6.08 (m, 1H), 6.57 (s, 2H), 6.93 (d, *J* = 8.80 Hz, 2H), 7.31 (d, *J* = 8.80 Hz, 2H). ^{13}C NMR (100 MHz, $CDCl_3$): δ 14.33, 55.55, 60.50, 60.94, 63.11, 63.43, 94.22, 114.65, 119.40, 126.83, 128.49, 130.14, 133.42, 133.90, 153.01, 158.81, 164.94 (C=O). HRMS: found 384.1819 (M^++H); $C_{22}H_{26}NO_5$ requires 384.1811.

4-(4-Butoxyphenyl)-1-(3,4,5-trimethoxyphenyl)-3-vinylazetidin-2-one (**7j**)

Preparation as described above from crotonyl chloride and (4-butoxybenzylidene)-3,4,5-trimethoxyphenylamine (**5j**) to afford a yellow solid, yield 40%, Mp 100–102 °C. IR (KBr) ν_{max}: 1749 (C=O) cm^{-1}. ^1H NMR (400 MHz, $CDCl_3$): δ 0.98 (t, *J* = 7.32 Hz, 3H), 1.45–1.54 (m, 2H), 1.74–1.81 (m, 2H), 3.72 (s, 6H), 3.73-3.74 (m, 1H), 3.77 (s, 3H), 3.97 (t, *J* = 6.84 Hz, 2H), 4.73 (d, *J* = 1.96 Hz,

1H), 5.31–5.40 (m, 2H), 6.00–6.05 (m, 1H), 6.56 (s, 2H), 6.92 (d, *J* = 7.84 Hz, 2H), 7.30 (d, *J* = 8.80 Hz, 2H). ^{13}C NMR (100 MHz, $CDCl_3$): δ 13.39, 18.77, 30.78, 55.53, 60.48, 60.93, 63.43, 67.33, 94.22, 114.66, 119.36, 126.80, 128.40, 130.15, 133.42, 133.89, 153.00, 159.03, 164.93. HRMS: found 412.2129 (M^++H); $C_{24}H_{30}NO_5$ requires 412.2124.

4-(4-Phenoxyphenyl)-1-(3,4,5-trimethoxyphenyl)-3-vinylazetidin-2-one (**7k**)

Preparation as described above from crotonyl chloride and (4-phenoxylbenzylidene)-(3,4,5-trimethoxyphenyl)amine (**5k**) to afford a pale yellow solid, yield 37%, Mp 128–130 °C. IR (KBr) ν_{max}: 1749 (C=O) cm^{-1}. ^{1}H NMR (400 MHz, $CDCl_3$): δ 3.75 (s, 6H), 3.77–3.78 (m, 1H), 3.79 (s, 3H), 4.78 (d, *J* = 2.52 Hz, 1H), 5.35–5.44 (m, 2H), 6.01–6.10 (m, 1H), 6.57 (s, 2H), 7.02–7.05 (m, 4H), 7.14–7.17 (m, 1H), 7.35–7.39 (m, 4H). ^{13}C NMR (100 MHz, $CDCl_3$): δ 55.58, 60.52, 60.77, 63.42, 94.26, 118.73, 118.77, 119.58, 123.37, 127.03, 129.44, 130.00, 131.27, 133.29, 134.18, 153.07, 156.09, 157.40, 164.74. HRMS: found 454.1610 (M^++Na); $C_{26}H_{25}NO_5Na$ requires 454.1630.

4-(4-Benzyloxyphenyl)-1-(3,4,5-trimethoxyphenyl)-3-vinylazetidin-2-one (**7l**)

Preparation as described above from crotonyl chloride and (4-benzyloxybenzylidene)-3,4,5-trimethoxyphenylamine (**5l**) to afford a cream solid, yield 37%, Mp 148–149 °C. IR (KBr) ν_{max}: 1746 (C=O) cm^{-1}. ^{1}H NMR (400 MHz, $CDCl_3$): δ 3.72 (s, 6H), 3.75–3.76 (m, 1H), 3.78 (s, 3H), 4.74 (d, *J* = 2.52 Hz, 1H), 5.09 (s, 2H), 5.33–5.42 (m, 2H), 5.99–6.08 (m, 1H), 6.56 (s, 2H), 7.02 (d, *J* = 8.56 Hz, 2H), 7.31–7.46 (m, 7H). ^{13}C NMR (100 MHz, $CDCl_3$): δ 56.03, 60.97, 61.36, 63.89, 70.08, 94.69, 115.57, 119.92, 127.36, 127.48, 128.14, 128.67, 129.44, 130.58, 133.86, 136.61, 139.50, 153.49, 159.05, 165.37. HRMS: found 468.1774 (M^++Na); $C_{27}H_{27}NO_5Na$ requires 468.1787.

4-Naphthalen-1-yl-1-(3,4,5-trimethoxyphenyl)-3-vinylazetidin-2-one (**7m**)

Preparation as described above from crotonyl chloride and naphthalen-1-ylmethylene-(3,4,5-trimethoxyphenyl)amine (**5m**) to afford the product as a yellow solid, yield 34%, Mp 121–122 °C. IR (KBr) ν_{max}: 1754 (C=O) cm^{-1}. ^{1}H NMR (400 MHz, $CDCl_3$): δ 3.71 (s, 6H), 3.76–3.78 (m, 1H), 3.82 (s, 3H), 5.44–5.49 (m, 2H), 5.60 (d, *J* = 2.00 Hz, 1H), 6.22–6.31 (m, 1H), 6.67 (s, 2H), 7.44–8.04 (m, 7H). ^{13}C NMR (100 MHz, $CDCl_3$): δ 55.69, 58.42, 60.54, 63.11, 94.49, 120.72, 122.29, 125.10, 125.74, 126.28, 127.86, 128.22, 128.75, 129.96, 130.67, 132.21, 133.45, 133.62, 134.13, 153.19, 164.82. HRMS: found 390.1715 (M^++H); $C_{24}H_{24}NO_4$ requires 390.1705.

4-Naphthalen-2-yl-1-(3,4,5-trimethoxyphenyl)-3-vinylazetidin-2-one (**7n**)

Preparation as described above from crotonyl chloride and naphthalen-2-ylmethylene-(3,4,5-trimethoxyphenyl)amine (**5n**) to afford the product as a yellow solid, yield 30%, Mp 145–146 °C. IR (KBr) ν_{max}: 1749 (C=O) cm^{-1}. ^{1}H NMR (400 MHz, $CDCl_3$): δ 3.69 (s, 6H), 3.77 (s, 3H), 3.84–3.87 (m, 1H), 4.97 (d, *J* = 2.52 Hz, 1H), 5.37–5.45 (m, 2H), 6.06–6.12 (m, 1H), 6.62 (s, 2H), 7.47–7.92 (m, 7H). ^{13}C NMR (100 MHz, $CDCl_3$): δ 55.58, 60.50, 61.38, 63.44, 94.25, 119.71, 122.47, 124.97, 126.13, 126.34, 127.39, 127.42, 129.01, 130.00, 132.86, 132.94, 133.45, 134.05, 134.33, 153.08, 164.80. HRMS: found 390.1714 (M^++H); $C_{24}H_{24}NO_4$ requires 390.1705.

4-(4-Methoxy-3-nitrophenyl)-1-(3,4,5-trimethoxyphenyl)-3-vinylazetidin-2-one (**7p**)

Preparation as described above from crotonyl chloride and (4-methoxy-3-nitrobenzylidene)-(3,4,5-trimethoxyphenyl)amine (**5p**) to afford a brown oil, yield 14%. IR (NaCl) ν_{max}: 1754 (C=O) cm^{-1}. ^{1}H NMR (400 MHz, $CDCl_3$): δ 3.75 (s, 6H), 3.78 (s, 3H), 3.85–3.86 (m, 1H), 3.99 (s, 3H), 4.80 (d, *J* = 2.00 Hz, 1H), 5.37–5.43 (m, 2H), 5.98–6.07 (m, 1H), 6.52 (s, 2H), 7.14–7.16 (m, 1H), 7.54–7.57 (m, 1H), 7.90 (br s, 1H). ^{13}C NMR (100 MHz, $CDCl_3$): δ 55.61, 56.27, 59.66, 60.52, 63.43, 94.23, 114.14, 120.19, 123.18, 129.23, 129.38, 130.74, 132.80, 134.36, 138.76, 152.65, 153.23, 164.19. HRMS: found 437.1326 (M^++Na); $C_{21}H_{22}N_2O_7Na$ requires 437.1325.

4-[4-Oxo-1-(3,4,5-trimethoxyphenyl)-3-vinyl-azetidin-2-yl]benzonitrile (**7q**)

Preparation as described above from 4-[(3,4,5-trimethoxyphenylimino)methyl]benzonitrile (**5q**) and *trans*-crotonyl chloride to afford the product as a colourless oil (31%). IR ν_{max} 1756.1(CO), 2312.0 (CN) cm^{-1}. ^{1}H NMR (400 MHz, $CDCl_3$): δ 3.76 (s, br, 10H), 4.86 (d, *J* = 2.52 Hz, 1H), 5.40 (m, 2H), 5.90–6.08 (m, 1H), 6.48 (s, 2H), 7.49 (d, 2H), 7.71 (d, 2H). HRMS: Found: 387.1335 (M^++Na); $C_{21}H_{20}N_2O_4Na$ requires 387.1321.

4-(4-Methylsulfanylphenyl)-1-(3,4,5-trimethoxyphenyl)-3-vinylazetidin-2-one (**7r**)

Preparation as described above from crotonyl chloride and *N*-(3,4,5-trimethoxybenzylidene) -4-methylsulfanylphenylamine (**5r**), yield 17%, brown oil [98]. IR (NaCl ν max): 1744 (C=O) cm^{-1}. ^{1}H NMR (400 MHz, $CDCl_3$): δ 2.48 (s, 3H), 3.72–3.76 (m, 10H, OMe), 4.75 (d, *J* = 2.33Hz, 1H), 5.31–5.40 (m, 2H), 5.98–6.05 (m, 1H), 6.54 (s, 2H), 7.25–7.31 (m, 4H). ^{13}C NMR (100 MHz, $CDCl_3$): δ15.55, 55.88, 55.61, 60.77, 60.47, 63.39, 94.23, 119.59, 125.98, 126.09, 129.96, 133.25, 133.49, 139.00, 141.19, 153.05, 164.70. HRMS: found 408.1230 (M^++Na); $C_{21}H_{23}NO_4SNa$, requires 408.1245.

1-(3,5-Dimethoxyphenyl)-4-(4-methoxyphenyl)-3-vinylazetidin-2-one (**7u**)

Preparation as described above from imine **5s** and crotonyl chloride to afford the product as brown oil; Yield: 17%, IR ν_{max}: 1748.72 cm^{-1} (C=O, β- lactam). δ ^{1}H NMR (400 MHz, $CDCl_3$): 3.69 (s, 7 H), 3.79 (s, 3 H), 4.68 (s, 1 H), 5.27–5.39 (m, 2 H), 5.94–6.06 (m, 1 H), 6.15 (s, 1 H), 6.48 (s, 2 H), 6.89 (d, *J* = 7.93 Hz, 2 H), 7.27 (d, *J* = 8.54 Hz, 2 H). ^{13}C NMR (100 MHz, $CDCl_3$): **δ** 55.31, 55.49, 61.24, 63.97, 95.66, 96.27, 114.58, 119.77, 127.14, 129.16, 130.54, 139.23, 159.79, 161.06, 165.63. HRMS: found 340.1540 (M^+ + H); $C_{20}H_{22}NO_4$ requires 340.1549.

4-(3,4,5-Trimethoxyphenyl)-1-(4-fluorophenyl)-3-vinylazetidin-2-one (**8a**)

Preparation as described above from crotonyl chloride and *N*-(3,4,5-trimethoxybenzylidene) -4-fluorophenylamine (**6a**) as a yellow oil, yield 18%. IR (NaCl) ν_{max}: 1751 (C=O) cm^{-1}. ^{1}H NMR (400 MHz, $CDCl_3$): δ 3.77–3.79 (m, 1H), 3.83 (s, 6H), 3.86 (s, 3H), 4.71 (d, *J* = 2.48 Hz, 1H), 5.35–5.43 (m, 2H), 6.00–6.09 (m, 1H), 6.54 (s, 2H), 6.96–7.00 (m, 2H), 7.29–7.32 (m, 2H). ^{13}C NMR (100 MHz, $CDCl_3$): δ 55.76, 60.43, 61.39, 63.73, 101.99, 115.34, 115.57, 117.98, 118.06, 119.84, 129.87, 132.18, 133.36, 137.63, 153.54, 159.88, 164.74. HRMS: found 358.1454 (M^++H); $C_{20}H_{21}FNO_4$ requires 358.1455.

4-(3,4,5-Trimethoxyphenyl)-1-(4-chlorophenyl)-3-vinylazetidin-2-one (**8b**)

Preparation as described above from crotonyl chloride and *N*-(3,4,5-trimethoxybenzylidene) -4-chlorophenylamine (**6b**) as a yellow solid, yield 32%, Mp 131–133 °C. IR (KBr) ν_{max}: 1753 (C=O) cm^{-1}. ^{1}H NMR (400 MHz, $CDCl_3$): δ 3.78–3.79 (m, 1H), 3.83 (s, 6H), 3.87 (s, 3H), 4.71 (d, *J* = 1.00 Hz, 1H), 5.36–5.43 (m, 2H), 6.02–6.08 (m, 1H), 6.54 (s, 2H), 7.24 (d, *J* = 5.88 Hz, 2H), 7.28 (d, *J* = 5.88 Hz, 2H). ^{13}C NMR (100 MHz, $CDCl_3$): δ 56.11, 60.70, 61.67, 64.09, 102.43, 118.11, 120.10, 129.04, 130.08, 130.24, 132.33, 135.94, 138.15, 153.91, 165.18. HRMS: found 396.0966 (M^++Na); $C_{20}H_{20}{}^{35}ClNO_4Na$ requires 396.0979.

4-(3,4,5-Trimethoxyphenyl)-1-(4-bromophenyl)-3-vinylazetidin-2-one (**8c**)

Preparation as described above from crotonyl chloride and *N*-(3,4,5-trimethoxy benzylidene) -4-bromophenylamine (**6c**) as a colourless solid, yield 32%, Mp 120–122 °C. IR (KBr) ν_{max}: 1754 (C=O) cm^{-1}. ^{1}H NMR (400 MHz, $CDCl_3$): δ 3.77–3.79 (m, 1H), 3.83 (s, 6H), 3.86 (s, 3H), 4.71 (d, *J* = 2.48 Hz, 1H), 5.36–5.44 (m, 2H), 6.00–6.07 (m, 1H), 6.53 (s, 2H), 7.22 (d, *J* = 8.56 Hz, 2H), 7.40 (d, *J* = 8.52 Hz, 2H). ^{13}C NMR (100 MHz, $CDCl_3$): δ 55.79, 60.43, 61.33, 63.82, 101.97, 116.38, 118.16, 119.93, 129.72, 131.67, 132.00, 136.05, 137.70, 153.58, 164.96. HRMS: found 440.0466 (M^++Na); $C_{20}H_{20}{}^{79}BrNO_4Na$ requires 440.0473.

4-(3,4,5-Trimethoxyphenyl)-1-(4-nitrophenyl)-3-vinylazetidin-2-one (**8d**)

Preparation as described above from crotonyl chloride and *N*-(3,4,5-trimethoxybenzylidene) -4-nitrophenylamine (**6d**) as a yellow oil, yield 42%. IR (NaCl) ν_{max}: 1762 (C=O) cm^{-1}. ^1H NMR (400 MHz, $CDCl_3$): δ 3.85 (s, 6H), 3.87 (s, 3H), 3.89–3.91 (m, 1H), 4.81 (d, *J* = 2.52 Hz, 1H), 5.40–5.47 (m, 2H), 6.01–6.10 (m, 1H), 6.54 (s, 2H), 7.45 (d, *J* = 9.04 Hz, 2H), 8.19 (d, *J* = 9.04 Hz, 2H). ^{13}C NMR (100 MHz, $CDCl_3$): δ 55.83, 60.45, 61.77, 64.16, 101.95, 116.45, 120.38, 124.85, 129.10, 131.32, 137.97, 142.11, 143.00, 153.73, 165.55. HRMS: found 383.1234 (M^+-H); $C_{20}H_{19}N_2O_6$ requires 383.1243.

4-(3,4,5-Trimethoxyphenyl)-1-(4-tert-butylphenyl)-3-vinylazetidin-2-one (**8e**)

Preparation as described above from crotonyl chloride and *N*-(3,4,5-trimethoxybenzylidene) -4-*tert*-butylphenylamine (**6e**) as a yellow solid, yield 22%, Mp 172–174 °C. IR (KBr) ν_{max}: 1746 (C=O) cm^{-1}. ^1H NMR (400 MHz, $CDCl_3$): δ 1.29 (s, 9H), 3.76–3.78 (m, 1H), 3.84 (s, 6H), 3.87 (s, 3H), 4.69 (d, *J* = 2.48 Hz, 1H), 5.33–5.42 (m, 2H), 6.98–6.07 (m, 1H), 6.58 (s, 2H), 7.27 (d, *J* = 9.04 Hz, 2H), 7.31 (d, *J* = 9.04 Hz, 2H). ^{13}C NMR (100 MHz, $CDCl_3$): δ 30.86, 33.96, 55.78, 60.43, 61.25, 63.56, 102.13, 116.27, 119.58, 125.45, 130.15, 132.77, 134.69, 137.51, 146.63, 153.45, 164.84. HRMS: found 396.2182 (M^++H); $C_{24}H_{30}NO_4$ requires 396.2175.

4-(3,4,5-Trimethoxyphenyl)-1-phenyl-3-vinylazetidin-2-one (**8f**)

Preparation as described above from crotonyl chloride and *N*-(3,4,5-trimethoxybenzylidene) phenylamine (**6f**) as a colourless solid, yield 34%, Mp 150–151 °C. IR (KBr) ν_{max}: 1752 (C=O) cm^{-1}. ^1H NMR (400 MHz, $CDCl_3$): δ 3.77–3.79 (m, 1H), 3.83 (s, 6H), 3.86 (s, 3H), 4.74 (d, *J* = 2.48 Hz, 1H), 5.35–5.44 (m, 2H), 6.01–6.10 (m, 1H), 6.56 (s, 2H), 7.07–7.11 (m, 1H), 7.27–7.33 (m, 4H). ^{13}C NMR (100 MHz, $CDCl_3$): δ 55.76, 60.43, 61.19, 63.57, 102.01, 116.60, 119.72, 123.67, 128.65, 130.02, 132.54, 137.12, 137.53, 153.49, 165.02. HRMS: found 362.1371 (M^++Na); $C_{20}H_{21}NO_4Na$ requires 362.1368.

4-(3,4,5-Trimethoxyphenyl)-1-p-tolyl-3-vinylazetidin-2-one (**8g**)

Preparation as described above from crotonyl chloride and *N*-(3,4,5-trimethoxybenzylidene) -4-methylphenylamine (**6g**) as a yellow oil, yield 16%. IR (NaCl) ν_{max}: 1749 (C=O) cm^{-1}. ^1H NMR (400 MHz, $CDCl_3$): δ 2.30 (s, 3H), 3.75–3.77 (m, 1H), 3.83 (s, 6H), 3.86 (s, 3H), 4.71 (d, *J* = 2.48 Hz, 1H), 5.34–5.43 (m, 2H), 6.00–6.09 (m, 1H), 6.55 (s, 2H), 7.09 (d, *J* = 8.04 Hz, 2H), 7.23 (d, *J* = 8.56 Hz, 2H). ^{13}C NMR (100 MHz, $CDCl_3$): δ 20.48, 55.75, 60.42, 61.16, 63.54, 102.03, 116.54, 119.62, 129.12, 130.15, 132.66, 133.29, 134.69, 137.48, 153.45, 164.76. HRMS: found 376.1534 (M^++Na); $C_{21}H_{23}NO_4Na$ requires 376.1525.

4-(3,4,5-Trimethoxyphenyl)-1-(4-ethylphenyl)-3-vinylazetidin-2-one (**8h**)

Preparation as described above from crotonyl chloride and *N*-(3,4,5-trimethoxybenzylidene) -4-ethylphenylamine (**6h**) as yellow crystals, yield 15%, Mp 110–112 °C. IR (KBr) ν_{max}: 1749 (C=O) cm^{-1}. ^1H NMR (400 MHz, $CDCl_3$): δ 1.21 (t, *J* = 7.48 Hz, 3H), 2.57–2.63 (q, *J* = 7.52 Hz, 2H), 3.75–3.78 (m, 1H), 3.84 (s, 6H), 3.87 (s, 3H), 4.71 (d, *J* = 2.52 Hz, 1H), 5.34–5.43 (m, 2H), 6.00–6.09 (m, 1H), 6.57 (s, 2H), 7.12 (d, *J* = 8.76 Hz, 2H), 7.25–7.29 (m, 2H). ^{13}C NMR (100 MHz, $CDCl_3$): δ 15.62, 28.34, 56.23, 60.89, 61.67, 64.00, 102.54, 117.07, 120.07, 128.42, 130.63, 133.18, 135.37, 137.98, 140.20, 153.93, 165.25. HRMS: found 390.1666 (M^++Na). $C_{22}H_{25}NO_4Na$ requires 390.1681.

4-(3,4,5-Trimethoxyphenyl)-1-(4-methoxyphenyl)-3-vinylazetidin-2-one (**8i**)

Preparation as described above from crotonyl chloride and *N*-(3,4,5-trimethoxybenzylidene) -4-methoxyphenylamine (**6i**) as a yellow oil, yield 18%. IR (NaCl) ν_{max}: 1744 (C=O) cm^{-1}. ^1H NMR (400 MHz, $CDCl_3$): δ 3.78 (s, 3H), 3.80–3.82 (m, 1H), 3.83 (s, 6H), 3.86 (s, 3H), 4.69 (d, *J* = 2.48 Hz, 1H), 5.34–5.43 (m, 2H), 6.03–6.05 (m, 1H), 6.55 (s, 2H), 6.83 (d, *J* = 9.00 Hz, 2H), 7.28 (d, *J* = 9.00 Hz, 2H). ^{13}C NMR (100 MHz, $CDCl_3$): δ 54.99, 55.75, 60.42, 61.30, 63.59, 102.06, 113.85, 117.92, 119.62, 130.20,

130.68, 132.62, 137.49, 153.46, 155.67, 164.44. HRMS: found 392.1479 (M^++Na); $C_{21}H_{23}NO_5Na$ requires 392.1474.

N-(4-(2-(3,4,5-Trimethoxyphenyl)-4-oxo-3-vinylazetidin-1-yl)phenyl)acetamide (**8j**)

Preparation as described above from crotonyl chloride and *N*-((*E*)-4-(3,4,5-trimethoxybenzylideneamino) phenyl)acetamide (**6j**) as a colourless solid, yield 14%, Mp 223–224 °C. IR (KBr) ν_{max}: 1742 (C=O) 1689 (C=O) cm^{-1}. ^{1}H NMR (400 MHz, $CDCl_3$): δ 2.16 (s, 3H), 3.76–3.78 (m, 1H), 3.82 (s, 6H), 3.86 (s, 3H), 4.71 (d, *J* = 2.52 Hz, 1H), 5.34–5.42 (m, 2H), 6.00–6.09 (m, 1H), 6.54 (s, 2H), 7.27 (d, J = 8.56 Hz, 2H), 7.43 (d, *J* = 8.56 Hz, 2H), 7.49 (s, 1H). ^{13}C NMR (100 MHz, $CDCl_3$): δ 23.99, 55.75, 60.43, 61.26, 63.63, 102.04, 117.16, 119.80, 120.27, 129.99, 132.36, 133.41, 133.70, 137.52, 153.49, 164.76, 167.92. HRMS: found 419.1579 (M^++Na); $C_{22}H_{24}N_2O_5Na$ requires 419.1583.

1-(4-(Methylthio)phenyl)-4-(3,4,5-trimethoxyphenyl)-3-vinylazetidin-2-one (**8k**)

Preparation as described above from crotonyl chloride and *N*-(3,4,5-trimethoxybenzylidene) -4-thiomethylphenylamine (**6k**) as a colourless solid, yield 41%, Mp 104–106 °C. IR (NaCl, film) ν_{max}: 1748.72 cm^{-1} (C=O, β-lactam). ^{1}H NMR (400 MHz, $CDCl_3$): δ ppm 2.41 (s, 3 H), 3.73 (d, *J* = 7.93, 1.22 Hz, 1 H), 3.77–3.85 (m, 9 H), 4.67 (d, *J* = 2.44 Hz, 1 H), 5.30–5.40 (m, 2 H), 5.98 (d, *J* = 10.07, 7.63 Hz, 1 H), 6.50 (s, 2 H), 7.13–7.18 (m, 2 H), 7.23 (d, *J* = 7.32 Hz, 2 H). ^{13}C NMR (100 MHz, $CDCl_3$): δ ppm 16.50, 56.21, 60.83, 61.70, 64.07, 102.52, 117.59, 120.12, 127.90, 130.40, 132.77, 133.52, 135.16, 153.95, 165.19. HRMS: found 408.1255 (M^++Na); $C_{21}H_{23}NNaO_4S$ requires 408.1246.

4.1.4. 4-[3-Hydroxy-4-methoxyphenyl]-1-(3,4,5-trimethoxyphenyl)-3-vinylazetidin-2-one (**7s**)

To a stirring, refluxing solution of the TBDMS protected imine **5o** (5 mmol) and triethylamine (6 mmol) in anhydrous dichloromethane (40 mL), a solution of crotonyl chloride (6 mmol) in anhydrous dichloromethane (10 mL) was added over 45 min under nitrogen. The reaction was kept at reflux for 5 h and then at room temperature overnight (16 h), until the starting material had disappeared as monitored by TLC in (1:1 *n*-hexane: ethyl acetate). The reaction mixture was washed with water (2 × 100 mL). The combined organic extract was dried over anhydrous Na_2SO_4 before the solvent was removed under reduced pressure. The crude product was purified by flash chromatography over silica gel (eluant: *n*-hexane: ethyl acetate, 4:1) to afford the β-lactam **7o** as an oil. To a stirring solution of the protected β-lactam **7o** (5 mmol) under N_2 and 0 °C in dry THF was added dropwise 1.5 equivalents of 1.0 M *tert*-butylammonium fluoride (*t*-BAF) solution in hexanes (5 mmol). The resulting solution was left to stir at 0 °C until reaction was complete as monitored by TLC. The reaction mixture was diluted with ethyl acetate (75 mL) and washed with 0.1M HCl (100 mL). The aqueous layer was further extracted with ethyl acetate (2 × 25 mL). All organic layers were combined and washed with water (100 mL) and saturated brine (100 mL) before being dried over anhydrous sodium sulphate. The solvent was removed under reduced pressure to yield the phenol which was further purified by flash chromatography over silica gel (eluent: *n*-hexane: ethyl acetate, 4:1) to afford the product as a yellow oil, yield 20%. IR (NaCl, film) ν_{max}: 3367 (OH), 1749 (C=O, β-lactam), 1587, 1501, 1235, 1127 cm^{-1}. ^{1}H NMR (400 MHz, $CDCl_3$): δ 3.74 (s, 6H), 3.74–3.75 (m, 1H), 3.78 (s, 3H), 3.91 (s, 3H), 4.69 (d, *J* = 2.52 Hz, 1H), 5.32–5.40 (m, 2H), 5.77 (br s, 1H), 5.98–6.05 (m, 1H), 6.57 (s, 2H), 6.87–6.96 (m, 3H). ^{13}C NMR (100 MHz, $CDCl_3$): δ 55.56, 55.58, 60.50, 60.86, 63.38, 94.24, 110.50, 111.54, 117.30, 119.44, 129.90, 130.08, 133.38, 133.91, 145.82, 146.36, 153.01, 164.86. HRMS: found 408.1434 (M^++Na); $C_{21}H_{23}NO_6Na$ requires 408.1423.

4.1.5. 4-(3-Amino-4-methoxyphenyl)-1-(3,4,5-trimethoxyphenyl)-3-vinylazetidin-2-one (**7t**)

To a flask containing the 4-(4-methoxy-3-nitrophenyl)-1-(3,4,5-trimethoxyphenyl)-3-vinylazetidin-2 -one (**7p**) (0.25 mmol) and zinc powder 10 μm (2.5 mmol) was added 15 mL of acetic acid at room temperature under N_2 and reaction left to stir for 7 days. The reaction was filtered through a celite pad and the filtrate collected. Solvent was removed under reduced pressure and purified by flash chromatography over silica gel (elutent: ethyl acetate: *n*-hexane, 1:1) to yield the title compound as a brown solid, yield 43%, Mp 100–101 °C. IR (KBr) ν_{max}: 3370 (NH_2), 1747 (C=O) cm^{-1}. ^{1}H NMR (400 MHz, $CDCl_3$): δ 3.75 (s, 6H), 3.79 (s, 3H), 3.87–3.88 (m, 1H), 3.88 (s, 3H), 4.65 (d, *J* = 2.52 Hz, 1H), 5.31–5.41 (m, 2H), 5.98–6.07 (m, 1H), 6.60 (s, 2H), 6.72–6.78 (m, 3H). ^{13}C NMR (100 MHz, $CDCl_3$): δ 55.11, 55.58, 60.50, 61.15, 63.35, 94.23, 109.93, 111.06, 115.86, 119.29, 129.26, 130.25, 133.53, 134.01, 136.50, 147.09, 152.99, 165.07. HRMS: found 407.1597(M^++Na); $C_{21}H_{24}N_2O_5Na$ requires 407.1583.

4.1.6. 4-(4-Methoxyphenyl)-1-(3,4,5-trimethoxyphenyl)azetidin-2-one (**9a**)

Zinc powder (9 mmol) was activated using trimethylchlorosilane (0.5 mmol) in anhydrous benzene (1 mL) by heating for 15 min at 40 °C and followed by 5 min at 100 °C in a microwave. After cooling, the imine **5h** (2 mmol) and ethyl bromoacetate (2.4 mmol) were added to the reaction vessel and the mixture was placed in the microwave for 30 min at 100 °C. The reaction mixture was filtered through Celite to remove the zinc catalyst and then diluted with dichloromethane. This solution was washed with saturated ammonium chloride solution (20 mL) and 25% ammonium hydroxide (20 mL) and then with dilute HCl (40 mL), followed by water (40 mL). The organic phase was dried over anhydrous sodium sulphate and the solvent was removed under reduced pressure. The crude product was purified by flash column chromatography over silica gel (eluent: *n*-hexane: ethyl acetate, 2:1) to afford the product as a yellow solid, 39%, 267 mg, Mp 60–62 °C [87]. Purity (HPLC): 99.6%. IR (KBr) ν_{max}: 2938, 1747 (C=O), 1603, 1507, 1246, 1126 cm^{-1}. ^{1}H NMR (400 MHz, $CDCl_3$): δ 2.96 (dd, *J* = 15.20, 2.50 Hz, 1H), 3.55 (dd, *J* = 15.18, 5.86 Hz, 1H), 3.73 (s, 6H), 3.77 (s, 3H), 3.83 (s, 3H), 4.94 (dd, *J* = 5.84, 2.36 Hz, 1H), 6.56 (s, 2H), 6.93 (d, *J* = 8.76 Hz, 2H), 7.34 (d, *J* = 8.76 Hz). ^{13}C NMR (100 MHz, $CDCl_3$): δ 46.49, 53.66, 54.88, 55.54, 60.49, 93.98, 114.09, 126.84, 129.53, 133.62, 133.93, 152.99, 159.34, 164.16. HRMS: found 344.1506 (M^++H); $C_{19}H_{22}NO_5$ requires 344.1498.

4.1.7. 4-(3-Hydroxy-4-methoxyphenyl)-1-(3,4,5-trimethoxyphenyl)-azetidin-2-one (**9c**)

(i) Zinc powder (458 mg, 7 mmol (method A) or 21 mmol (method B)) and chlorotrimethylsilane (0.32 mL, 2.5 mmol) were refluxed for 3 min in anhydrous benzene (10 mL) under N_2 and then allowed to cool. To the cooled stirring solution, the appropriately substituted imine (**5o**) (5 mmol) and ethylbromoacetate (0.66 mL, 6 mmol) were added and refluxed for 7 h. The reaction was cooled to 0 °C and poured onto NH_4Cl (sat), (10 mL) and 30% NH_4OH (10 mL). The resulting solution was extracted with DCM (2 × 20 mL) and the organic layer further washed with 0.1N HCl (20 mL) and water (20 mL) before being dried over Na_2SO_4, filtered and the solvent removed under reduced pressure to afford the protected product (**9b**), yield 37%, 876 mg (method A), 77%, 1.823 g (method B) as a pale brown resin which was used immediately in the following reaction. IR (NaCl $_{\gamma}$max): 1749 (C=O) cm^{-1}. ^{1}H NMR (400 MHz, $CDCl_3$): δ 0.07 (s, 3H, OTBDMS), δ0.09 (s, 3H), 2.91–2.95 (dd, *J* = 2.47 Hz, 15.04, 1H), 3.48–3.53 (dd, *J* = 5.52 Hz, 15.55 Hz, 1H), 3.71 (s, 6H), 3.76 (s, 3H), 3.80 (s, 3H), 4.86–4.88 (dd, *J* = 2.52 Hz, 5.52, 1H), 6.54 (s, 2H), 6.83–6.94 (m, 3H). ^{13}C NMR (100 MHz, $CDCl_3$): −5.19, −5.17, 17.98, 25.02, 46.41, 53.59, 55.03, 60.46, 55.49, 94.04, 111.82, 117.99, 119.05, 129.98, 133.57, 133.74, 145.15, 150.74, 152.95, 164.14. (ii) To a stirring solution of the silyl ether β-lactam (**9b**) (4 mmol) in dry THF (30 mL) was added a solution of 1.0M tBAF in hexanes (4 mL, 4 mmol) under N_2 at 0 °C. The reaction mixture was stirred for a further 90 min. Reaction was diluted with ethyl acetate (150 mL) and washed with 0.1M HCl (200 mL). The aqueous layer was further extracted with ethyl acetate (2 × 50 mL). All the organic layers were collected and washed with water (200 mL) and saturated brine (200 mL) before being dried over Na_2SO_4. Solvent was removed under reduced pressure and the phenol was isolated by flash chromatography over silica gel (eluent: *n*-hexane: ethyl actetate, 1:1) to afford the desired product, yield 73%, 1.05 g, as a yellow solid, Mp 78–80 °C [87]. IR (NaCl $_{\gamma}$max): 1741 cm^{-1}, 3443 cm^{-1}, 2937 cm^{-1}. ^{1}H NMR (400 MHz, $CDCl_3$): δ2.88–2.93 (dd, *J* = 2.48 Hz, 15.06 Hz, 1H), 3.45–3.50 (dd, *J* = 5.52 Hz, 15.56Hz, 1H), 3.67 (s, 6H), 3.72 (s, 3H), 3.84 (s, 3H), 4.84–4.86 (dd, *J* = 2.52 Hz, 5.52 Hz, 1H), 6.14 (s, 1H), 6.53 (s, 2H), 6.81–6.93 (m, 3H). ^{13}C NMR (100 MHz, $CDCl_3$): δ 46.27, 53.68, 60.44,

55.52, 94.04, 110.57, 111.63, 117.36, 130.61, 133.56, 133.75, 145.90, 146.48, 152.94, 164.27. HRMS: Found 382.1251 (M^++Na); $C_{19}H_{21}NO_6Na$ requires 382.1267.

4.1.8. 3-(1-Hydroxyethyl)-4-(3-hydroxy-4-methoxyphenyl)-1-(3,4,5-trimethoxyphenyl) azetidin-2-one (**10a**)

To a solution of the TBDMS protected 3-unsubstituted β-lactam (**9b**) (125 mg, 0.264 mmol) in dry THF (3 mL) under N_2 at −78 °C (dry ice and acetone) was added 2.0 M LDA solution (0.264 mL, 0.528 mmol). The resulting solution was left to stir for 5 min before a solution of acetaldehyde (49 mg, 0.396 mmol) in dry THF (1.5 mL) was added. The reaction was left to stir for 30 min at −78 °C, then poured onto saturated NaCl solution (25 mL). The resulting solution was extracted with ethyl acetate (50 mL) and the solvent was dried over Na_2SO_4 before being removed under reduced pressure. Preliminary purification was achieved by passage through a short pad (5 cm) of silica (eluent: DCM) to yield the OTBDMS protected ether **10i** as an oil. To a stirring solution of the OTBDMS protected ether **10i** (2 mmol) in dry THF (10 mL) was added a solution of 1.0 M TBAF in hexanes (2 mL, 2 mmol) under N_2 at 0 °C. The reaction mixture was stirred for a further 90 min then diluted with ethyl acetate (75 mL) and washed with 0.1 M HCl (100 mL). The aqueous layer was further extracted with ethyl acetate (2 × 25 mL). All the organic extracts were collected and washed with H_2O (100 mL), and saturated brine (100 mL) before being dried over Na_2SO_4 and solvent was removed under reduced pressure. Purification was carried out by chromatography using a Biotage SP1 chromatography system using a +12M column and detection set at 280 nM and a fraction volume of 12 mL. A gradient elution of 2% ethyl acetate in *n*-hexane to 100% ethyl acetate over 15 column volumes was used. The desired product was obtained as a brown oil, 36 mg, yield 17% [99] IR (NaCl $_{\gamma}$max): 1738 (C=O), 3427 (OH) cm^{-1}. ^1H NMR (400 MHz, $CDCl_3$): δ1.33 (d, *J* = 6.28 Hz, 1H), 1.40 (d, *J* = 6.52 Hz, 2H), 2.58 (br s, 1H), 3.14 (m, 1H), 3.72 (s, 6H), 3.76 (s, 3H), 3.89 (s, 3H), 4.24 (q, *J* = 6.04 Hz, 0.66H), 4.36 (q, *J* = 5.76 Hz, 0.33H), 4.77 (d, *J* = 2.28 Hz, 0.6H), 4.99 (d, *J* = 2.28, 0.4H), 5.95 (s, 0.6H), 5.96 (s, 0.4H), 6.54 (s, 2H), 6.83–7.01 (m, 3H). ^{13}C NMR (100 MHz, $CDCl_3$): δ 21.34, 21.52, 55.99, 56.06, 57.64 57.68, 56.68, 60.93, 64.94, 66.05, 66.10, 94.70, 94.75, 111.05, 112.16, 112.22, 117.88, 130.50, 130.97, 133.67, 134.32, 146.25, 146.32, 146.88, 153.43, δ165.89, 166.06. HRMS: Found 426.1540 (M^++Na); $C_{21}H_{25}NO_7Na$ requires 426.1529.

4.1.9. 3-((E)-1-Hydroxybut-2-enyl)-1-(3,4,5-trimethoxyphenyl)-4-(4-methoxyphenyl) azetidin-2-one (**10b**)

Following the procedure described above for compound **10a**, using the β-lactam **9a** and crotonaldehyde, the product was obtained as a colourless solid, 82 mg, yield 25%, Mp 143–144 °C. IR (KBr) ν_{max}: 3455 (OH), 1745 (C=O), 1591, 1502, 1248, 1127 cm^{-1}. ^1H NMR (400 MHz, $CDCl_3$): δ 1.73–1.77 (m, 2H), 3.25–3.28 (m, 1H), 3.73 (s, 6H), 3.77 (s, 3H), 3.83 (s, 3H), 4.69–4.72 (m, 1H), 4.83 (d, *J* = 2.52 Hz, 1H), 5.57–5.62 (m, 1H), 5.80–5.88 (m, 1H), 6.56 (s, 2H), 6.91–6.94 (m, 2H), 7.28–7.32 (m, 2H). ^{13}C NMR (100 MHz, $CDCl_3$): δ 17.28, 54.86, 55.52, 55.90, 60.49, 64.70, 68.68, 94.25, 114.06, 114.11, 126.96, 127.81, 129.27, 129.37, 129.75, 133.31, 152.97, 159.16, 165.00. HRMS: found 436.1740 (M^++Na); $C_{23}H_{27}NO_6Na$ requires 436.1736.

4.1.10. 3-(1-Hydroxybut-2-enyl)-4-(3-hydroxy-4-methoxyphenyl)-1-(3,4,5-trimethoxyphenyl) azetidin-2-one (**10c**)

Following the procedure described above for compound **10a**, using the β-lactam (**9b**) and crotonaldehyde, the title compound was obtained as a brown oil, 73 mg, yield 32%. IR (NaCl $_{\gamma}$max): 1732 (C=O), 3427 (OH) cm^{-1}. ^1H NMR (400 MHz, $CDCl_3$): δ1.72 (d, *J* = 7.0 Hz, 1.8H), 1.74 (d, *J* = 1.0Hz, 1.2H), 2.50 (br, s, 1 H), 3.24 (m, 1H), 3.73–3.79 (overlapping singlets, 9H), 3.89 (s, 3H), 4.51 (t, *J* = 6.53Hz, 0.4H), 4.67 (t, *J* = 6.80 Hz, 0.6H), 4.76 (d, *J* = 2.48 Hz, 0.4H), 4.96 (d, *J* = 2.0 Hz, 0.6H), 5.78–5.85 (m, 2H). ^{13}C NMR (100 MHz, $CDCl_3$): δ17.25, 55.53, 55.84, 64.38, 60.47, 64.65, 68.42, 70.60, 94.26, 110.50, 111.75, 111.82, 117.42, 117.48, 127.62, 129.22, 129.78, 130.47, 133.25, 133.27, 146.17, 146.32, 152.93, 165.21. HRMS: Found 452.1707 (M^++Na); $C_{23}H_{27}NO_7Na$ requires 452.1685.

4.1.11. 4-(3-Hydroxy-4-methoxyphenyl)-3-(1-hydroxy-1-methylethyl)-1-(3,4,5-trimethoxy-phenyl) azetidin-2-one (**10d**)

Following the procedure described above for compound **10a**, using the β-lactam (**9b**) and acetone, the title compound was obtained as a brown oil, 51 mg, yield 23%. IR (NaCl ν max): 1732 (C=O), 3429 (OH) cm^{-1}. ^1H NMR (400 MHz, $CDCl_3$): δ1.35 (s, 3H), 1.48 (s, 3H), 1.91 (br, s, 1H), 3.13 (d, *J* = 2.52 Hz, 1H), 3.72 (s, 6H), 3.76 (s, 3H), 3.89 (s, 3H), 4.89 (d, *J* = 2.52 Hz, 1H), 5.90 (br, s, 1H), 6.56 (s, 2H), 6.83–6.96 (m, 3H). ^{13}C NMR (100 MHz, $CDCl_3$): δ 27.36, 27.62, 55.50, 55.53, 56.73, 60.47, 69.50, 94.27, 110.57, 111.78, 117.48, 130.51, 133.18, 133.79, 145.80, 146.25, 152.93, 165.29. HRMS: found 440.1671 (M^++Na); $C_{22}H_{27}NO_7Na$ requires 440.1685.

4.1.12. 3-((E)-1-Hydroxy-3-phenylallyl)-1-(3,4,5-trimethoxyphenyl)-4-(4-methoxyphenyl) azetidin-2-one (**10e**)

Following the procedure described above for compound **10a**, using the β-lactam **9a** and cinnamaldehyde, the product was obtained as a brown oil, 88 mg, yield 23%. IR (NaCl, film) ν_{max}: 3456 (OH), 1746 (C=O), 1579, 1503, 1266, 1123 cm^{-1}. ^1H NMR (400 MHz, $CDCl_3$): δ 3.38–3.39 (m, 1H), 3.73 (s, 6H), 3.78 (s, 3H), 3.82 (s, 3H), 4.53–4.56 (m, 1H), 4.78 (br s, 1H), 6.26–6.33 (m, 1H), 6.57 (s, 2H), 6.71–6.80 (m, 1H), 6.89–7.35 (m, 9H). HRMS: found 498.1885 (M^++Na); $C_{28}H_{29}NO_6Na$ requires 498.1893.

4.1.13. 4-(3-Hydroxy-4-methoxy-phenyl)-3-(1-hydroxy-3-phenyl-allyl)-1-(3,4,5-trimethoxy-phenyl) -azetidin-2-one (**10f**)

Following the procedure described above for compound **10a**, using 3-unsubstituted β-lactam (**9b**) and cinnamaldehyde, the title compound was obtained as a brown oil, 99 mg, yield 38%. IR (NaCl ν max): 1732 (C=O) 3418 (OH) cm^{-1}. ^1H NMR (400 MHz, $CDCl_3$): δ3.21 (br, s, 1H), 3.34 (dd, *J* = 2.55 Hz, 5.63 Hz, 0.53H), 3.37 (dd, *J* = 2.55 Hz, 5.62 Hz, 0.57H), 3.69 (s, 6H), 3.76 (s, 3H), 3.85 (s, 3H), 4.75 (dd, *J* = 6.13 Hz, 12.40 Hz, 0.43H), 4.86 (d, *J* = 2.45 Hz, 0.43H), 4.91 (dd, *J* = 3.82 Hz, 7.63 Hz, 0.57H), 5.03 (d, *J* = 2.45 Hz, 0.53H), 5.81–5.98 (m, 1H), 6.24 (dd, *J* = 5.54 Hz, 16.28 Hz, 0.57H), 6.41 (dd, *J* = 5.54 Hz, 16.28 Hz, 0.43H), 6.58 (s, 2H), 6.72–6.96 (m, 3H), 7.35–7.39 (m, 5H). ^{13}C NMR (100 MHz, $CDCl_3$): 53.32, 55.84, 56.17, 60.75, 57.35, 57.41, 64.81, 68.41, 70.77, 94.81, 94.86, 95.12, 110.61, 110.95, 110.98, 117.84, 117.91, 126.37, 126.61, 128.03, 128.46, 129.49, 130.33, 131.45, 133.12, 134.48, 136.20, 146.16, 146.61, 148.29, 153.29, 153.31, 165.48, 165.48. HRMS: found 514.1826 (M^++Na); $C_{28}H_{29}NO_7Na$ requires 514.1842.

4.1.14. 4-(3-Hydroxy-4-methoxyphenyl)-3-(1-hydroxyallyl)-1-(3,4,5-trimethoxy phenyl) azetidin-2-one (**10g**)

Following the procedure described above for compound **10a**, using 3-unsubstituted β-lactam (**9b**) and acrolein, the title compound was obtained as a brown oil, 48 mg, yield 22%. IR (NaCl ν max): 1732 (C=O), 3428 (OH) cm^{-1}. ^1H NMR (400 MHz, $CDCl_3$): δ 1.78 (br, s, 1H), 2.42 (br, s, 1H), 3.24–3.30 (m, 1H), 3.73 (s, 6H), 3.77 (s, 3H), 3.91 (s, 3H), 6.60 (t, *J* = 6.4 Hz, 6.6 Hz, 0.58H), 4.74 (dd, *J* = 6.4 Hz, 6.5 Hz, 0.32H), 4.80 (d, *J* = 2.3 Hz, 0.58H), 4.96 (d, *J* = 2.7 Hz, 0.32H), 5.28–5.44 (m, 2H), 5.78 (br, s, 1H), 5.90–5.98 (m, 0.32H), 6.02–6.10 (m, 0.68H), 6.56 (s, 2H), 6.84–7.28 (m, 3H). ^{13}C NMR (100 MHz, $CDCl_3$): δ 55.53, 55.55, 55.62, 60.48, 56.85, 63.99, 68.28, 70.76, 94.34, 110.47, 110.52, 111.74 111.81, 115.56, 117.47, 117.51, 129.93, 130.20, 133.20, 136.59, 136.80, 145.79, 146.14, 146.33, 152.96, 164.89. HRMS: found 438.1547 (M^++Na); $C_{22}H_{25}NO_7Na$ requires 438.1529.

4.1.15. 4-(3-Hydroxy-4-methoxy-phenyl)-3-(1-hydroxy-1-methylallyl)-1-(3,4,5-trimethoxy-phenyl) -azetidin-2-one (**10h**)

Following the procedure described above for compound **10a**, using 3-unsubstituted β-lactam (**9b**) and 3-buten-2-one, the title compound was obtained as a brown oil, 41mg, yield 18%. IR (NaCl ν max): 1734 (C=O), 3433 (OH) cm^{-1}. ^1H NMR (400 MHz, $CDCl_3$): δ1.46 (s, 1.53H), 1.56 (s, 1.34H), 1.8 (br, s, 1H), 3.17 (d, *J* = 2.40 Hz, 0.45H), 3.25 (d, *J* = 2.42 Hz, 0.42H), 3.71 (s, 6H), 3.76 (s, 3H), 3.88 (s, 3H), 4.81 (d, *J* = 2.40 Hz, 0.47H), 4.86 (d, *J* = 2.41 Hz, 0.44H), 5.17–5.23 (m, 1H), 5.31–5.42 (m, 1H), 5.81–6.81 (m,

1H), 5.81–5.83 (overlapping singlets, 1H), 6.54 (s, 2H), 6.83–6.96 (m, 3H). ^{13}C NMR (100 MHz, $CDCl_3$): δ 26.06, 26.19, 53.00, 56.01, 60.46, 55.51, 55.54, 67.47, 68.46, 71.70, 71.76, 94.28, 110.46, 110.54, 111.84, 111.92, 117.51, 117.60, 130.35, 133.17, 133.81, 140.73, 141.39, 141.46, 145.66, 146.13, 152.94, 164.45, δ164.91. HRMS: found 452.1691 (M^+Na); $C_{23}H_{27}NO_7Na$ requires 452.1685.

4.1.16. 3-Acetyl-4-(3-hydroxy-4-methoxyphenyl)-1-(3,4,5-trimethoxyphenyl)azetidin-2-one (**11**)

Method A: To a stirring solution of pyridinium chlorochromate (132 mg, 0.57 mmol) in dry DCM (2 mL) under N_2 at room temperature was added quickly a solution of the silyl protected β-lactam (**10i**) (195 mg, 0.38 mmol). The reaction was stirred at room temperature for 18 h and then diluted with diethyl ether (25 mL) and the resulting suspension allowed to settle and the diethyl ether layer decanted off. The remaining solid was washed and decanted twice with two further 25 mL portions of diethylether. The organic extracts were combined and dried over $MgSO_4$, filtered, and the solvent removed under reduced pressure. The *t*BDMS ether was removed by treatment with tBAF as previously described, to afford the title compound as an oil, 7%, 11mg. **Method B:** The 3-unsubstituted β-lactam (**9b**) (378 mg, 0.80 mmol) was dissolved in THF (7 mL) in a dry flask flushed with N_2 and cooled to −78 °C. To this stirring solution LDA (1.0 M solution, 0.8 mL, 0.8 mmol) was added all at once and the reaction left to stir for 5 min prior to the dropwise addition of acetyl chloride (0.085 mL, 1.2 mmol), in THF (2 mL). The reaction mixture was allowed to stir at −78 °C for 30 min then stirred at room temperature for 5 min before being poured into saturated brine (50 mL). The brine solution was extracted with ethyl acetate (2 × 50 mL), the organic layers combined, dried over $MgSO_4$, filtered, and the solvent removed under reduced pressure. Purification by flash column chromatography over silica gel (eluent: *n*-hexane: ethyl acetate, 1:1) followed by removal of the TBDMS ether by treatment with tBAF as previously described afforded the title compound as an oil, 35 mg, yield 11%. IR (NaCl ν max): 1731 (C=O), 1739, (C=O) 3434 (OH) cm^{-1}. ^{1}H NMR (400 MHz, $CDCl_3$): δ1.99 (s, 3H), 3.73 (s, 6H), 3.75 (s, 3H), 3.81 (s, 3H), 4.23 (d, *J* = 1.98 Hz, 1H), 5.12 (d, *J* = 1.99 Hz, 1H), 6.08 (s, 2H), 6.37–6.57 (m, 3H). ^{13}C NMR (100 MHz, $CDCl_3$): δ 23.14, 53.93, 55.71, 60.87, 65.03, 61.71, 93.81, 111.21, 113.02, 118.21, 130.98, 131.02, 134.27, 147.12, 147.34, 153.27, 164.45, 181.23. HRMS: found 402.1463 (M^++H); $C_{21}H_{24}NO_7$ requires 402.1553.

4.1.17. 3-Ethylidene-4-(3-hydroxy-4-methoxy-phenyl)-1-(3,4,5-trimethoxy-phenyl)-azetidin-2-one (**12**)

To a solution of the silyl ether protected β-lactam **10i** (1 mmol) in DCM (10 mL), stirring at 0 °C under N_2, was added PPh_3 (1 mmol) and DEAD (1.2 mmol). Stirring at 0 °C was continued for a further 3 min before the reaction was allowed to warm to room temperature. Diethyl ether (30 mL) was added to the reaction mixture to precipitate the triphenylphosphine oxide side product which was removed by filtration. The filtrate was collected and evaporated to dryness under reduced pressure to afford the product. Separation of the *E*/*Z* isomers was carried out on a Biotage SP1 system using a gradient elution from 2% ethyl acetate in hexanes to 100% ethyl acetate over 20 column volumes, and detection at 280 nm. The product was obtained as a colourless resin, [99], [100], 87 mg, yield 52%. IR (NaCl ν max): 1738 (C=O), 2935 (CH), 3327 (OH) cm^{-1}. ^{1}H NMR (400 MHz, $CDCl_3$): *E isomer*, δ 1.62 (d, *J* = 4.40 Hz, 3H), 3.76 (s, 6H), 3.78 (s, 3H), 3.92 (s, 3H), 5.32 (s, 1H), 5.68, s, 1H), 6.32 (m, 1H), 6.61 (s, 2H), 6.86 (d, *J* = 8.2 Hz, 1H), 7.03 (d, *J* = 1.96 Hz, 1H), 6.99 (m, 1H). *Z isomer*, δ 2.05 (d, *J* = 4.16 Hz, 3H), 3.76 (s, 6H), 3.79 (s, 3H), 3.92 (s, 3H), 5.19 (s, 1H), 5.65–5.66 (m, 2H), 6.63 (s, 2H), 6.85–6.90 (m, 3H). ^{13}C NMR (100 MHz, $CDCl_3$): *E isomer* δ 13.26, 55.80, 55.88, 60.76, 62.72, 94.47, 110.68, 113.04, 118.87, 123.32, 129.72, 133.94, 134.20, 142.32, 146.04, 146.74, 153.33, 161.19. *Z isomer* δ 14.30, 55.81, 55.82, 60.81, 62.80, 94.57, 110.61, 112.73, 118.48, 126.89, 130.37, 133.93, 134.15, 141.71, 146.11, 146.72, 153.38, 161.79. HRMS: found 408.1411(M^++Na); $C_{21}H_{23}NO_6Na$ requires 408.1423.

4.1.18. 3-(1,2-Dihydroxyethyl)-4-(3-hydroxy-4-methoxyphenyl)-1-(3,4,5-trimethoxyphenyl) azetidin-2-one (**13**)

To a solution of the silyl ether protected azetidin-2-one (**7o**) (156 mg, 0.312 mmol) in pyridine (0.5 mL) stirring under N_2 at room temperature was added osmium tetroxide, OsO_4 (80 mg, 0.312 mmol). The reaction darkened in colour and became hot to the touch upon completion of the addition. The flask was immersed in ice-water for 60 s, then left to stir at room temperature under N_2 for 22 h. A solution of $Na_2(SO_3)_2$ (1.343 g, 6.8 mmol) in a 1:4 mixture of pyridine/water (20 mL) was added and the reaction was stirred at room temperature for a further 7 h. The reaction mixture was extracted with warm ethyl acetate (100 mL). The organic layer was collected and washed with 0.1M HCl (100 mL), saturated $NaHCO_3$ (100 mL), and water (100 mL). The organic layer was collected and dried over $MgSO_4$, filtered and the solvent removed under reduced pressure. The product was purified by passage through a short silica column (5 cm) and eluted with DCM. The tBDMS group was cleaved by treatment with tBAF as described above, to afford the product as a colourless resin, yield 39%, 51 mg. IR (NaCl ν max): 1727 (C=O), 3454 (OH) cm^{-1}. ^1H NMR (400 MHz, $CDCl_3$): δ 2.72 (br s, 1H, OH), 3.16 (dd, 0.72H, *J* = 2.42 Hz, 5.55 Hz), 3.19 (dd, 0.29H, *J* = 2.46 Hz, 4.56 Hz), 3.60-3.67 (m, 8H), 3.74 (s, 3H), 3.83 (s, 3H), 4.10 (dd, *J* = 4.05 Hz, 0.26H), 4.19 (dd, *J* = 5.50 Hz, 0.75H), 4.25 (br s, 0.5H), 4.90 (d, *J* = 2.37 Hz, 0.31H), 5.00 (d, *J* = 2.36 Hz, 0.69H), 6.25 (br, s, 0.30H), 6.46 (br, s, 0.70H), 6.53 (s, 2H), 6.77–6.94 (m, 3H). ^{13}C NMR (100 MHz, $CDCl_3$): δ 55.79, 55.85, 56.80, 56.97, 60.73, 62.18, 64.46, 64.76, 68.54, 69.30, 94.92, 111.06, 111.11, 112.23, 112.43, 117.76, 117.90, 129.92, 130.29, 133.17, 133.33, 146.07, 146.22, 146.85, 146.98, 153.27, 165.76, 165.96. HRMS: found 442.1490 (M^++Na); $C_{21}H_{25}NO_8Na$ requires 442.1478.

4.1.19. (1-((2-Methoxy-5-(4-oxo-1-(3,4,5-trimethoxyphenyl)-3-vinylazetidin-2-yl)phenyl)-amino)-1 -oxopropan-2-yl) carbamaic acid 9H-fluoren-9-ylmethyl ester (**14**)

To a stirred solution of β-lactam **7t** (4.76 mmol) in anhydrous DMF (30 mL) were added DCC (5.7 mmol), Fmoc-protected alanine (5.6 mmol) and HOBt.H_2O (7.3 mmol) at room temperature. The mixture was stirred for 24 h, then ethyl acetate (50 mL) was added and the reaction mixture was filtered. The DMF was removed by washing with water (5 × 50 mL). The organic solvent was removed under reduced pressure, and the product was isolated by flash column chromatography over silica gel (eluent: dichloromethane: methanol gradient) as a brown oil, yield, 58%, 173 mg. IR (NaCl, film) ν_{max}: 3323 (NH), 1723 (C=O), 1640 (C=O), 1598 cm^{-1}. H NMR (400 MHz, $CDCl_3$): δ 1.52 (br s, 3H), 3.74 (s, 6H), 3.77 (s, 4H), 3.83 (s, 3H), 4.25 (t, *J* = 6.78 Hz, 1H), 4.45–4.47 (m, 3H), 4.76 (br s, 1H), 5.31–5.34 (m, 1H), 5.37–5.41 (m, 1H), 5.98–6.07 (m, 1H), 6.59 (s, 2H), 6.86–7.79 (m, 11H), 8.39–8.44 (br s, 1H), 8.50 (s, 1H). ^{13}C NMR (100 MHz, $CDCl_3$): δ 20.62, 46.63, 55.47, 55.64, 60.49, 59.96, 60.93, 63.32, 66.83, 94.30, 110.15, 117.70, 119.50, 120.58, 124.52, 126.64, 127.35, 128.39, 128.80, 128.84, 129.31, 130.03, 133.38, 133.91, 137.63, 140.85, 143.22, 153.03, 164.91, 169.98, 170.76. HRMS: Found 700.2632 (M^++Na); $C_{39}H_{39}N_3O_8Na$ requires 700.2635.

4.1.20. 2-Amino-N-(2-methoxy-5-(1-(3,4,5-trimethoxyphenyl)-4-oxo-3-vinylazetidin-2-yl)phenyl) propanamide (**15**)

To amino acid amide **14** (1.56 mmol) in methanol (10 mL)/CH_2Cl_2 (10 mL) was added 2N NaOH (3.4 mmol) at room temperature and the mixture was stirred for 24 h. Saturated aq. $NaHCO_3$ was added and the mixture was extracted with CH_2Cl_2 three times. The organic solution was dried and evaporated. The product was dissolved diethyl ether and extracted with 2N HCl (5 × 50 mL). 2N NaOH was added to the HCl mixture solution and the mixture was washed with diethyl ether (5 × 50 mL). The organic solution was dried and the solvent was removed under reduced pressure to afford the product as an off-yellow oil, yield 57%. IR (NaCl) ν_{max}: 3307 cm^{-1} (NH_2), 1741 (C=O), 1679 (C=O) cm^{-1}. ^1H NMR (400 MHz, $CDCl_3$): δ 1.61–1.64 (m, 3H), 3.76 (s, 9H), 3.68–3.69 (m, 1H), 3.78 (br s, 1H), 3.79 (s, 3H), 5.40 (br s, 1H), 6.33–6.35 (m, 1H), 6.65 (s, 2H), 6.83–6.90 (m, 2H), 7.08–7.20 (m, 3H). ^{13}C NMR (100 MHz, $CDCl_3$): δ 21.65, 51.69, 55.87, 55.90, 60.92, 62.95, 65.87, 94.47, 109.81, 119.33, 121.61,

123.70, 127.72, 133.57, 133.69, 134.14, 148.34, 153.45, 161.44, 167.06. HRMS: found 456.2137 (M^++H); $C_{24}H_{30}N_3O_6$ requires 456.2135.

4.1.21. General procedure III: Preparation of dibenzyl phosphates **16a**, **16b**

To a solution of phenol **7s**, **9a** (17 mmol) in acetonitrile (100 mL cooled to 0 °C) was added carbon tetrachloride (85 mmol). The resulting solution was stirred for 10 min prior to adding diisopropylethylamine (35 mmol) and dimethylaminopyridine (1.7 mmol). The dibenzyl phosphite (24.5 mmol) was then added dropwise to the mixture. When the reaction was complete, 0.5M KH_2PO_4 (aq) was added and the reaction mixture was allowed to warm to room temperature. An ethyl acetate extract (3 × 50 mL) was washed with saturated sodium chloride (aqueous, 100 mL) followed by water (100 mL) and dried using anhydrous sodium sulfate. The organic solvent was removed under reduced pressure and the product was isolated by flash column chromatography over silica gel (*n*-hexane: ethyl acetate gradient).

2-Methoxy-5-(1-(3,4,5-trimethoxyphenyl)-4-oxoazetidin-2-yl)phenyl dibenzyl phosphate (**16a**)

Preparation as described in the general method above from β-lactam **9a**. Yield: 60%, 507 mg, brown oil. IR (NaCl, film) ν_{max}: 2940, 1730 (C=O, β-lactam), 1507, 1300 (P=O), 1235, 1127 cm^{-1}. ^1H NMR (400 MHz, $CDCl_3$): δ 2.90 (dd, *J* = 15.08 Hz, 2.52 Hz, 1H), 3.50 (dd, *J* = 15.56 Hz, 5.52 Hz, 1H), 3.76 (s, 6H), 3.76 (s, 3H), 3.81 (s, 3H), 4.84 (dd, *J* = 5.04 Hz, 2.52 Hz, 1H), 5.15–5.18 (m, 4H), 6.53 (s, 2H), 6.93–7.23 (m, 3H), 7.31–7.36 (m, 10H). ^{13}C NMR (100 MHz, $CDCl_3$): δ 46.44, 53.23, 55.54, 55.61, 60.47, 69.44, 69.48, 69.54, 93.97, 112.77, 119.36, 122.59, 127.43, 127.47, 128.14, 128.16, 130.14, 133.47, 133.89, 135.10, 139.47, 139.54, 150.35, 153.06, 163.87. HRMS: found 642.1838 (M^++Na); $C_{33}H_{34}NO_9PNa$ requires 642.1869.

2-Methoxy-5-(1-(3,4,5-trimethoxyphenyl)-4-oxo-3-vinylazetidin-2-yl)phenyl dibenzyl phosphate (**16b**)

Preparation as described in the general method above from β-lactam **7s**. Yield: 61%, 502 mg, brown oil. IR (NaCl, film) ν_{max}: 2946, 1749 (C=O, β-lactam), 1502, 1300 (P=O), 1240, 1127 cm^{-1}. ^1H NMR (400 MHz, $CDCl_3$): δ 3.70 (br s, 1H), 3.71 (s, 6H), 3.76 (s, 3H), 3.82 (s, 3H), 4.65 (d, *J* = 2.00 Hz, 1H), 5.14–5.18 (m, 4H), 5.33–5.40 (m, 2H), 5.97–6.02 (m, 1H), 6.53 (s, 2H), 6.94–7.20 (m, 3H), 7.28–7.35 (m, 10H). ^{13}C NMR (100 MHz, $CDCl_3$): δ 55.56, 55.61, 60.43, 60.48, 63.29, 69.48, 69.50, 94.19, 112.79, 119.27, 119.62, 122.75, 127.41, 127.49, 128.15, 128.22, 129.29, 129.85, 133.22, 134.00, 135.07, 135.12, 139.57, 150.52, 153.07, 164.69. HRMS: found 668.2017 (M^++Na); $C_{35}H_{36}NO_9PNa$ requires 668.2025.

4.1.22. Phosphoric acid 2-methoxy-5-[4-oxo-1-(3,4,5-trimethoxyphenyl)azetidin-2-yl]phenyl ester dimethyl ester (**16c**)

A solution of β-lactam phenol **7s** (280 mg, 0.64 mmol), acetonitrile (5 mL) and carbon tetrachloride (0.62 mL, 0.64 mmol) was cooled to −10 °C and stirred under a nitrogen atmosphere for ten minutes. Diisopropyl ethylamine (1.28 mmol) and dimethylaminopyridine (0.06 mmol) were added. After one minute, dimethyl phosphite (0.96 mmol) was added over three minutes. The mixture was stirred for a further 3 h allowing the reaction to come to ambient temperature slowly. The reaction was terminated via the addition of 0.5 M potassium dihydrogen phosphate. The mixture was extracted with ethyl acetate. The organic phases were combined and evaporated to dryness under reduced pressure. The residue was purified by flash chromatography on silica gel to afford the product (155 mg, 52%). IR (KBr) ν_{max}: 3437.4, 2960.9, 1752.1, 1603.4, 1509.2, 1466.2, 1281.4, 1239.3, 1185.6, 1130.0, 1052.1, 999.4, 855.8. ^1H-NMR (400 MHz, $CDCl_3$): δ 2.94 (dd, 1H, *J* = 2.8 Hz, 15.3 Hz), 3.52 (dd, 1H, *J* = 5.5 Hz, 15.3 Hz), 3.72 (s, 6H), 3.74 (s, 3H), 3.82–3.87 (m, 9H, OCH_3), 4.92 (m, 1H), 6.52 (s, 2H), 6.95–6.96 (m, 1H), 7.16–7.18 (m, 1H), 7.29–7.30 (m, 1H). ^{13}C NMR (100 MHz, $CDCl_3$): δ 46.80, 53.61, 54.91, 54.97, 55.98, 56.05, 60.83, 94.40, 113.29, 119.61, 119.64, 123.21, 130.61, 133.84, 134.23, 139.81, 139.89, 150.72, 150.76, 153.43, 164.37. HRMS: Found 468.1425 (M^++H), $C_{21}H_{27}NO_9P$ requires 468.1423.

4.1.23. Phosphoric acid diethyl ester 2-methoxy-5-[4-oxo-1-(3,4,5-trimethoxyphenyl)azetidin-2-yl]phenyl ester (**16d**)

Preparation as described above for β-lactam **16c** using diethyl phosphite (0.96 mmol). Yield 250 mg, 79%. IR (KBr) ν_{max}: 3487.5, 2988.0, 1756.3, 1603.4, 1586.6, 1507.1, 1451.5, 1292.0, 1238.7, 1127.0, 1035.6, 1000.2, 988.1, 823.1. ^{1}H-NMR (400 MHz, $CDCl_3$): δ 1.29 (t, 6H), 2.90 (dd, 1H, *J* = 2.5 Hz, 15.3 Hz), 3.49 (dd, 1H, *J* = 5.8 Hz, 15.3 Hz), 3.69 (s, 6H), 3.71 (s, 3H), 3.83 (s, 3H), 4.03 –4.07 (m, 4H), 6.50 (s, 2H), 6.92 (m, 1H), 7.12–7.15 (m, 1H), 7.29–7.30 (m, 1H). ^{13}C NMR (100 MHz, $CDCl_3$): δ: 15.96, 16.03, 46.84, 53.65, 56.00, 60.84, 63.45, 63.50, 94.38, 113.17, 119.49, 119.51, 123.07, 130.53, 133.88, 134.24, 140.06, 140.13, 150.80, 150.85, 153.45, 164.36. HRMS: Found 496.1734 (M^++H); $C_{23}H_{31}NO_9P$ requires 496.1736.

4.1.24. 2-Methoxy-5-(1-(3,4,5-trimethoxyphenyl)-4-oxoazetidin-2-yl)phenyl dihydrogen phosphate (**17a**)

Dibenzyl phosphate ester (**16a**) (0.27 mmol) was dissolved in dry dichloromethane (5 mL) under nitrogen at 0 °C. Bromotrimethylsilane (0.59 mmol) was added to the reaction mixture and allowed to stir for 45 min. Sodium thiosulfate solution (10%, 5 mL) was added to the reaction and stirring was continued for 5 min. The aqueous phase was extracted with ethyl acetate (3 × 25 mL). The combined organic phases were concentrated under reduced pressure and the crude product was purified by flash chromatography on silica gel (eluent: *n*-hexane: ethyl acetate, 1:1) to afford the product as a brown solid. Yield: 91%, 289 mg, Mp 207–209 °C. Purity (HPLC): 100.0%. IR (KBr) ν_{max}: 3497 (OH), 1730 (C=O, β-lactam), 1303 (P=O), 1237, 1128 cm^{-1}. ^{1}H NMR (400 MHz, DMSO-d_6): δ 2.91 (dd, *J* = 15.04 Hz, 2.52 Hz, 1H), 3.51 (dd, *J* = 15.64 Hz, 5.52 Hz, 1H), 3.58 (s, 3H), 3.64 (s, 6H), 3.74 (s, 3H), 5.08 (br s, 1H), 6.52 (s, 2H), 7.03–7.48 (m, 3H). ^{13}C NMR (100 MHz, DMSO-d_6): δ 45.88, 52.92, 55.64, 55.72, 60.06, 94.30, 113.02, 118.96, 121.91, 130.08, 130.71, 133.53, 133.68, 150.19, 153.09, 164.47. HRMS: found 438.0947 (M-H)$^-$; $C_{19}H_{21}NO_9P$ requires 438.0954

4.1.25. 2-Methoxy-5-(1-(3,4,5-trimethoxyphenyl)-4-oxo-3-vinylazetidin-2-yl)phenyl dihydrogen phosphate (**17b**)

Following the preparation described above for compound **16a**, using dibenzyl phosphate ester (**16b**) (0.27 mmol) and bromotrimethylsilane (0.59 mmol). Purification by flash chromatography on silica gel (eluent: *n*-hexane: ethyl acetate, 1:1) afforded the product as a yellow oil, yield 63%. IR (NaCl) ν_{max}: 3483 (OH), 1749 (C=O), 1307 (P=O) cm^{-1}. ^{1}H NMR (400 MHz, $CDCl_3$): δ 3.70 (s, 6H), 3.76 (s, 3H), 3.79 (s, 3H), 4.68–4.70 (m, 1H), 5.14 (br s, 1H), 5.28–5.38 (m, 2H), 5.94–6.00 (m, 1H), 6.51 (s, 2H), 6.91–7.35 (m, 3H). ^{13}C NMR (100 MHz, $CDCl_3$): δ 55.49, 55.58, 60.43, 60.50, 63.07, 94.31, 112.69, 119.18, 119.55, 122.70, 129.81, 133.08, 133.99, 134.67, 135.23, 150.52, 153.02, 165.14. HRMS: found 488.1106 (M^++Na); $C_{21}H_{24}NO_9PNa$ requires 488.1086.

4.1.26. 5-(3-Ethyl-1-(3,4,5-trimethoxyphenyl)-4-oxoazetidin-2-yl)-2-methoxyphenyl dihydrogen phosphate (**17c**)

The dibenzylphosphate ester protected compound **16b** (2 mmol) was dissolved in ethanol: ethyl acetate (50 mL; 1:1 mixture) and hydrogenated over 1.2 g of 10% palladium on carbon until complete on TLC, typically less than 3 h. The catalyst was filtered, the solvent was removed under reduced pressure and the product was isolated by flash column chromatography over silica gel (eluent: *n*-hexane: ethyl acetate gradient) to afford the product as a brown oil, 140 mg, 98%. Purity (HPLC): 100%. IR (NaCl, film) ν_{max}: 3483 (OH), 1742 (C=O), 1272 (P=O), 1236, 1126 cm^{-1}. ^{1}H NMR (400 MHz, $CDCl_3$): δ 0.97 (br s, 3H), 1.76–1.83 (m, 2H), 3.09 (s, 1H), 3.66 (s, 6H), 3.71 (s, 6H), 4.56 (br s, 1H), 6.51 (s, 2H), 6.82–7.38 (m, 3H). ^{13}C NMR (100 MHz, $CDCl_3$): δ 13.74, 20.62, 55.47, 55.55, 59.67, 59.99, 60.39, 94.33, 112.48, 118.69, 122.27, 130.12, 133.16, 133.86, 135.64, 150.06, 152.97, 168.22. HRMS: found 490.1239 (M^++Na); $C_{21}H_{26}NO_9PNa$ requires 490.1243.

4.2. Biochemical Evaluation

All biochemical assays were performed in triplicate on at least three independent occasions for the determination of mean values reported.

4.2.1. Cell Culture

The human breast carcinoma cell line MCF-7, was purchased from the European Collection of Animal Cell Cultures (ECACC) and was cultured in Eagle's minimum essential medium with 10% fetal bovine serum, 2 mM L-glutamine and 100 µg/mL penicillin/streptomycin. The medium was supplemented with 1% non-essential amino acids. The human breast carcinoma cell line MDA-MB-231 was purchased from the European Collection of Animal Cell Cultures (ECACC). MDA-MB-231 cells were maintained in Dulbecco's modified Eagle's medium (DMEM) supplemeted with 10% (*v*/*v*) fetal bovine serum, 2 mM L-glutamine and 100 µg/mL penicillin/streptomycin (complete medium). All media contained 100 U/mL penicillin and 100 µg/mL streptomycin. Triple negative breast cancer Hs578T cells and its invasive variant Hs578Ts(i)$_8$ were obtained as a kind gift from Dr. Susan McDonnell, School of Chemical and Bioprocess Engineering, University College Dublin and were cultured in Dulbecco's Modified Eagle's Media (DMEM) with GlutaMAX^{TM}-I, with the same supplement as for MDA-MB-231 cells in the absence of non-essential amino acids. HEK-293T normal epithelial embryonic kidney cells were cultured in Dulbecco's Modified Eagle's Medium (DMEM) with GlutaMAX^{TM}-I in the absence of non-essential amino acids. K562 and HL-60 cells were originally obtained from the European Collection of Cell Cultures (Salisbury, UK).The K562 cells were derived from a patient in the blast crisis stage of CML HL-60 cells were derive from a patient with acute myeloid leukaemia. Cells were cultured in RPMI-1640 Glutamax medium supplemented with 10% FCS media, and 100 µg/mL penicillin/streptomycin. Cells were maintained at 37 °C in 5% CO_2 in a humidified incubator. All cells were sub-cultured three times/week (adherent cells by trypsinisation).

4.2.2. Cell Viability Assay

Cells were seeded at a density of 5×10^3 cells/well (MCF-7), in triplicate in 96-well plates. After 24 h, cells were then treated with either medium alone, vehicle [1% ethanol (*v*/*v*)] or with serial dilutions of CA-4 or β-lactam analogue. Cell viability for MCF-7 and MDA-MB-231 was analysed using the Alamar Blue assay (Invitrogen Corp, Thermo Fisher Scientific, 168 Third Avenue, Waltham, MA, USA) according to the manufacturer's instructions. After 72 h, Alamar Blue [10% (*v*/*v*)] was added to each well and plates were incubated for 3–5 h at 37 °C in the dark. Fluorescence was read using a 96-well fluorimeter with excitation at 530 nm and emission at 590 nm. Results were expressed as percentage viability relative to vehicle control (100%). Dose response curves were plotted and IC_{50} values (concentration of drug resulting in 50% reduction in cell survival) were obtained using the commercial software package Prism (GraphPad Software, Inc., 2365 Northside, Suite 560, San Diego, CA, USA). Experiments were performed in triplicate on at least three separate occasions.

4.2.3. Lactate Dehydrogenase Assay for Cytotoxicity

Cytotoxicity was determined using the CytoTox 96 non-radioactive cytotoxicity assay (Promega Corporation; 2800 Woods Hollow Road, Madison, WI, USA) [101] following the manufacturer's protocol. Briefly, MCF-7 cells were seeded in 96-well plates, incubated for 24 hr and then treated with test compounds (**7d**, **7h**, **7i**, **7q**, **7r**, **7u**, **7t**, **10d**, **10f**, **12**) as described in the cell viability assay above. After 72 h, 20 µL of 'lysis solution (10X)' was added to control wells and the plate was incubated for a further 1 hr to ensure 100% death. 50 µL of supernatant was carefully removed from each well and transferred to a new 96-well plate. 50 µL of reconstituted 'substrate mix' was added and the plate was placed in the dark at room temperature for 30 min. After this period, 50 µL of 'stop solution' was added to each well and the absorbance was read at a wavelength of 490 nm using a Dynatech MR5000 plate reader. The percentage cell death at 10 µM was calculated.

4.2.4. Cytotoxicity Assay

As previously reported [45,74,75] mammary glands from 14–18 day pregnant CD-1 mice were used as source and primary mammary epithelial cell cultures were prepared from these. The isolated mammary epithelial cells were seeded at two concentrations (25,000 cells/mL and 50,000 cells/mL). Initially a third concentration of 100,000 cells/mL was also used, but this proved to be too high to give meaningful results. After 24 h, the cells were treated with 2 µL volumes of test compound **7s** which had been pre-prepared as stock solutions in ethanol to furnish the concentration range of study, 1 nM–100 µM, and re-incubated for a further 72 h. Control wells contained the equivalent volume of the vehicle ethanol (1% *v*/*v*). The cytotoxicity was assessed using alamar blue dye.

4.2.5. Cell Cycle Analysis

MCF-7 cells (adherent and detached) were treated with the appropriate concentration of compound **7s** and incubated for the designated time. Cells were collected, trypsinised and centrifuged at 800× *g* for 15 min. Cells were washed twice with ice-cold PBS and fixed in ice-cold 70% ethanol overnight at −20 °C. Fixed cells were centrifuged at 800× *g* for 15 min and stained with 50 µg/mL of PI, containing 50 µg/mL of DNase-free RNase A, at 37 °C for 30 min. The DNA content of cells (10,000 cells/experimental group) was analysed by flow cytometer at 488 nm using a FACSCalibur flow cytometer (BD Biosciences, 2350 Qume Dr, San Jose, CA, USA) all data were recorded and analysed using the CellQuest^{TM} software, (BD Biosciences, 2350 Qume Dr, San Jose, CA, USA)

4.2.6. Annexin V/PI Apoptotic Assay

Apoptotic cell death was detected by flow cytometry using Annexin V and propidium iodide (PI). MCF-7 Cells were seeded in 6 well plated at density of 1×10^5 cells/mL and treated with either vehicle (0.1% (*v*/*v*) EtOH), CA-4 or β-lactam compound **7s** at different concentrations for selected time. Cells were then harvested and prepared for flow cytometric analysis. Cells were washed in 1X binding buffer (20X binding buffer: 0.1M HEPES, pH 7.4; 1.4 M NaCl; 25 mM $CaCl_2$ diluted in dH_2O) and incubated in the dark for 30 min on ice in Annexin V-containing binding buffer [1:100]. Cells were then washed once in binding buffer and then re-suspended in PI-containing binding buffer [1:1000]. Samples were analysed immediately using the BD accuri flow cytometer (BD Biosciences, 2350 Qume Dr, San Jose, CA, USA) and prism software for analysis the data (GraphPad Software, Inc., 2365 Northside Dr., Suite 560, San Diego, CA, USA). Four populations are produced during the assay Annexin V and PI negative (Q4, healthy cells), Annexin V positive and PI negative (Q3, early apoptosis), Annexin V and PI positive (Q2, late apoptosis) and Annexin V negative and PI positive (Q1, necrosis). Paclitaxel was used as a positive control for cell death

4.2.7. Tubulin Polymerization Assay

The assembly of purified bovine tubulin was monitored using a kit, BK006, purchased from Cytoskeleton Inc., 1830 S Acoma St, Denver, CO, 80223, USA. [78]. The assay was carried out in accordance with the manufacturer's instructions in the tubulin polymerisation assay kit manual using the standard assay conditions. The values reported represent the average values from two independent assays. Purified (>99%) bovine brain tubulin (3 mg/mL) in a buffer consisting of 80 mM PIPES (pH 6.9), 0.5 mM EGTA, 2 mM $MgCl_2$, 1 mM GTP and 10% glycerol was incubated at 37 °C in the presence of either vehicle (2% (*v*/*v*) ddH_2O) or compounds **7h**, **7i**, **7s**, **7t** (initially 10 µM in EtOH); CA-4 and Paclitaxel were used as controls. Light is scattered proportionally to the concentration of polymerised microtubules in the assay. Therefore, tubulin assembly was monitored turbidimetrically at 340 nm at 37 °C in a Spectramax 340 PC spectrophotometer (Molecular Devices, 3860 N 1st St, San Jose, CA, USA). The absorbance was measured at 30 s intervals for 60 min.

4.2.8. Colchicine-Binding Site Assay

MCF-7 cells were seeded at a density of 5×10^4 cells/well in 6-well plates and incubated overnight. Cells were treated with vehicle control [ethanol (0.1% *v/v*)] or compound **7s** (10 μM) for 2 h. After this time, selected wells were treated with *N,N′*-ethylene-bis(iodoacetamide)(EBI) (100 μM) (Santa Cruz Biotechnology Inc. 10410 Finnell Street, Dallas, Texas, USA) for 1.5 h. Following treatment, cells were twice washed with ice-cold PBS and lysed by addition of Laemmli buffer. Samples were separated by SDS-PAGE, trasnsferred to polyvinylidene difluoride membranes and probed with β-tubulin antibodies (Sigma-Aldrich, 2033 Westport Center Dr, St. Louis, MO, USA) [85].

4.2.9. Immunofluorescence Microscopy

Confocal microscopy was used to study the effects of drug treatment on MCF-7 cytoskeleton. For immunofluorescence, MCF-7 cells were seeded at 1×10^5 cells/mL on eight chamber glass slides (BD Biosciences, 2350 Qume Dr, San Jose, CA, USA). Cells were either untreated or treated with vehicle [1% ethanol (*v/v*)], paclitaxel (1 μM), combretastatin A-4 (100 nM) or compound **7s** (100 nM) for 16 h. Following treatment cells were gently washed in PBS, fixed for 20 min with 4% paraformaldehyde in PBS and permeabilised in 0.5% Triton X-100. Following washes in PBS containing 0.1% Tween (PBST), cells were blocked in 5% bovine serum albumin diluted in PBST. Cells were then incubated with mouse monoclonal anti-α-tubulin–FITC antibody (clone DM1A) (Sigma-Aldrich, 2033 Westport Center Dr, St. Louis, MO, USA) (1:100) for 2 h at room temperature. Following washes in PBST, cells were incubated with Alexa Fluor 488 dye (1:450) for 1 h at room temperature. Following washes in PBST, the cells were mounted in Ultra Cruz Mounting Media (Santa Cruz Biotechnology Inc., 10410 Finnell Street, Dallas, TX, USA) containing 4,6-diamino-2-phenolindol dihydrochloride (DAPI). Images were captured by Leica SP8 confocal microscopy with Leica application suite X software (Leica Microsystems CMS GmbH Am Friedensplatz 3 D-68165 Mannheim, Germany). All images in each experiment were collected on the same day using identical parameters. Experiments were performed on three independent occasions.

4.3. Stability Study of Compounds 7s, 17b and 17c

Analytical high-performance liquid chromatography (HPLC) stability studies were performed using a Symmetry® column (C_{18}, 5 μm, 4.6 × 150 mm), a Waters 2487 Dual Wavelength Absorbance detector, a Waters 1525 binary HPLC pump and a Waters 717 plus Autosampler (Waters Corporation, 34 Maple St, Milford, MA, USA). Samples were detected at wavelength of 254 nm. All samples were analysed using acetonitrile (80%) and water (20%) as the mobile phase over 10 min and a flow rate of 1 mL/min. Stock solutions were prepared by dissolving 5 mg of compound **7s, 17b** and **17c** in 10 mL of mobile phase. Phosphate buffers at the desired pH values (4, 7.4 and 9) were prepared in accordance with the British Pharmacopoeia monograph 2015. 30 μL of stock solution was diluted with 1 mL of appropriate buffer, shaken and injected immediately. Samples were withdrawn and analysed at time intervals of $t = 0$ min, 5 min, 30 min, 60 min, 90 min, 120 min, 24 h and 48 h. **Plasma stability studies**: 360 μL stock solution of compounds **7s, 17b** and **17c** were transferred to buffered plasma (plasma: buffer = 1:9, 4 mL in total) at 37 °C in screw cap container. Immediately a 250 μL aliquot was withdrawn and added to the Eppendorf tube containing 500 μL $ZnSO_4.7H_2O$ solution (2% w/v $ZnSO_4$ solution in acetonitrile: water, 1:1). The samples were then centrifuged at 10,000 rpm for 3 min and filtered through a 0.2-micron filter and injected according to the HPLC conditions listed above. Further samples were taken in the same manner every 1 h thereafter up to 6 h. A final sample was taken after 24 h. **Whole blood stability studies**. A 360 μL aliquot of stock solution of compounds **17b** and **17c** in acetonitrile was added in whole blood (4 mL, treated with 2% sodium citrate) at 37 °C and 300 μL aliquots were withdrawn at approptiate intervals. Samples were transferred to 1.5 mL Eppenddorf tubes containing 1 mL of $ZnSO_4$. $7H_2O$ solution (2% w/v $ZnSO_4$ solution in acetonitrile: water, 1:1), vortexed and then centrifuged for 5 min at 14,000 rpm. The sample filtered through a 0.2-micron filter and injected according to the HPLC conditions listed above.

4.4. X-Ray Crystallography

Data for samples **6k**, **7h** and **8i**, **8k** were collected on a Bruker APEX DUO and Bruker D8 Quest ECO respectively using Cu Kα (λ = 1.54178 Å; **7h**) and Mo Kα radiation (λ = 0.71073 Å; **6k**, **8i**, **8k**), (Bruker, 40 Manning Road, Billerica, MA, USA) Each sample was mounted on a Mitegen cryoloop and data collected at 100(2) K (Oxford Cobra and Cryostream cryosystems, Oxford Cryosystems, 3 Blenheim Office Park, Long Hanborough, Oxford OX29 8LN, UK). Bruker APEX [102] software was used to collect and reduce data and determine the space group. The structures were solved using direct methods (XS) [103] or intrinsic phasing (XT) [104] and refined with least squares minimization (XL) [105] in Olex2 [106]. Absorption corrections were applied using SADABS 2014 [107]. Data for sample **8h** were collected on a Rigaku Saturn 724 at 150(2) K (X-Stream), (Rigaku, Tokyo, Tōkyō Prefecture, JP 151-0051) and CrystalClear [108,109] was used for cell refinement and data reduction and absorption corrections. Bruker APEX software as well as XT, XL were used to determine the space group, solve and refine the structure in Olex2 [106]. Crystal data, details of data collections and refinement are given in Table 1. CCDC 1820354-1820359 contains the supplementary crystallographic data for this paper. These data can be obtained free of charge from The Cambridge Crystallographic Data Centre (www.ccdc.cam.ac.uk/data_request/cif).

All non-hydrogen atoms were refined anisotropically. Hydrogen atoms were assigned to calculated positions using a riding model with appropriately fixed isotropic thermal parameters. Some structures have multiple independent molecules in the asymmetric unit: **7h** has 4 independent molecules with chirality C3: R, C4: S, C30: R, C31: S, C57: S, C58: R, C84: S and C85: R; **8i** has 2 independent molecules with chirality: C3: R, C4: S, C30: R and C3: S.

4.5. Computational Procedure: Molecular Docking Study

For ligand preparation, all compounds were built using ChemBioDraw 13.0, (PerkinElmer Inc., 940 Winter Street, Waltham, MA 02451, USA) saved as mol files and opened in MOE (Molecular Operating Environment (MOE) Version 2015.10, Chemical Computing Group Inc., 1010 Sherbrooke St W, Montreal, QC, Canada). For the receptor preparation, the PDB entry1SA0 was downloaded from the Protein Data Bank PDB [5]. A UniProt Align analysis confirmed a 100% sequence identity between human and bovine beta tubulin. All waters were retained in both isoforms. Addition and optimisation of hydrogen positions for these waters was carried out using MOE 2015.10 ensuring all other atom positions remained fixed [110]. For both enantiomers of each compound, MMFF94x partial charges were calculated and each was minimised to a gradient of 0.001 kcal/mol/Å. Default parameters were used for docking except that 500 poses were sampled for each enantiomer and the top 50 docked poses were retained for subsequent analysis. The crystal structure was prepared using QuickPrep (minimised to a gradient of 0.001 kcal/mol/Å), Protonate 3D, Residue pKa and Partial Charges protocols in MOE 2016 with the MMFF94x force field.

Supplementary Materials: The following are available online at http://www.mdpi.com/1424-8247/12/2/56/s1, Experimental procedures and spectroscopic data for intermediate compounds **5a–i**, **5m–s**, **6a–c**, **6f–k**, additional cytotoxicity data in normal murine epithelial cells for compound **7s**, Tier-1 Profiling Screen of Selected β-Lactams, results of comparative antitumor evaluations of compounds **7h**, **7s**, **7t**, **17b**, **17c** in the NCI60 cell line in vitro primary screen, NCI 60 cell line mean screening results for selected compounds and results of standard COMPARE analysis of **7h** and **7s**.

Author Contributions: S.W. synthesised and characterised compounds in the studies according to Schemes 1, 2 and 4 performed cell studies and generated data in Tables 3–5, performed the HPLC analytical study and the stability study. and performed data analysis and interpreted data. A.M.M. synthesised and characterised some molecules in Schemes 1 and 2, performed cell studies and generated the the data for Figures 4–6 and 9. T.F.G. synthesised compounds in Schemes 1–4, characterised these compounds, performed the cell studies and generated data in Tables 3–5 and Figure 7, and performed HPLC analytical and stability studies. N.M.O. performed biochemical experiments and generated the data in Figure 8. D.F. performed the molecular modelling studies in Figures 10 and 11. S.M.N. performed biochemical experiments and generated data in Figure 7. X-Ray Crystallographic structures were determined by B.T. (Figure 2A,B and Figure 3A,B), and T.M. (Figure 3C), Tables 1 and 2. N.O.K. synthesised compounds in Scheme 4. D.M.Z. assisted with the design of the biochemical studies. M.J.M. designed the studies, wrote drafts of the manuscript and submitted the manuscript.

Funding: A postgraduate research scholarship from King Abdulaziz University (KAU) is gratefully acknowledged (A.M.M.). This work was also supported by the Irish Research Council Postdoctoral Fellowship (GOIPD/2013/188; N.M.O.). Postgraduate research scholarships from Trinity College Dublin (T.F.G., S.W.) and the Irish Research Council (N.O.K.) are also gratefully acknowledged.

Acknowledgments: We thank Gavin McManus for assistance with confocal microscopy and Orla Woods for assistance with biochemical experiments. We thank Orla Bergin, UCD Conway Institute and School of Biomolecular and Biomedical Science, University College Dublin, Belfield, Dublin4, Ireland, Triple negative breast cancer Hs578T cells and its invasive variant Hs578Ts(i)8 were obtained as a kind gift from Susan McDonnell, School of Chemical and Bioprocess Engineering, University College Dublin. The Trinity Biomedical Sciences Institute (TBSI) is supported by a capital infrastructure investment from Cycle 5 of the Irish Higher Education Authority's Programme for Research in Third Level Institutions (PRTLI). DF thanks the software vendors for their continuing support of academic research efforts, in particular the contributions of the Chemical Computing Group, Biovia and OpenEye Scientific. The support and provisions of Dell Ireland, the Trinity Centre for High Performance Computing (TCHPC) and the Irish Centre for High-End Computing (ICHEC) are also gratefully acknowledged.

Conflicts of Interest: The authors declare no conflict of interest.

Abbreviations

The following abbreviations are used in this manuscript:

CA-4	Combretastatin A-4
DBU	1,8-Diazabicyclo[5.4.0]undec-7-ene
DCC	*N,N′*-Dicyclohexyl carbodiimide
DCM	Dichloromethane
DCTD	Division of Cancer Treatment and Diagnosis
DEAD	Diethyl azodicarboxylate
DIPEA	*N,N*-diisopropylethylamine
DMAP	4-Dimethylaminopyridine
DMF	*N,N*-Dimethylformamide
DTP	Development Therapeutics Program
Et_3N	Triethylamine
EBI	*N,N′*-Ethylene-bis(iodoacetamide)
ESI	Electrospray ionisation
FMOC	Fluorenylmethyloxycarbonyl
HPLC	High-performance liquid chromatography
HRMS	High Resolution Mass Spectrometry
IC	Inhibitory concentration
IR	Infrared
MIC	Minimum inhibitory concentration
MTD	Maximum tolerated dose
MS	Mass spectrometry
NCI	National Cancer Institute
NIH	National Institute of Health
NMR	Nuclear Magnetic Resonance
PBS	Phosphate-buffered saline
SAR	Structure-activity relationship
SERM	Selective Estrogen Receptor Modulator
TBAF	Tetrabutylammonium fluoride
TBDMS	*tert*-Butyldimethylchlorosilane
TEA	Triethylamine
TLC	Thin layer chromatography
TMS	Tetramethylsilane
TMCS	Tetramethylchlorosilane
UV	Ultraviolet
VDA	Vascular disrupting agent

References

1. Bates, D.; Eastman, A. Microtubule destabilising agents: Far more than just antimitotic anticancer drugs. *Br. J. Clin. Pharmcol.* **2017**, *83*, 255–268. [CrossRef] [PubMed]
2. Rohena, C.C.; Mooberry, S.L. Recent progress with microtubule stabilizers: New compounds, binding modes and cellular activities. *Nat. Prod. Rep.* **2014**, *31*, 335–355. [CrossRef]
3. Van Vuuren, R.J.; Visagie, M.H.; Theron, A.E.; Joubert, A.M. Antimitotic drugs in the treatment of cancer. *Cancer Chemother. Pharmcol.* **2015**, *76*, 1101–1112. [CrossRef]
4. Gigant, B.; Wang, C.; Ravelli, R.B.; Roussi, F.; Steinmetz, M.O.; Curmi, P.A.; Sobel, A.; Knossow, M. Structural basis for the regulation of tubulin by vinblastine. *Nature* **2005**, *435*, 519–522. [CrossRef] [PubMed]
5. Ravelli, R.B.; Gigant, B.; Curmi, P.A.; Jourdain, I.; Lachkar, S.; Sobel, A.; Knossow, M. Insight into tubulin regulation from a complex with colchicine and a stathmin-like domain. *Nature* **2004**, *428*, 198–202. [CrossRef] [PubMed]
6. De Filippis, B.; Ammazzalorso, A.; Fantacuzzi, M.; Giampietro, L.; Maccallini, C.; Amoroso, R. Anticancer activity of stilbene-based derivatives. *ChemMedChem* **2017**, *12*, 558–570. [CrossRef] [PubMed]
7. Tron, G.C.; Pirali, T.; Sorba, G.; Pagliai, F.; Busacca, S.; Genazzani, A.A. Medicinal chemistry of combretastatin a4: Present and future directions. *J. Med. Chem.* **2006**, *49*, 3033–3044. [CrossRef] [PubMed]
8. Hsieh, H.P.; Liou, J.P.; Mahindroo, N. Pharmaceutical design of antimitotic agents based on combretastatins. *Curr. Pharm. Des.* **2005**, *11*, 1655–1677. [CrossRef]
9. Tozer, G.M.; Kanthou, C.; Baguley, B.C. Disrupting tumour blood vessels. *Nat. Rev. Cancer* **2005**, *5*, 423–435. [CrossRef]
10. Kanthou, C.; Greco, O.; Stratford, A.; Cook, I.; Knight, R.; Benzakour, O.; Tozer, G. The tubulin-binding agent combretastatin a-4-phosphate arrests endothelial cells in mitosis and induces mitotic cell death. *Am. J. Pathol.* **2004**, *165*, 1401–1411. [CrossRef]
11. Rustin, G.J.; Shreeves, G.; Nathan, P.D.; Gaya, A.; Ganesan, T.S.; Wang, D.; Boxall, J.; Poupard, L.; Chaplin, D.J.; Stratford, M.R.; et al. A phase ib trial of ca4p (combretastatin a-4 phosphate), carboplatin, and paclitaxel in patients with advanced cancer. *Br. J. Cancer* **2010**, *102*, 1355–1360. [CrossRef]
12. Bilenker, J.H.; Flaherty, K.T.; Rosen, M.; Davis, L.; Gallagher, M.; Stevenson, J.P.; Sun, W.; Vaughn, D.; Giantonio, B.; Zimmer, R.; et al. Phase i trial of combretastatin a-4 phosphate with carboplatin. *Clin. Cancer Res.* **2005**, *11*, 1527–1533. [CrossRef] [PubMed]
13. Liu, P.; Qin, Y.; Wu, L.; Yang, S.; Li, N.; Wang, H.; Xu, H.; Sun, K.; Zhang, S.; Han, X.; et al. A phase i clinical trial assessing the safety and tolerability of combretastatin a4 phosphate injections. *Anticancer Drugs* **2014**, *25*, 462–471. [CrossRef] [PubMed]
14. Grisham, R.; Ky, B.; Tewari, K.S.; Chaplin, D.J.; Walker, J. Clinical trial experience with ca4p anticancer therapy: Focus on efficacy, cardiovascular adverse events, and hypertension management. *Gynecol. Oncol. Res. Pract.* **2018**, *5*, 1. [CrossRef]
15. Combretastatin A4 Phosphate in Treating Patients with Advanced Anaplastic Thyroid Cancer. Available online: https://clinicaltrials.Gov/ct2/show/nct00060242 (accessed on 16 January 2019).
16. Pazofos: Phase IB and Phase II Trial of Pazopanib +/− Fosbretabulin in Advanced Recurrent Ovarian Cancer (pazofos)clinicaltrials.Gov; a Service of the U.S. National Institutes of Health. Available online: https://www.Clinicaltrials.Gov/ct2/show/nct02055690 (accessed on 16 January 2019).
17. Nathan, P.; Zweifel, M.; Padhani, A.R.; Koh, D.M.; Ng, M.; Collins, D.J.; Harris, A.; Carden, C.; Smythe, J.; Fisher, N.; et al. Phase i trial of combretastatin a4 phosphate (ca4p) in combination with bevacizumab in patients with advanced cancer. *Clin. Cancer Res.* **2012**, *18*, 3428–3439. [CrossRef] [PubMed]
18. Aboubakr, E.M.; Taye, A.; Aly, O.M.; Gamal-Eldeen, A.M.; El-Moselhy, M.A. Enhanced anticancer effect of combretastatin a-4 phosphate when combined with vincristine in the treatment of hepatocellular carcinoma. *Biomed. Pharmcol.* **2017**, *89*, 36–46. [CrossRef]
19. Ng, Q.S.; Mandeville, H.; Goh, V.; Alonzi, R.; Milner, J.; Carnell, D.; Meer, K.; Padhani, A.R.; Saunders, M.I.; Hoskin, P.J. Phase ib trial of radiotherapy in combination with combretastatin-a4-phosphate in patients with non-small-cell lung cancer, prostate adenocarcinoma, and squamous cell carcinoma of the head and neck. *Ann. Oncol.* **2012**, *23*, 231–237. [CrossRef] [PubMed]
20. Siemann, D.W.; Chaplin, D.J.; Walicke, P.A. A review and update of the current status of the vasculature-disabling agent combretastatin-a4 phosphate (ca4p). *Expert Opin. Investig. Drugs* **2009**, *18*, 189–197. [CrossRef] [PubMed]

21. Greene, L.M.; Meegan, M.J.; Zisterer, D.M. Combretastatins: More than just vascular targeting agents? *J. Pharmacol. Exp. Ther.* **2015**, *355*, 212–227. [CrossRef]
22. Pettit, G.R.; Toki, B.; Herald, D.L.; Verdier-Pinard, P.; Boyd, M.R.; Hamel, E.; Pettit, R.K. Antineoplastic agents. 379. Synthesis of phenstatin phosphate. *J. Med. Chem.* **1998**, *41*, 1688–1695. [CrossRef] [PubMed]
23. Lu, Y.; Chen, J.; Xiao, M.; Li, W.; Miller, D.D. An overview of tubulin inhibitors that interact with the colchicine binding site. *Pharm. Res.* **2012**, *29*, 2943–2971. [CrossRef]
24. Pettit, G.R.; Rhodes, M.R.; Herald, D.L.; Hamel, E.; Schmidt, J.M.; Pettit, R.K. Antineoplastic agents. 445. Synthesis and evaluation of structural modifications of (z)- and (e)-combretastatin a-41. *J. Med. Chem.* **2005**, *48*, 4087–4099. [CrossRef]
25. Theeramunkong, S.; Caldarelli, A.; Massarotti, A.; Aprile, S.; Caprioglio, D.; Zaninetti, R.; Teruggi, A.; Pirali, T.; Grosa, G.; Tron, G.C.; et al. Regioselective suzuki coupling of dihaloheteroaromatic compounds as a rapid strategy to synthesize potent rigid combretastatin analogues. *J. Med. Chem.* **2011**, *54*, 4977–4986. [CrossRef]
26. Hadimani, M.B.; Macdonough, M.T.; Ghatak, A.; Strecker, T.E.; Lopez, R.; Sriram, M.; Nguyen, B.L.; Hall, J.J.; Kessler, R.J.; Shirali, A.R.; et al. Synthesis of a 2-aryl-3-aroyl indole salt (oxi8007) resembling combretastatin a-4 with application as a vascular disrupting agent. *J. Nat. Prod.* **2013**, *76*, 1668–1678. [CrossRef]
27. Macdonough, M.T.; Strecker, T.E.; Hamel, E.; Hall, J.J.; Chaplin, D.J.; Trawick, M.L.; Pinney, K.G. Synthesis and biological evaluation of indole-based, anti-cancer agents inspired by the vascular disrupting agent 2-(3′-hydroxy-4′-methoxyphenyl)-3-(3″,4″,5″-trimethoxybenzoyl)-6-methoxyindole (oxi8006). *Bioorg. Med. Chem.* **2013**, *21*, 6831–6843. [CrossRef]
28. Romagnoli, R.; Baraldi, P.G.; Prencipe, F.; Oliva, P.; Baraldi, S.; Tabrizi, M.A.; Lopez-Cara, L.C.; Ferla, S.; Brancale, A.; Hamel, E.; et al. Design and synthesis of potent in vitro and in vivo anticancer agents based on 1-(3′,4′,5′-trimethoxyphenyl)-2-aryl-1h-imidazole. *Sci. Rep.* **2016**, *6*, 26602. [CrossRef]
29. Lee, S.; Kim, J.N.; Lee, H.K.; Yoon, K.S.; Shin, K.D.; Kwon, B.M.; Han, D.C. Biological evaluation of kribb3 analogs as a microtubule polymerization inhibitor. *Bioorg. Med. Chem. Lett.* **2011**, *21*, 977–979. [CrossRef]
30. Odlo, K.; Fournier-Dit-Chabert, J.; Ducki, S.; Gani, O.A.; Sylte, I.; Hansen, T.V. 1,2,3-triazole analogs of combretastatin a-4 as potential microtubule-binding agents. *Bioorg. Med. Chem.* **2010**, *18*, 6874–6885. [CrossRef]
31. Romagnoli, R.; Baraldi, P.G.; Salvador, M.K.; Preti, D.; Aghazadeh Tabrizi, M.; Brancale, A.; Fu, X.H.; Li, J.; Zhang, S.Z.; Hamel, E.; et al. Synthesis and evaluation of 1,5-disubstituted tetrazoles as rigid analogues of combretastatin a-4 with potent antiproliferative and antitumor activity. *J. Med. Chem.* **2012**, *55*, 475–488. [CrossRef]
32. Rasolofonjatovo, E.; Provot, O.; Hamze, A.; Rodrigo, J.; Bignon, J.; Wdzieczak-Bakala, J.; Lenoir, C.; Desravines, D.; Dubois, J.; Brion, J.D.; et al. Design, synthesis and anticancer properties of 5-arylbenzoxepins as conformationally restricted isocombretastatin a-4 analogs. *Eur. J. Med. Chem.* **2013**, *62*, 28–39. [CrossRef]
33. Xu, Q.L.; Qi, H.; Sun, M.L.; Zuo, D.Y.; Jiang, X.W.; Wen, Z.Y.; Wang, Z.W.; Wu, Y.L.; Zhang, W.G. Synthesis and biological evaluation of 3-alkyl-1,5-diaryl-1h-pyrazoles as rigid analogues of combretastatin a-4 with potent antiproliferative activity. *PLoS ONE* **2015**, *10*, e0128710. [CrossRef]
34. Zheng, S.; Zhong, Q.; Mottamal, M.; Zhang, Q.; Zhang, C.; Lemelle, E.; McFerrin, H.; Wang, G. Design, synthesis, and biological evaluation of novel pyridine-bridged analogues of combretastatin-a4 as anticancer agents. *J. Med. Chem.* **2014**, *57*, 3369–3381. [CrossRef]
35. Prota, A.E.; Danel, F.; Bachmann, F.; Bargsten, K.; Buey, R.M.; Pohlmann, J.; Reinelt, S.; Lane, H.; Steinmetz, M.O. The novel microtubule-destabilizing drug bal27862 binds to the colchicine site of tubulin with distinct effects on microtubule organization. *J. Mol. Biol.* **2014**, *426*, 1848–1860. [CrossRef]
36. Rajak, H.; Dewangan, P.K.; Patel, V.; Jain, D.K.; Singh, A.; Veerasamy, R.; Sharma, P.C.; Dixit, A. Design of combretastatin a-4 analogs as tubulin targeted vascular disrupting agent with special emphasis on their cis-restricted isomers. *Curr. Pharm. Des.* **2013**, *19*, 1923–1955. [CrossRef]
37. Zhou, P.; Liu, Y.; Zhou, L.; Zhu, K.; Feng, K.; Zhang, H.; Liang, Y.; Jiang, H.; Luo, C.; Liu, M.; et al. Potent antitumor activities and structure basis of the chiral beta-lactam bridged analogue of combretastatin a-4 binding to tubulin. *J. Med. Chem.* **2016**, *59*, 10329–10334. [CrossRef]
38. Zhou, P.L.; Liang, Y.; Zhang, H.; Jiang, H.; Feng, K.; Xu, P.; Wang, J.; Wang, X.; Ding, K.; Luo, C.; et al. Design, synthesis, biological evaluation and cocrystal structures with tubulin of chiral b-lactam bridged combretastatin a-4 analogues as potent antitumor agents. *Eur. J. Med. Chem.* **2018**, *144*, 817–842. [CrossRef]

39. Galletti, P.; Soldati, R.; Pori, M.; Durso, M.; Tolomelli, A.; Gentilucci, L.; Dattoli, S.D.; Baiula, M.; Spampinato, S.; Giacomini, D. Targeting integrins alphavbeta3 and alpha5beta1 with new beta-lactam derivatives. *Eur. J. Med. Chem.* **2014**, *83*, 284–293. [CrossRef]
40. Geesala, R.; Gangasani, J.K.; Budde, M.; Balasubramanian, S.; Vaidya, J.R.; Das, A. 2-azetidinones: Synthesis and biological evaluation as potential anti-breast cancer agents. *Eur. J. Med. Chem.* **2016**, *124*, 544–558. [CrossRef]
41. Arya, N.; Jagdale, A.Y.; Patil, T.A.; Yeramwar, S.S.; Holikatti, S.S.; Dwivedi, J.; Shishoo, C.J.; Jain, K.S. The chemistry and biological potential of azetidin-2-ones. *Eur. J. Med. Chem.* **2014**, *74*, 619–656. [CrossRef]
42. Fu, D.J.; Fu, L.; Liu, Y.C.; Wang, J.W.; Wang, Y.Q.; Han, B.K.; Li, X.R.; Zhang, C.; Li, F.; Song, J.; et al. Structure-activity relationship studies of beta-lactam-azide analogues as orally active antitumor agents targeting the tubulin colchicine site. *Sci. Rep.* **2017**, *7*, 12788. [CrossRef]
43. Kamath, A.; Ojima, I. Advances in the chemistry of beta-lactam and its medicinal applications. *Tetrahedron* **2012**, *68*, 10640–10664. [CrossRef]
44. O'Boyle, N.M.; Pollock, J.K.; Carr, M.; Knox, A.J.; Nathwani, S.M.; Wang, S.; Caboni, L.; Zisterer, D.M.; Meegan, M.J. Beta-lactam estrogen receptor antagonists and a dual-targeting estrogen receptor/tubulin ligand. *J. Med. Chem.* **2014**, *57*, 9370–9382. [CrossRef]
45. O'Boyle, N.M.; Carr, M.; Greene, L.M.; Bergin, O.; Nathwani, S.M.; McCabe, T.; Lloyd, D.G.; Zisterer, D.M.; Meegan, M.J. Synthesis and evaluation of azetidinone analogues of combretastatin a-4 as tubulin targeting agents. *J. Med. Chem.* **2010**, *53*, 8569–8584. [CrossRef] [PubMed]
46. Greene, T.F.; Wang, S.; Greene, L.M.; Nathwani, S.M.; Pollock, J.K.; Malebari, A.M.; McCabe, T.; Twamley, B.; O'Boyle, N.M.; Zisterer, D.M.; et al. Synthesis and biochemical evaluation of 3-phenoxy-1,4-diarylazetidin-2-ones as tubulin-targeting antitumor agents. *J. Med. Chem.* **2016**, *59*, 90–113. [CrossRef] [PubMed]
47. Nathwani, S.M.; Hughes, L.; Greene, L.M.; Carr, M.; O'Boyle, N.M.; McDonnell, S.; Meegan, M.J.; Zisterer, D.M. Novel cis-restricted beta-lactam combretastatin a-4 analogues display anti-vascular and anti-metastatic properties in vitro. *Oncol. Rep.* **2013**, *29*, 585–594. [CrossRef] [PubMed]
48. Singh, G.S.; Sudheesh, S. Advances in synthesis of monocyclic beta-lactams. *Arkivoc* **2014**, 337–385. [CrossRef]
49. Gaspari, R.; Prota, A.E.; Bargsten, K.; Cavalli, A.; Steinmetz, M.O. Structural basis of cis- and trans-combretastatin binding to tubulin. *Chem* **2017**, *2*, 102–113. [CrossRef]
50. Zamboni, R.; Just, G. Beta-lactams. 7. Synthesis of 3-vinyl and 3-isopropenyl 4-substituted azetidinones. *Can. J. Chem.* **1979**, *57*, 1945–1948. [CrossRef]
51. Neary, A.D.; Burke, C.M.; O'Leary, A.C.; Meegan, M.J. Transformation of 4-acetoxy-3-vinylazetidin-2-ones to 3-(1-hydroxyethyl)azetidin-2-ones and 3-ethylideneazetidin-2-ones: Intermediates for carbapenem antibiotics. *J. Chem. Res.* **2001**, *2001*, 166–169. [CrossRef]
52. Chang, J.Y.; Yang, M.F.; Chang, C.Y.; Chen, C.M.; Kuo, C.C.; Liou, J.P. 2-amino and 2′-aminocombretastatin derivatives as potent antimitotic agents. *J. Med. Chem.* **2006**, *49*, 6412–6415. [CrossRef]
53. Tripodi, F.; Pagliarin, R.; Fumagalli, G.; Bigi, A.; Fusi, P.; Orsini, F.; Frattini, M.; Coccetti, P. Synthesis and biological evaluation of 1,4-diaryl-2-azetidinones as specific anticancer agents: Activation of adenosine monophosphate activated protein kinase and induction of apoptosis. *J. Med. Chem.* **2012**, *55*, 2112–2124. [CrossRef]
54. O'Boyle, N.M.; Greene, L.M.; Bergin, O.; Fichet, J.B.; McCabe, T.; Lloyd, D.G.; Zisterer, D.M.; Meegan, M.J. Synthesis, evaluation and structural studies of antiproliferative tubulin-targeting azetidin-2-ones. *Bioorg. Med. Chem.* **2011**, *19*, 2306–2325. [CrossRef]
55. Mayrhofer, R.; Otto, H.H. Simple preparation of 3-benzylidene-2-azetidinones. *Synthesis* **1980**, *1980*, 247–248. [CrossRef]
56. Kano, S.; Ebata, T.; Funaki, K.; Shibuya, S. New and facile synthesis of 3-alkylideneazetidin-2-ones by reactions of 3-trimethylsilylazetidin-2-one with carbonyl-compounds. *Synthesis* **1978**, *1978*, 746–747. [CrossRef]
57. Plantan, I.; Selic, L.; Mesar, T.; Anderluh, P.S.; Oblak, M.; Prezelj, A.; Hesse, L.; Andrejasic, M.; Vilar, M.; Turk, D.; et al. 4-substituted trinems as broad spectrum beta-lactamase inhibitors: Structure-based design, synthesis, and biological activity. *J. Med. Chem.* **2007**, *50*, 4113–4121. [CrossRef]
58. O'Boyle, N.M.; Greene, L.M.; Keely, N.O.; Wang, S.; Cotter, T.S.; Zisterer, D.M.; Meegan, M.J. Synthesis and biochemical activities of antiproliferative amino acid and phosphate derivatives of microtubule-disrupting beta-lactam combretastatins. *Eur. J. Med. Chem.* **2013**, *62*, 705–721. [CrossRef]
59. Spek, A.L.; Vandersteen, F.H.; Jastrzebski, J.T.B.H.; Vankoten, G. Trans-3-amino-1-methyl-4-phenyl-2-azetidinone, C10H12N2O. *Acta Crystallogr. C* **1994**, *50*, 1933–1935. [CrossRef]

60. Kabak, M.; Senoz, H.; Elmali, A.; Adar, V.; Svoboda, I.; Dusek, M.; Fejfarova, K. Synthesis and x-ray crystal structure determination of n-p-methylphenyl-4-benzoyl-3,4-diphenyl-2-azetidinone. *Crystallogr. Rep.* **2010**, *55*, 1220–1222. [CrossRef]
61. Lara-Ochoa, F.; Espinosa-Perez, G. A new synthesis of combretastatins a-4 and ave-8062a. *Tetrahedron Lett.* **2007**, *48*, 7007–7010. [CrossRef]
62. Combes, S.; Barbier, P.; Douillard, S.; McLeer-Florin, A.; Bourgarel-Rey, V.; Pierson, J.T.; Fedorov, A.Y.; Finet, J.P.; Boutonnat, J.; Peyrot, V. Synthesis and biological evaluation of 4-arylcoumarin analogues of combretastatins. Part 2. *J. Med. Chem.* **2011**, *54*, 3153–3162. [CrossRef]
63. Messaoudi, S.; Treguier, B.; Hamze, A.; Provot, O.; Peyrat, J.F.; De Losada, J.R.; Liu, J.M.; Bignon, J.; Wdzieczak-Bakala, J.; Thoret, S.; et al. Isocombretastatins a versus combretastatins a: The forgotten isoca-4 isomer as a highly promising cytotoxic and antitubulin agent. *J. Med. Chem.* **2009**, *52*, 4538–4542. [CrossRef]
64. Cushman, M.; Nagarathnam, D.; Gopal, D.; He, H.M.; Lin, C.M.; Hamel, E. Synthesis and evaluation of analogues of (z)-1-(4-methoxyphenyl)-2-(3,4,5-trimethoxyphenyl)ethene as potential cytotoxic and antimitotic agents. *J. Med. Chem.* **1992**, *35*, 2293–2306. [CrossRef]
65. Flynn, B.L.; Flynn, G.P.; Hamel, E.; Jung, M.K. The synthesis and tubulin binding activity of thiophene-based analogues of combretastatin a-4. *Bioorg. Med. Chem. Lett.* **2001**, *11*, 2341–2343. [CrossRef]
66. Chaudhary, A.; Pandeya, S.N.; Kumar, P.; Sharma, P.P.; Gupta, S.; Soni, N.; Verma, K.K.; Bhardwaj, G. Combretastatin a-4 analogs as anticancer agents. *Mini Rev. Med. Chem.* **2007**, *7*, 1186–1205. [CrossRef]
67. Devkota, L.; Lin, C.M.; Strecker, T.E.; Wang, Y.; Tidmore, J.K.; Chen, Z.; Guddneppanavar, R.; Jelinek, C.J.; Lopez, R.; Liu, L.; et al. Design, synthesis, and biological evaluation of water-soluble amino acid prodrug conjugates derived from combretastatin, dihydronaphthalene, and benzosuberene-based parent vascular disrupting agents. *Bioorg. Med. Chem.* **2016**, *24*, 938–956. [CrossRef]
68. Mousset, C.; Giraud, A.; Provot, O.; Hamze, A.; Bignon, J.; Liu, J.M.; Thoret, S.; Dubois, J.; Brion, J.D.; Alami, M. Synthesis and antitumor activity of benzils related to combretastatin a-4. *Bioorg. Med. Chem. Lett.* **2008**, *18*, 3266–3271. [CrossRef]
69. Hughes, L.; Malone, C.; Chumsri, S.; Burger, A.M.; McDonnell, S. Characterisation of breast cancer cell lines and establishment of a novel isogenic subclone to study migration, invasion and tumourigenicity. *Clin. Exp. Metastasis* **2008**, *25*, 549–557. [CrossRef]
70. National Cancer Institute Division of Cancer Treatment and Diagnosis. Available online: https://dtp.Cancer.Gov (accessed on 25 February 2019).
71. *National Cancer Institute Biological Testing Branch*; National Cancer Institute: Bethesda, MD, USA. Available online: https://dtp.Nci.Nih.Gov/branches/btb/hfa.Html (accessed on 16 January 2019).
72. Vichai, V.; Kirtikara, K. Sulforhodamine b colorimetric assay for cytotoxicity screening. *Nat. Protoc.* **2006**, *1*, 1112–1116. [CrossRef]
73. Smith, S.M.; Wunder, M.B.; Norris, D.A.; Shellman, Y.G. A simple protocol for using a ldh-based cytotoxicity assay to assess the effects of death and growth inhibition at the same time. *PLoS ONE* **2011**, *6*, e26908. [CrossRef]
74. Furlong, E.E.; Keon, N.K.; Thornton, F.D.; Rein, T.; Martin, F. Expression of a 74-kda nuclear factor 1 (nf1) protein is induced in mouse mammary gland involution. Involution-enhanced occupation of a twin nf1 binding element in the testosterone-repressed prostate message-2/clusterin promoter. *J. Biol. Chem.* **1996**, *271*, 29688–29697. [CrossRef]
75. Murtagh, J.; McArdle, E.; Gilligan, E.; Thornton, L.; Furlong, F.; Martin, F. Organization of mammary epithelial cells into 3d acinar structures requires glucocorticoid and jnk signaling. *J. Cell Biol.* **2004**, *166*, 133–143. [CrossRef]
76. Shen, C.H.; Shee, J.J.; Wu, J.Y.; Lin, Y.W.; Wu, J.D.; Liu, Y.W. Combretastatin a-4 inhibits cell growth and metastasis in bladder cancer cells and retards tumour growth in a murine orthotopic bladder tumour model. *Br. J. Pharmcol.* **2010**, *160*, 2008–2027. [CrossRef]
77. Greene, L.M.; O'Boyle, N.M.; Nolan, D.P.; Meegan, M.J.; Zisterer, D.M. The vascular targeting agent combretastatin-a4 directly induces autophagy in adenocarcinoma-derived colon cancer cells. *Biochem. Pharmcol.* **2012**, *84*, 612–624. [CrossRef]
78. *Tubulin Polymerization Assay Kit Manual (CDS03 and BK006)*; Cytoskeleton: Denver, CO, USA, 2009; pp. 1–18.
79. Barbier, P.; Tsvetkov, P.O.; Breuzard, G.; Devred, F. Deciphering the molecular mechanisms of anti-tubulin plant derived drugs. *Phytochem. Rev.* **2014**, *13*, 157–169. [CrossRef]

80. Castedo, M.; Perfettini, J.-L.; Roumier, T.; Andreau, K.; Medema, R.; Kroemer, G. Cell death by mitotic catastrophe: A molecular definition. *Oncogene* **2004**, *23*, 2825–2837. [CrossRef]
81. Vitale, I.; Antoccia, A.; Cenciarelli, C.; Crateri, P.; Meschini, S.; Arancia, G.; Pisano, C.; Tanzarella, C. Combretastatin ca-4 and combretastatin derivative induce mitotic catastrophe dependent on spindle checkpoint and caspase-3 activation in non-small cell lung cancer cells. *Apoptosis* **2007**, *12*, 155–166. [CrossRef]
82. Cenciarelli, C.; Tanzarella, C.; Vitale, I.; Pisano, C.; Crateri, P.; Meschini, S.; Arancia, G.; Antoccia, A. The tubulin-depolymerising agent combretastatin-4 induces ectopic aster assembly and mitotic catastrophe in lung cancer cells h460. *Apoptosis* **2008**, *13*, 659–669. [CrossRef]
83. Simoni, D.; Romagnoli, R.; Baruchello, R.; Rondanin, R.; Rizzi, M.; Pavani, M.G.; Alloatti, D.; Giannini, G.; Marcellini, M.; Riccioni, T.; et al. Novel combretastatin analogues endowed with antitumor activity. *J. Med. Chem.* **2006**, *49*, 3143–3152. [CrossRef]
84. O'Boyle, N.M.; Carr, M.; Greene, L.M.; Knox, A.J.S.; Lloyd, D.G.; Zisterer, D.M.; Meegan, M.J. Synthesis, biochemical and molecular modelling studies of antiproliferative azetidinones causing microtubule disruption and mitotic catastrophe. *Eur. J. Med. Chem.* **2011**, *46*, 4595–4607. [CrossRef]
85. Fortin, S.; Lacroix, J.; Cote, M.F.; Moreau, E.; Petitclerc, E.; Gaudreault, R.C. Quick and simple detection technique to assess the binding of antimicrotubule agents to the colchicine-binding site. *Biol. Proced. Online* **2010**, *12*, 113–117. [CrossRef]
86. Canela, M.D.; Perez-Perez, M.J.; Noppen, S.; Saez-Calvo, G.; Diaz, J.F.; Camarasa, M.J.; Liekens, S.; Priego, E.M. Novel colchicine-site binders with a cyclohexanedione scaffold identified through a ligand-based virtual screening approach. *J. Med. Chem.* **2014**, *57*, 3924–3938. [CrossRef]
87. Carr, M.; Greene, L.M.; Knox, A.J.; Lloyd, D.G.; Zisterer, D.M.; Meegan, M.J. Lead identification of conformationally restricted beta-lactam type combretastatin analogues: Synthesis, antiproliferative activity and tubulin targeting effects. *Eur. J. Med. Chem.* **2010**, *45*, 5752–5766. [CrossRef]
88. Molecular Operating Environment (MOE); C.C.G.I.; (1010 Sherbooke St. West, Suite #910, Montreal, QC, Canada). Personal communications, 2016.
89. Elmeligie, S.; Taher, A.T.; Khalil, N.A.; El-Said, A.H. Synthesis and cytotoxic activity of certain trisubstituted azetidin-2-one derivatives as a cis-restricted combretastatin a-4 analogues. *Arch. Pharm. Res.* **2017**, *40*, 13–24. [CrossRef]
90. Georg, G.I.; He, P.; Kant, J.; Mudd, J. N-vinyl and n-unsubstituted beta-lactams from 1-substituted 2-aza-1,3-butadienes. *Tetrahedron Lett.* **1990**, *31*, 451–454. [CrossRef]
91. Arroyo, Y.; Sanz-Tejedor, M.A.; Alonso, I.; Garcia-Ruano, J.L. Synthesis of optically pure vic-sulfanyl amines mediated by a remote sulfinyl group. *Org. Lett.* **2011**, *13*, 4534–4537. [CrossRef]
92. Sandhar, R.K.; Sharma, J.R.; Manrao, M.R. Reaction of acetylacetone with benzal-4-fluoroanilines and antifungal potential of the products. *J. Indian Counc. Chem.* **2005**, *22*, 32–34.
93. Dehno Khalaji, A.; Fejfarova, K.; Dusek, M. *N,N'*-bis(3,4-dimethoxy-benzyl-idene)butane-1,4-diamine. *Acta Crystallogr. Sect. E Struct. Rep. Online* **2009**, *65*, o1773. [CrossRef]
94. Khalaji, A.D.; Weil, M.; Gotoh, K.; Ishida, H. 4-bromo-*N*-(3,4,5-trimethoxy-benzyl-idene)aniline. *Acta Crystallogr. Sect. E Struct. Rep. Online* **2009**, *65*, o436. [CrossRef]
95. Yang, Z. Synthesis and in vitro biological activity evaluation of the derivatives of combretastatin a-4. *Lett. Drug Des. Discov. 2006* *3*, 544–546. [CrossRef]
96. Cushman, M.; He, H.M.; Lin, C.M.; Hamel, E. Synthesis and evaluation of a series of benzylaniline hydrochlorides as potential cytotoxic and antimitotic agents acting by inhibition of tubulin polymerization. *J. Med. Chem.* **1993**, *36*, 2817–2821. [CrossRef]
97. Gaidhane, M.K.; Ghatole, A.M.; Lanjewar, K.R. Novel synthesis and antimicrobial activity of novel schiff base derived quinoline and their beta-lactam derivatives. *Int. J. Pharm. Pharm. Sci.* **2013**, *5*, 421–426.
98. Malebari, A.M.; Greene, L.M.; Nathwani, S.M.; Fayne, D.; O'Boyle, N.M.; Wang, S.; Twamley, B.; Zisterer, D.M.; Meegan, M.J. Beta-lactam analogues of combretastatin a-4 prevent metabolic inactivation by glucuronidation in chemoresistant ht-29 colon cancer cells. *Eur. J. Med. Chem.* **2017**, *130*, 261–285. [CrossRef]
99. Meegan, M.J.; Zisterer, D.M.; Carr, M.; Greene, T.; O'Boyle, N.; Greene, L. Combretastatin Derivatives and Uses Therefor. European Patent WO 2011073211, 23 June 2011.
100. Wang, Y.L.; Liu, M.; Zhou, P.; Feng, K.; Ding, K.; Wang, X. Diaryl-B-Lactam Compound and Preparation Method and Pharmaceutical Use Thereof. Chinese Patent WO 2017167183, 5 October 2017.

101. Promega Corporation. *Cytotox 96® Non-Radioactive Cytotoxicity Assay*; Promega Cytotox 96 Nonradioactive Cytotoxicity Assay Protocol; Promega Corporation: Fitchburg, WI, USA, 2016.
102. *Bruker Apex2 v2012.12-0*; Bruker Axs Inc.: Madison, Wi, USA, 2012.
103. Sheldrick, G.M. A short history of shelx. *Acta Crystallogr. A* **2008**, *64*, 112–122. [CrossRef]
104. Sheldrick, G.M. Shelxt—Integrated space-group and crystal-structure determination. *Acta Crystallogr. A Found. Adv.* **2015**, *71*, 3–8. [CrossRef]
105. Sheldrick, G.M. Crystal structure refinement with shelxl. *Acta Crystallogr. C Struct. Chem.* **2015**, *71*, 3–8. [CrossRef]
106. Dolomanov, O.V.; Bourhis, L.J.; Gildea, R.J.; Howard, J.A.K.; Puschmann, H. Olex2: A complete structure solution, refinement and analysis program. *J. Appl. Crystallogr.* **2009**, *42*, 339–341. [CrossRef]
107. Sadabs; (Bruker Axs Inc., Madison, WI, USA); Sheldrick, G.M.; (University of Göttingen, Göttingen, Germany). Personal communications, 2014.
108. Crystalclear Rigaku Molecular Structure Corporation Inc.; (The Woodlands, TX, USA). Personal communications, 2000.
109. Pflugrath, J.W. The finer things in x-ray diffraction data collection. *Acta Crystallogr. D Biol. Crystallogr.* **1999**, *55*, 1718–1725. [CrossRef]
110. *Molecular Operating Environment (MOE) Version 2015.10*; Chemical Computing Group Inc.: Montreal, QC, Canada, 2016.

pharmaceuticals

MDPI

Article

Novel 11-Substituted Ellipticines as Potent Anticancer Agents with Divergent Activity against Cancer Cells

Charlotte M. Miller, Elaine C. O'Sullivan and Florence O. McCarthy *

School of Chemistry, Analytical and Biological Chemistry Research Facility, University College Cork, Western Road, T12 K8AF Cork, Ireland; charlotte.herstad@dynea.com (C.M.M.); elosullivan@hotmail.com (E.C.O.)

* Correspondence: f.mccarthy@ucc.ie; Tel.: +353-21-4901695

Received: 19 May 2019; Accepted: 12 June 2019; Published: 14 June 2019

Abstract: Ellipticines have well documented anticancer activity, in particular with substitution at the 1-, 2-, 6- and 9-positions. However, due to limitations in synthesis and coherent screening methodology the full SAR profile of this anticancer class has not yet been achieved. In order to address this shortfall, we have set out to explore the anticancer activity of this potent natural product by substitution. We currently describe the synthesis of novel 11-substituted ellipticines with two specific derivatives showing potency and diverging cellular growth effects.

Keywords: ellipticine; anticancer; heterocyclic chemistry; indole; NCI screen; topoisomerase II

1. Introduction

Cancer is a collection of diseases defined by the proliferation of cells in an unregulated and inappropriate manner leading to tumours and eventual mortality. Within this broad definition it is evident that the control of cell growth is a key mechanism as cell growth can be restricted, proliferation can be stopped and cells can be killed by multiple anticancer agents, one of which (ellipticine) is explored further here [1].

Ellipticine **1** (5,11-dimethyl-6*H*-pyrido [4,3-*b*]carbazole, Figure 1) is a natural product which was isolated in 1959 from a small tropical evergreen tree (*Ochrosia elliptica*) by Goodwin et al. [2]. The extract also contained a number of other alkaloids, including the related 9-methoxyellipticine **2**. Since its isolation, the planar tetracyclic structure of ellipticine has been the focus of extensive chemical and pharmacological research [3]. Over the last 60 years, ellipticine and its derivatives have been identified with potent anticancer activity and been subject to clinical trials. Celiptium (9-hydroxy-*N*-methylellipticinium acetate) **3** and 9-hydroxyellipticine **4** both progressed to phase II clinical trials though these were subsequently discontinued due to side effects and efficacy [4–7].

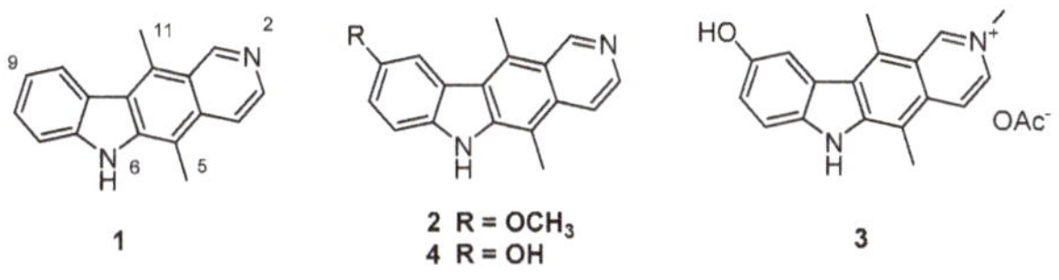

Figure 1. Structures of Ellipticine **1** and related anticancer agents.

The mechanisms by which ellipticine exerts its anticancer activity are particularly diverse. These include topoisomerase II inhibition with associated DNA intercalation, well established in the literature and clinically relevant [8–10]. Cytotoxic ellipticine metabolites via biooxidation at a number of positions on the tetracycle and subsequent adduct formation have also been identified as responsible for some of the effects [11]. Recently, ellipticines have been described to interact with kinases such as c-Kit, AKT and CK2, and to influence the p53 tumour suppressor, all of which have key roles in cell growth and progression [12–14]. Ellipticines have also been discovered to disrupt RNA polymerase I transcription and stabilize pharmaceutically relevant G-quadruplexes and so there is significant and continued interest in the biological effects of this compound class [15,16].

It is therefore evident that ellipticine and its derivatives exhibit multimodal activity with simple substitutions on this template eliciting diverse effects. Despite their potency, there has been little exploration of the functional space in this natural product outside of the 1-, 2-, 6- and 9-positions in order to answer fundamental questions in pharmacology and effect on cells. A programme of research has been initiated in this group in order to evaluate the effect of novel substitution patterns on the ellipticine framework. This has led to the recent discoveries of substituted ellipticine and isoellipticines as new investigational probes with diverse pharmacology and exceptional in vivo activity (**5** and **6**, Figure 2) [17–20].

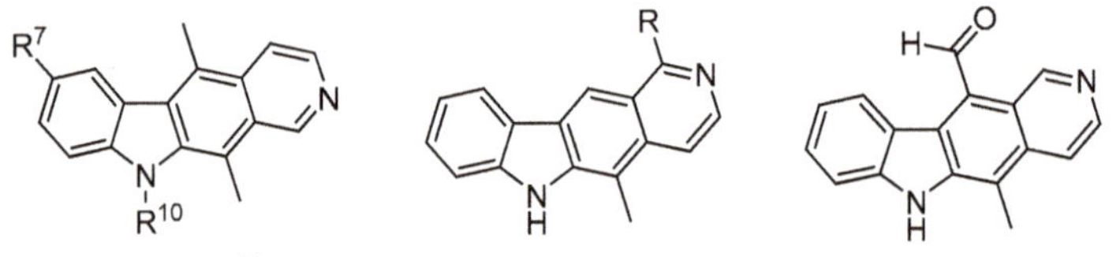

5 R^7 = OH, R^{10} = H
6 R^7 = CHO, R^{10} = CH_3
7
8

Figure 2. Substituted isoellipticines (**5** and **6**) with in vivo activity, Olivacine **7** and 11-formylellipticine **8**.

The 11-position of ellipticine has received little attention from medicinal chemists despite evidence that it may be a key position in order to affect the bioactivity and crucially selectivity of pharmacology [21]. The activity of the closely related olivicine series of compounds signifies that removal of the methyl group does little to affect the potency of the template especially in regard to topoisomerase activity and DNA intercalation (**7**, R = CH_3, Figure 2) [22,23]. An olivacine derivative, S16020 (**7**, R = carboxamide) has also progressed to phase I clinical trials before being discontinued [24]. Despite synthesis of 11-formyl ellipticine **8** (Figure 2) almost 30 years ago, no concerted effort to functionalise this position is recorded in literature other than a carboxamide and a methyl ketone (only four reported compounds in total with carbonyl at 11-position).

Molecular modelling of ellipticine in the active site of biological targets has postulated that 11-substitution with bulky or mobile functional groups would inhibit the intercalation process and may reduce a number of undesirable effects associated with treatment [25]. This position has also been implicated in the process of DNA adduct formation via oxidation [11].

To this end, we set out to functionalise the parent heterocycle and to exploit its known anticancer activity: it has obvious potency across numerous spheres of biology and affects cells from development to apoptosis [4]. Substitution of 11-position is an important step towards full SAR profiling of the cellular effects of ellipticine derivatives. We document here the initial scoping of this chemical space and probe of the anticancer activity through known ellipticine mechanisms.

2. Results and Discussion

2.1. Synthesis of 11-Substituted Ellipticine Derivatives

Since its isolation in 1959, the total synthesis of ellipticine has been accomplished many times and most recent work in the area has focused on preparation of analogues and derivatives of ellipticine [3]. At the outset of this work there existed relatively few examples of 11-substituted ellipticines. Gribble et al. had published a very versatile and efficient route in 1989, giving access to 5- and 11-substituted ellipticines [26–29]. This was further elaborated by Modi et al. to give 11-formylellipticine 8 and this compound was chosen as the starting point for the current synthetic work [30,31].

2.1.1. Modification of 11-formylellipticine

11-Formylellipticine 8 was synthesised as previously described and initially the focus was to provide a carboxylic acid handle for modification (Scheme 1) [30,31]. Hence, 8 was subjected to oxidation under a number of conditions with the most successful conversion to carboxylic acid 9 achieved using sodium chlorite and dimethylsulfoxide (73% yield). Subsequent conversion to acid chloride 10 allowed for introduction of amide functionality which was a key target in this series and the benzylamine derivative 11 was prepared in two steps in 30% yield. The methyl ester 12 was also prepared via similar methodology using carbonyldiimidazole.

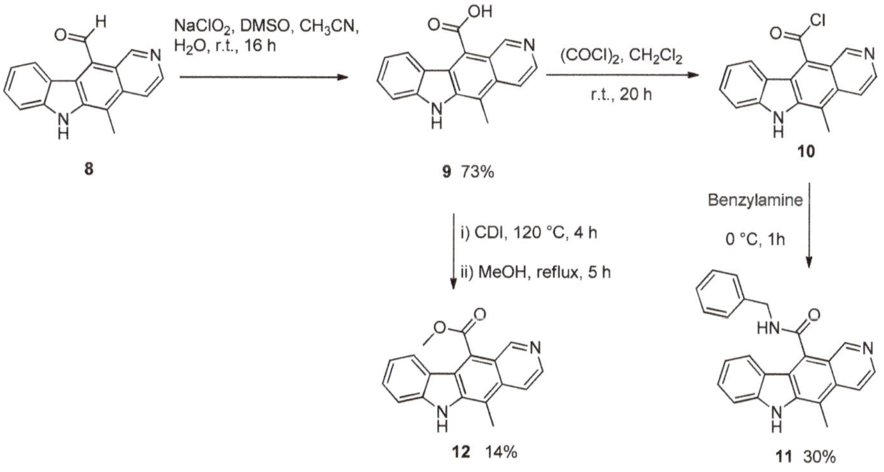

Scheme 1. Formation of 11-substituted ellipticine amide **11** and ester **12**.

Interestingly, while attempting to form the acid initially with other oxidants the expected product was not isolated. On treatment of 8 with potassium permanganate under standard conditions the reaction resulted in base condensation of acetone and isolation of the novel α,β-unsaturated ketone 13 in 87% yield (Scheme 2).

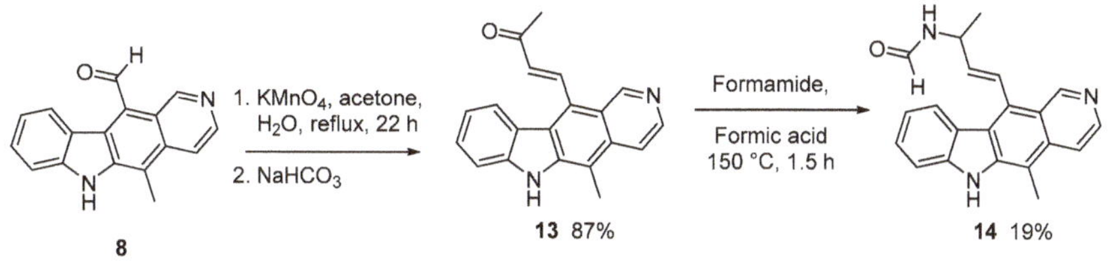

Scheme 2. α,β-Unsaturated ketone condensation product **13** from acetone solvent.

Attempts at cyclisation of compound 13 using aluminium chloride in dichloromethane or chloroform to form a new ring system were unsuccessful and unreacted starting material was recovered. However, a Leuckart reaction gave the formamide 14 in 19% yield, the low yield owing to difficulties in purification. However, the unsaturated ketone 13 provides an interesting template for potential covalent adduct formation and will be revisited in the future.

2.1.2. Modification of the 9-position of 11-substituted Ellipticines

Given the extensive literature background in 9-substituted ellipticines and the recent developments in this area we next turned our focus to functionalization of this position. Initially, carboxylic acid 9 was derivatised via a Duff reaction to give the aldehyde 15 in 82% yield (Scheme 3) [32].

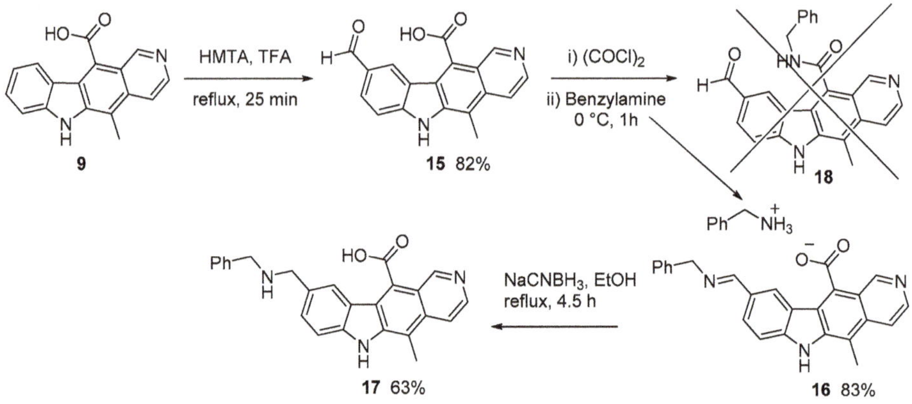

Scheme 3. Synthesis of 9- and 11-substituted ellipticines.

Subsequent reaction of 15 with nucleophiles opens up opportunities for potential synthesis at either the 9- or the 11-position (Scheme 3). To probe the 11-position further, acid chloride formation prior to the addition of benzylamine (as seen in Scheme 1) was undertaken with the aim of generating amide 18. In this reaction, the product isolated was the imine 16 (83% yield) which was identified after full characterization. Confirmation of structure was given by subsequent treatment with aqueous acid which hydrolysed the product to starting material 15.

Additional conformation of the imine 16 was provided by reduction of the imine with sodium cyanoborohydride in ethanol to give the novel amine 17.

2.1.3. 1H NMR Analysis of 11-Substituted Ellipticines

A summary of the ^{1}H NMR analysis is provided in Supplementary Materials (Figures S1–S3). Of note is the influence of conversion from aldehyde to carboxylic acid at the 11-position with corresponding upfield shift of C1 and C10 protons (reversed on formylation of the 9-position). The shift of the C10 proton is again evident on conversion of carboxylic acid to amide and ester.

2.2. Biological Evaluation of 11-Substituted Ellipticines

Given the interest in new ellipticines, several of the novel 9- and 11-substitued ellipticines were evaluated for their biological activity in cellular screens and by gel electrophoresis. In the first instance, inhibition of topoisomerase II (a well-known target of ellipticines) was assessed.

2.2.1. Inhibition of Topoisomerase II

Topoisomerase II inhibition is a clinically used cancer treatment and is considered to be a key mechanism of action for ellipticines [9]. Topoisomerase II has key functions in the change of topological structure of DNA and hence cell replication which can be evaluated using a decatenation assay. As expected, the planar ellipticine 1 and the simple 9-substituted ellipticines (2,4,19) all displayed excellent inhibition of topoisomerase II at 100 μM (Figure 3). On assessment of the 11-substituted ellipticines, the majority were inactive against topoisomerase II but compounds 13 and 16 showed the most promise. α,β-Unsaturated ketone 13 and 9-substituted imine 16 both represent new templates for discovery. Both compounds were evaluated in a subsequent three-fold dilution assay (at 100, 10 and 1μM) where it became apparent that activity reduced significantly below the initial test concentration.

Notwithstanding this, the emergence of two diverse templates for topoisomerase inhibition will be of keen interest to the field and future efforts will aim to increase the potency of this interaction.

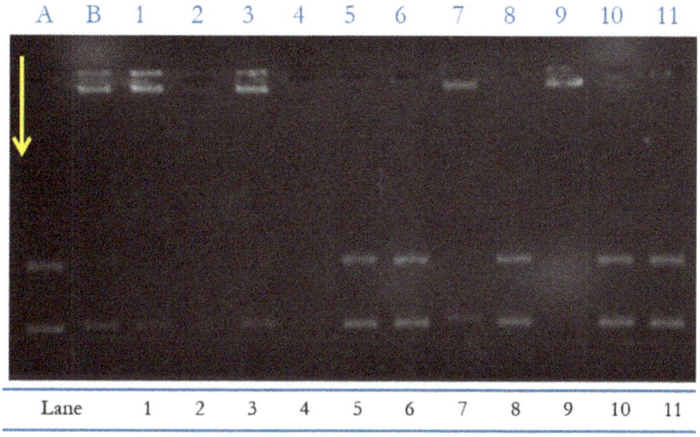

Figure 3. Screen of topoisomerase II inhibitory activity of the ellipticine derivatives at 100 μM. A = Positive Control (kDNA + ATP + Topo II); B = Negative Control (kDNA + ATP + Topo II + 100 μM Ellipticine); Consequent lanes all screened at 100 μM: 1 = Ellipticine 1; 2 = 9-Methoxyellipticine 2; 3 = 9-Formylellipticine 19; 4 = 9-Hydroxyellipticine 4; 5 = 8; 6 = 9; 7 = 13; 8 = 15; 9 = 16; 10 = 17; 11 = 11.

2.2.2. Inhibition of Cancer Cell Growth

Having identified some limited topoisomerase activity, screening of the 11-substituted ellipticine test set was next conducted by assessment of inhibition of cancer cell growth. Initial evaluation of anticancer activity at the National Cancer Institute focuses on the effect of each individual compound on the growth of up to 60 cancer cell lines at a specific concentration (10 μM). The results are summarised in Table 1 (see Supplementary Material for full data, Figures S5–S10).

Table 1. 11-Substituted ellipticine topoisomerase activity and National Cancer Institute (NCI) mean growth percent (single dose).

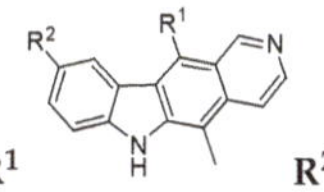

	R^1	R^2	Topo II Inhibition [a]	NSC No	NCI Mean Growth %
8	CHO	H	−		Not tested
9	COOH	H	−	762124	99.92
11	$CONHCH_2Ph$	H	−	762144	21.22
13	CH=CH-C(O)Me	H	+	762123	17.83
15	COOH	CHO	−	762141	95.56
16	$COO^{-}\ {}^{+}NH_3CH_2Ph$	$CH{=}NCH_2Ph$	+	762142	106.19
17	COOH	CH_2NHCH_2Ph	−	762143	101.72

[a] R^1 = C-9 substituent; R^2 = C11 substituent (+) Inhibition observed at 100 μM; (−) no activity observed at 100 μM.

Inhibition of Cancer Cell Growth—One Dose Assay

National Cancer Institute (NCI) evaluation of 11-substituted ellipticines identifies significant effects on the growth of the 60-cell line panel with mean growth values ranging from 18% to 106%. The Mean Growth percent is a reference tool whereby screening at 10 μM concentration is used to filter active anticancer compounds. Of the six compounds tested, two (11-substituted amide 11 and conjugated ketone 13) achieved Mean Growth percentages of <25% and fulfilled the requirements for progression to the five dose assay (Table 1). Of the other four compounds growth percentages were between 96% and 106% and hence have no effect on the growth as an average across the 60 cell lines. Compounds 9, 15, 16 and 17 elicited very similar effects being most active against renal cancer cell line UO-31 (range 63%–76% growth) and breast cancer cell lines MCF7 and MDA-MB-231/ATCC (range 68%–87% growth) but have little effect on the other cell lines of the screen (Figures S5, S8–S10).

In contrast, benzylamide 11 and ketone 13 had significant anticancer effects with differing cellular profiles. Ketone 13 is associated with a non-specific pattern with the range of cell growths (lowest to highest) of 77% whereas benzylamide 11 has a range of 165% and there is an evident difference in cell line effects. At 10 µM, compound 11 is cytotoxic (negative growth percentage) to 15 of the 60 cell lines whereas compound 13 to only four cell lines. It is noticeable that a large number of cell lines are refractory to benzylamide 11 which suggests there may be a targeted effect. It is also obvious from this preliminary screen that there is chemical space at the 11-position of ellipticine to accommodate anticancer activity.

Inhibition of Cancer Cell Growth—Five Dose Assay

The progression to evaluation at five dose assay confirmed the potency of both 11-substituted ellipticines 11 and 13 and their specific effects on cells seen in the one dose screen. Benzylamide 11 exerts a broad range of activity from cytostatic to cytotoxic at dose ranges from 1 to 100 µM (Table 2; Figure S11). In specific, the activity of this compound against HOP62, SNB75, OVCAR-3, OVCAR-4 and 786-0 is exceptional with more than 50% cytotoxicity measured after 48 h incubation (at 10 µM). Growth is restricted across the other cell lines but there is clear selective cytotoxicity. In addition it can be seen (Figure S12) that a number of cell lines are refractory with no evident effect on cell growth of cancer subtypes, in particular melanoma: Leukaemia (HL-60), Lung (EKVX), CNS (SF-295, SNB-19), Melanoma (MALME-3M, M14, SK-MEL-2, SK MEL-28, UACC-257), Ovarian (OVCAR-5, NCI/ADR-RES) and Breast (T-47D).

Table 2. Selected GI50 and LC50 of the NCI 60 cell line panel for compounds **11** and **13** [1].

Cell Line	Cancer Subtype	11		13	
		GI50	LC50	GI50	LC50
HOP-62	Lung	2.15	>100	1.77	26.0
SW-620	Colon	2.86	>100	1.65	44.0
SNB-75	CNS	2.05	>100	2.65	34.8
OVCAR-3	Ovarian	2.33	<10	2.53	28.0
OVCAR-4	Ovarian	1.71	6.19	2.88	41.5
786-0	Renal	2.79	72.0	2.79	29.8
A498	Renal	50.5	>100	0.386	7.48
UO-31	Renal	2.73	>100	1.25	33.8
MCF7	Breast	2.71	>100	1.74	52.3
MDA-MB-231/ATCC	Breast	2.43	>100	1.74	41.3
HS578T	Breast	2.61	>100	1.96	48.4

[1] data reported in µM values from NCI 60 cell line five dose assay; GI50: Growth Inhibition 50%; LC50: Lethal concentration 50%.

Ketone 13 exerts a far more cytotoxic effect across all cell lines with consistent cell death evident at 10 µM as in the one dose screen (Table 2, LC50 column; Figures S13 and S14). Aside the exception of the leukaemia cell panel, all cells are killed by 100 µM of 13 which suggests a potent and common mechanism of action. The compound is exceptionally potent against the growth of A498 renal cancer cells with a GI50 of 386 nM and merits future investigation. In the design of compound 13, the Michael acceptor moiety is presumably involved in alkylation of the essential machinery of the cell and development of this is the subject of current work.

In comparing the global effect of both 11 and 13 (Figures S13 and S16) it is evident that they affect cell growth by different mechanisms as would be expected from their structures. In specific, compound

11 has the potential for use in ovarian cancers given its exceptional toxicity against the OVCAR-3 and OVCAR-4 phenotypes (LC50 6.2 and <10 μM respectively; OVCAR-4 value assigned due to inflection of graph). OVCAR-3 and OVCAR-4 are both mutant p53 status but have individual profiles with OVCAR-3 having known upregulation of BRCA2-interacting transcriptional repressor and cyclin E1. OVCAR-4 in turn has been identified as a good model cell line for High Grade Serious Ovarian Cancer (HGSOC) which make these findings significant from a clinical perspective [33].

2.3. COMPARE Analysis of Compounds 11 and 13

COMPARE analysis was performed on the NCI COMPARE algorithm in order to identify correlations with known anticancer agents within the NCI database. Both compound 11 and 13 were analysed and with a specific focus on two subsets of the database: synthetic compounds and mechanistic set. Compound 13 gave a number of correlations as high as 0.74 with the most relevant mechanistic hit being to Chrysanthemic acid (NSC 11779) but this must be seen in the overall non-specific profile of activity of 13 and its limited potency.

However, on analysis of 11 in the synthetic compounds set, the top ranked correlation (0.6) is to SCH1473759 (NSC 761691) which has recently been reported as a picomolar inhibitor of Aurora kinases [34]. Again, while an important finding and a good match of cellular activity profile, this result must be seen in the context of potency with SCH1473759 having >100 the potency of 11 in the NCI assay (Figure S17). Compound 11 also gave rise to a correlation of 0.58 to Aclarubicin (Aclacinomycin A, NSC 208734) being the top hit of the mechanistic compound set. Aclarubicin has known topoisomerase inhibitory and recently reported histone eviction from open chromatin activity so despite the lack of evident topoisomerase activity of 11, this result merits further evaluation in respect of its interaction with DNA and DNA interacting enzymes [35].

3. Materials and Methods

Solvents were distilled prior to use as follows: dichloromethane was distilled from phosphorous pentoxide; ethyl acetate was distilled from potassium carbonate; ethanol and methanol were distilled from magnesium in the presence of iodine; toluene was distilled from sodium and benzophenone; hexane was distilled prior to use; tetrahydrofuran was freshly distilled from sodium and benzophenone. Diethyl ether was obtained pure from Riedel-de Haën. Organic phases were dried using anhydrous magnesium sulphate. All commercial reagents were used without further purification unless otherwise stated. All samples were confirmed as >95% pure by use of high resolution LCMS analysis.

Infrared spectra were recorded as a thin film on sodium chloride plates for liquids or potassium bromide (KBr) disc for solids on a Perkin Elmer Spectrum 100 FT-IR spectrometer.

^{1}H (300 MHz) and ^{13}C (75 MHz) NMR spectra were recorded on a Bruker Avance 300 NMR spectrometer. ^{1}H (600 MHz) and ^{13}C (150.9 MHz) NMR spectra were recorded on a Bruker Avance III 600 MHz NMR spectrometer equipped with a dual CH cryoprobe. All spectra were recorded at room temperature (~20 °C) in deuterated dimethylsulfoxide (DMSO-d_6) were assigned using the DMSO-d_6 peak as the reference peak. Chemical shifts (δH and δC) are expressed in parts per million (ppm) relative to the reference peak. Coupling constants (J) are expressed in Hertz (Hz). Splitting patterns in ^{1}H NMR spectra are designated as s (singlet), br s (broad singlet), d (doublet), br d (broad doublet), t (triplet), q (quartet), dd (doublet of doublets), dt (doublet of triplets), ddd (doublet of doublet of doublets), ddt (doublet of doublet of triplets) and m (multiplet).

Low resolution mass spectra were recorded on a Waters Quattro Micro triple quadrupole spectrometer (QAA1202) in electrospray ionisation (ESI) mode using 50% acetonitrile:water containing 0.1% formic acid as eluent. High resolution mass spectra (HRMS) were recorded on a Waters LCT Premier Time of Flight spectrometer (KD-160) in electrospray ionisation (ESI) mode using 50% acetonitrile:ater containing 0.1% formic acid as eluent.

Melting points were measured in a uni-melt Thomas Hoover capillary melting point apparatus and are uncorrected. Thin layer chromatography (TLC) was carried out on precoated silica gel plates

(Merck 60 PF254) or aluminium oxide TLC paltes (Sigma). Visualisation was achieved by UV light detection (254 nm).

5-Methyl-6*H*-pyrido[4,3-*b*]carbazole-11-carboxylic acid 9. 5-Methyl-6*H*-pyrido[4,3-*b*]carbazole -11-carbaldehyde **8** (92 mg, 0.353 mmol) in acetonitrile (9 mL) was treated with dimethylsulfoxide (0.03 mL, 0.423 mmol) and conc. sulfuric acid (0.3 mL, 0.622 mmol). A solution of sodium chlorite (48 mg, 0.530 mmol) in water (3 mL) was added dropwise and the reaction mixture was stirred at room temperature overnight. The reaction was quenched with sodium sulfite (22 mg, 0.177 mmol) in water (1 mL). The acetonitrile was evaporated to leave an aqueous solution, which was carefully adjusted to pH 5 with saturated aqueous sodium bicarbonate to precipitate the product. The mixture was cooled to 0 °C, filtered and washed with water (3 mL), to give 5-methyl-6*H*-pyrido[4,3-*b*]carbazole-11-carboxylic acid **9**. The orange solid was dried at 0.02 mbar for 24 h (71 mg, 73.2%). m.p. >300 °C; vmax/cm^{-1} (KBr): 3161 (NH), 3010 (OH broad), 1689 (C=O), 1648 (C=C arom.), 1597 (C=C arom.), 1488, 1463, 1417, 1241 (C-O stretch), 1109; δH (300 MHz, DMSO-d_6): 2.88 [3H, s, C(5)CH_3], 7.26 [1H, t, *J* = 7.9, C(9)H], 7.55–7.62 [2H, m, C(7)H, C(8)H], 8.03 [1H, d, *J* = 5.9, C(3)H], 8.21 [1H, d, *J* = 7.8, C(10)H], 8.47 [1H, d, *J* = 5.9, C(4)H], 9.43 [1H, s, C(1)H], 11.64 [1H, s, N(6)H]; δC (75.5 MHz, DMSO-d_6): 12.3 [3H, s, C(5)CH_3], 111.5 [CH, C(7)H], 113.3 (C, aromatic C), 117.7 [CH, C(3)H], 118.5 (C, aromatic C), 120.0 [CH, C(9)H], 120.3 (C, aromatic C), 122.3 (C, aromatic C), 123.1 [CH, C(10)H], 124.9 (C, aromatic C), 129.1 [CH, C(8)H], 132.2 (C, aromatic C), 136.1 [CH, C(4)H], 141.9 (C, aromatic C), 143.1 (C, aromatic C), 147.9 [CH, C(1)H], 168.8 [C, C(11)COOH]; m/z (ESI+): 277 [$(M+H)^+$ 40%], 115 (100%); HRMS (ESI+): Exact mass calculated for $[C_{17}H_{13}N_2O_2]^+$ 277.0977. Found 277.0977.

5-Methyl-6*H*-pyrido[4,3-*b*]carbazole-11-carbonylchloride 10. 5-Methyl-6*H*-pyrido[4,3-*b*]carbazole -11-carboxylic acid **9** (99 mg, 0.358 mmol) in dichloromethane (50 mL), under N_2, was treated with oxalyl chloride (0.04 mL, 0.459 mmol). Slight fizzing was observed on addition and mixture was stirred at room temperature for 20 h. The bright orange suspension was evaporated under reduced pressure. IR analysis showed the carbonyl peak at 1785 cm^{-1} indicating acid chloride formation.

***N*-Benzyl-5-methyl-6*H*-pyrido[4,3-*b*]carbazole-11-carboxamide 11.** 5-Methyl-6*H*-pyrido[4,3-*b*] carbazole-11-carboxylic acid **9** (99 mg, 0.358 mmol) in dichloromethane (50 mL), under N_2, was treated with oxalyl chloride (0.04 mL, 0.459 mmol) and stirred at room temperature for 20 h. The mixture was evaporated under reduced pressure, cooled to 0 °C under N_2, and treated drop-wise with benzylamine (2 mL, 18.3 mmol). After stirring for 1 h, diethyl ether (40 mL) was added, the mixture was cooled and filtered to give a cream solid (220 mg) containing the desired product and residual benzylamine. This was stirred with diethyl ether and decanted (3 × 40 mL). Purification by column chromatography, eluting with dichloromethane:methanol (100:0–95:5), gave product **11** as a yellow solid (39 mg, 30%). m.p. 294–296 °C; vmax/cm^{-1} (KBr): 3159 (NH), 3051 (CH) 1731 (C=O), 1621 (C=C arom.), 1600 (C=C arom.), 1542, 1466, 1410, 1245; δH (600 MHz, DMSO-d_6): 2.79 [3H, s, C(5)CH_3], 4.65–4.70 [2H, m, $CONHCH_2$], 6.98 [1H, t, *J* = 7.4, C(9)H], 7.28 [1H, t, *J* = 7.2, N-benzyl-C(4)H], 7.36 [2H, t, *J* = 7.3, *N*-benzyl-C(2)H, C(6)H], 7.43–7.50 [4H, m, C(7)H, C(8)H, *N*-benzyl-C(3)H, C(5)H], 7.72 [1H, d, *J* = 7.8, C(10)H], 7.93 [1H, d, *J* = 5.9, C(3)H], 8.37 [1H, d, *J* = 5.1, C(4)H], 9.19 [1H, s, C(1)H], 9.41 [1H, t, *J* = 5.9, C(11)CONH], 11.46 [1H, s, N(6)H]; δC (150.9 MHz, DMSO-d_6): 12.2 [CH_3, C(5)CH_3], 43.1 [CH_2, C(11)$CONHCH_2$], 110.9 (CH, aromatic CH), 111.3 (C, aromatic C), 116.0 [CH, C(3)H], 119.1 [CH, C(9)H], 119.8 (C, aromatic C), 120.9 (C, aromatic C), 121.1 (C, aromatic C), 122.8 [CH, C(10)H], 127.1 [CH, N-benzyl-C(4)H], 127.2 (C, aromatic C), 127.9 (CH, aromatic CH), 128.0 (CH, aromatic CH), 128.2 (CH, aromatic CH), 128.4 (CH, aromatic CH), 128.5 (CH, aromatic CH), 131.7 (C, aromatic C), 138.9 (C, aromatic C), 140.4 (C, aromatic C), 140.7 [CH, C(4)H], 142.7 (C, aromatic C), 150.1 [CH, C(1)H], 167.1 [C, C(11)CONH]; m/z (ESI+): 366 [$(M+H^+)$, 100%]; HRMS (ESI+): Exact mass calculated for $[C_{24}H_{20}N_3O]^+$ 366.1606. Found 366.1615.

Methyl 5-methyl-6*H*-pyrido[4,3-*b*]carbazole-11-carboxylate 12. 5-Methyl-6*H*-pyrido[4,3-*b*]carbazole -11-carboxylic acid **9** (99 mg, 0.358 mmol) in dimethylformamide (8 mL) under N_2, was heated gently until the acid dissolved. Carbonyldiimidazole (70 mg, 0.430 mmol) was added and the solution was heated at 120 °C for 4 h. The mixture was cooled to 0 °C and diethyl ether (20 mL) was added. The resulting precipitate was filtered and washed (diethyl ether 10 mL). The solid was cooled to 0 °C and treated dropwise with methanol (10 mL). The mixture was stirred at r.t. for 1 h and heated to reflux for 5 h. On cooling, a precipitate formed which was filtered to give the methyl ester, methyl 5-methyl-6*H*-pyrido[4,3-*b*]carbazole-11-carboxylate **12** (14 mg, 14%). m.p. 247–250 °C; vmax/cm^{-1} (KBr): 3147 (NH), 3008 (CH), 1742 (C=O), 1634 (C=C arom.), 1589 (C=C arom.), 1457, 1422, 1246 (C-O stretch), 1095; δH (300 MHz, DMSO-d_6): 2.89 [3H, s, C(5)CH_3], 4.22 [3H, s, C(11)$COOCH_3$], 7.27 [1H, overlapping ddd, *J* = 8.0, 5.8, 2.3, C(9)H], 7.57–7.63 [2H, m, C(7)H, C(8)H], 7.99 [1H, d, *J* = 8.0, C(10)H], 8.04 [1H, d, *J* = 6.1, C(3)H], 8.50 [1H, br s, C(4)H], 9.38 [1H, br s, C(1)H], 11.73 [1H, s, N(6)H]; δC (150.9 MHz, DMSO-d_6): 12.4 [CH_3, C(5)CH_3], 53.1 [CH_3, C(11)$COOCH_3$], 111.3 [CH, C(7)H or C(8)H], 113.7 (C, aromatic C), 116.2 [CH, C(3)H], 119.6 [CH, C(9)H], 120.2 (C, aromatic C), 121.3 (C, aromatic C), 121.8 (C, aromatic C), 122.5 [CH, C(10)H], 128.7 [CH, C(7)H or C(8)H], 131.6 (C, aromatic C), 140.2 (C, aromatic C), 140.9 [CH, C(4)H], 143.1 (C, aromatic C), 149.8 [CH, C(1)H], 168.4 [C, C(11)C=O]; m/z (ESI+): 291 [(M+H)$^+$, 100%]. HRMS (ESI+): Exact mass calculated for [$C_{18}H_{15}N_2O_2$]$^+$ 291.1134. Found 291.1121.

(*E*)-4-(5-methyl-6*H*-pyrido[4,3-*b*]carbazol-11-yl)but-3-en-2-one 13. A stirred solution of 5-methyl -6*H*-pyrido[4,3-*b*]carbazole-11-carbaldehyde **8** (300 mg, 1.15 mmol) in acetone (70 mL) was treated drop-wise with potassium permanganate (364 mg, 2.30 mmol) in water (70 mL). The mixture was stirred at r.t. for 1 h and heated to reflux for 22 h. Sodium bicarbonate (244 mg, 2.30 mmol) was added and stirred for 20 min. The mixture was filtered through celite and washed with water (100 mL) and acetone (200 mL). The filtrate was concentrated under reduced pressure to remove the acetone and then acidified to pH 5 with 20% aqueous HCl. The aqueous layer was extracted with chloroform:methanol (90:10, 3 × 100 mL). Organic extracts were combined and washed with water (1 × 100 mL) and brine (1 × 100 mL), dried over magnesium sulphate and evaporated under reduced pressure to give an orange solid (300 mg). Analysis showed that the desired carboxylic acid **9** had not formed but instead the condensation product (*E*)-4-(5-methyl-6*H*-pyrido[4,3-*b*]carbazol-11-yl)but-3-en-2-one **13** (87.0%). m.p. 263–265 °C; vmax/cm^{-1} (KBr): 3149(NH), 3087 (CH), 2982 (asymm. CH_3 stretch), 2883 (symm. CH_3 stretch), 1664 (C=O), 1620 (C=C), 1592 (C=C arom.), 1464, 1404, 1383, 1243; δH (300 MHz, DMSO-d_6): 2.61 [3H, s, $COCH_3$], 2.84 [3H, s, C(5)CH_3], 6.75 [1H, d, *J* = 16.6, C(11)CH=CH], 7.25 [1H, overlapping ddd, *J* = 8.0, 6.6, 1.5, C(9)H], 7.53–7.61 [2H, m, C(7)H, C(8)H], 7.98 [1H, dd, *J* = 6.1, 0.7, C(3)H], 8.14 [1H, d, *J* = 8.0, C(10)H], 8.47 [1H, d, *J* = 6.1, C(4)H], 8.59 [1H, d, *J* = 16.6, C(11)CH=CH], 9.58 [1H, s, C(1)H], 11.57 [1H, s, N(6)H]; δC (75.5 MHz, DMSO-d_6): 12.2 [CH_3, C(5)CH_3], 27.8 (CH_3, $COCH_3$), 111.1 [CH, C(7)H], 111.7 (C, aromatic C), 115.9 [CH, C(3)H], 119.4 [CH, C(9)H], 120.5 (C, aromatic C), 121.9 (C, aromatic C), 122.4 (C, aromatic C), 123.6 [CH, C(10)H], 126.0 (C, aromatic C), 127.9 [CH, C(8)H], 132.3 (C, aromatic C), 135.9 [CH, C(11)CH=CH], 138.4 [CH, C(11)CH=CH], 140.2 (C, aromatic C), 140.9 [CH, C(4)H], 143.0 (C, aromatic C), 150.1 [CH, C(1)H], 197.8 (C, C=O); m/z (ESI+): 301[(M+H)+ 100%]; HRMS (ESI+): Exact mass calculated for [$C_{20}H_{17}N_2O$]$^+$ 301.1341. Found 301.1348.

(*E*)-*N*-(4-(5-methyl-6*H*-pyrido[4,3-*b*]carbazol-11-yl)but-3-en-2-yl)formamide 14. (*E*)-4-(5-Methyl -6*H*-pyrido[4,3-*b*]carbazol-11-yl)but-3-en-2-one **13** (91 mg, 0.303 mmol), formamide (0.2 mL, 5.03 mmol) and formic acid (0.1 mL, 2.65 mmol) were heated to 150 °C for 1.5 h, at which point TLC analysis indicated consumption of the starting material. On cooling, saturated aqueous sodium bicarbonate (8 mL) was added and extraction was attempted with dichloromethane:methanol (90:10), however the organic extracts contained no material. The aqueous layer was treated with 20% aqueous HCl to pH 1, stirred for 20 min and then adjusted to pH 10 with 20% aqueous NaOH. The aqueous layer was extracted with dichloromethane–methanol (90:10 3 × 30 mL and 80:20 4 × 30 mL), dried and evaporated under reduced pressure to give an orange solid (64 mg). Purification by column chromatography on alumina, eluting with dichloromethane:methanol (97:3–90:10) gave three fractions. The largest of these (34 mg) was repurified by chromatography on silica to give an orange solid (19 mg). This was found to be the formamide, (*E*)-*N*-(4-(5-methyl-6*H*-pyrido[4,3-*b*]carbazol-11-yl)but-3-en-2-yl)formamide **14**. δH (300 MHz, DMSO-d_6): 1.47 [3H, d, *J* = 6.9, C(11)CH=CH–CH(CH_3)], 2.83 [3H, s, C(5)CH_3], 4.88–4.95 [1H, m, C(11)CH=CH–CH(CH_3)], 6.14 [1H, dd, *J* = 16.2, 5.6, C(11)CH=CH], 7.21 [1H, overlapping ddd,

J = 8.0, 6.7, 1.4, C(9)H], 7.36 [1H, d, *J* = 16.5, C(11)CH=CH], 7.52 [1H, td, *J* = 7.4, 1.1, C(8)H], 7.56–7.59 [1H, m, C(7)H], 7.99 [1H, br s, NHCHO], 8.23 [1H, br s, C(3)H], 8.33 [1H, d, *J* = 7.7, C(10)H], 8.43 [1H, br s, NHCHO], 8.54 [1H, d, *J* = 7.5, C(4)H], 9.58 [1H, br s, C(1)H], 11.51 [1H, s, N(6)H]; m/z (ESI+): 330 [$(M+H)^+$ 60%], 169 (100%); HRMS (ESI): Exact mass calculated for $[C_{21}H_{20}N_3O]^+$ 330.1606. Found 330.1619.

9-Formyl-5-methyl-6*H*-pyrido[4,3-*b*]carbazole-11-carboxylic acid 15. 5-Methyl-6*H*-pyrido[4,3-*b*] carbazole-11-carboxylic acid **9** (497 mg, 1.80 mmol) in trifluoroacetic acid (60 mL), was treated with hexamethylenetetramine (2.522 g, 18.0 mmol) portionwise over 5 min and heated to reflux for 25 min. On cooling, the reaction mixture was concentrated to approx. one quarter volume, water (30 mL) was added and the solution was transferred to a large conical flask (500 mL). The solution was cooled to 0 °C and neutralized with solid sodium bicarbonate while stirring vigorously. The mixture was stirred at 0 °C for 1 h, readjusted to pH 7 and filtered to give a brown solid which was dried at 0.02 mbar for 2 days (449 mg, 81.9%). m.p. 315–317 °C; vmax/cm^{-1} (KBr): 3069 (OH broad), 1677 (C=O × 2, broad), 1583 (C=C arom.), 1472, 1404, 1349, 1242 (C-O stretch), 1128, 808; δH (600 MHz, DMSO-d_6): 2.88 [3H, s, $C(5)CH_3$], 7.72 [1H, d, *J* = 8.3, C(7)H], 8.04 [1H, d, *J* = 6.0, C(3)H], 8.10 [1H, d, *J* = 8.4, C(8)H], 8.50 [1H, d, *J* = 6.0, C(4)H], 8.80 [1H, s, C(10)H], 9.51 [1H, s, C(1)H], 10.04 [1H, s, C(9)CHO], 12.14 [1H, s, N(6)H]; δC (150.9 MHz, DMSO-d_6): 12.3 [3H, s, $C(5)CH_3$], 111.4 [CH, C(7)H], 113.0 (C, aromatic C), 116.2 [CH, C(3)H], 119.7 (C, aromatic C), 120.4 (C, aromatic C), 121.3 (C, aromatic C), 125.7 [CH, C(10)H], 128.5 (C, aromatic C), 129.8 [CH, C(8)H], 129.9 (C, aromatic C), 132.4 (C, aromatic C), 140.8 [CH, C(4)H], 141.1 (C, aromatic C), 146.9 (C, aromatic C), 150.7 [CH, C(1)H], 169.2 [C, C(11)COOH], 191.6 [CH, C(9)CHO]; m/z (ESI+): 305 [$(M+H)^+$ 70%], 155 (40%), 64 (100%); HRMS (ESI+): Exact mass calculated for $[C_{18}H_{13}N_2O_3]^+$ 305.0926. Found 305.0940.

Benzylammonium 9-((benzylimino)methyl)-5-methyl-6H-pyrido[4,3-b]carbazole-11-carboxylate 16. A suspension of 9-formyl-5-methyl-6*H*-pyrido[4,3-*b*]carbazole-11-carboxylic acid **15** (194 mg, 0.638 mmol) in dichloromethane (65 mL), under N_2, was treated with oxalyl chloride (0.08 mL, 0.917 mmol) and stirred at room temperature overnight. Additional oxalyl chloride (0.08 mL, 0.917 mmol), was added and the reaction was stirred for 4 h. The mixture was evaporated under reduced pressure, cooled to 0 °C under N_2, and treated drop-wise with benzylamine (2 mL, 18.3 mmol). After stirring for 1 h, diethyl ether (40 mL) was added, the mixture was cooled and filtered to give a yellow solid. Crude analysis showed this to contain residual benzylamine. Recrystallisation from dichloromethane followed by a second recrystallisation from methanol gave product still containing benzylamine in 1:1 ratio with product. To investigate whether an amide or imine had formed, the product (27 mg) was dissolved in dichloromethane:methanol (90:10, 10 mL) and washed with 1M HCl (10 mL). The organic layer was dried and evaporated under reduced pressure. NMR and MS analysis showed that the compound had hydrolysed to the starting material **15**, indicating imine rather than amide formation. Full analysis (along with subsequent reduction of the imine) confirmed the product as the imine salt, benzylammonium 9-((benzylimino)methyl)-5-methyl-6*H*-pyrido[4,3-*b*]carbazole-11-carboxylate **16** (208 mg, 82.9%). m.p. 241–243 °C; vmax/cm^{-1} (KBr): 3029 (NH), 2864 (OH, broad), 1598 (C=O), 1572 (C=C arom.), 1494, 1450, 1402, 1347, 1278, 1244 (C-O stretch); δH (300 MHz, DMSO-d_6): 2.81 [3H, s, $C(5)CH_3$], 4.06 [2H, s, benzylammmonium-CH_2], 4.74 [2H, s, $C(9)CH{=}NCH_2$], 7.23–7.29 [1H, m, iminobenzyl-C(4)H], 7.33–7.42 [7H, m, iminobenzyl-C(2)H, C(3)H, C(5)H, C(6)H, benzylammmonium-C(3)H, C(4)H, C(5)H], 7.48 [2H, dd, *J* = 7.7, 1.7, benzylammmonium-C(2)H, C(6)H], 7.56 [1H, d, *J* = 8.3, C(7)H], 7.91 [1H, dd, *J* = 6.1, 0.7, C(3)H], 7.97 [1H, dd, *J* = 8.4, 1.6, C(8)H], 8.38 [1H, d, *J* = 6.1, C(4)H], 8.52 [1H, s, C(9)CH=N], 8.73 [1H, d, *J* = 1.1, C(10)H], 9.50 [1H, s, C(1)H], 11.64 [1H, s, N(6)H]; δC (75.5 MHz, DMSO-d_6): 12.0 [CH_3, $C(5)CH_3$], 42.3 [CH_2, benzylammonium CH_2], 64.1 [CH_2, $C(9)CH{=}N{-}CH_2$], 110.6 (CH, aromatic CH), 115.7 (CH, aromatic CH), 119.2 (C, aromatic C), 119.4 (C, aromatic C), 122.2 (C, aromatic C), 124.3 (CH, aromatic CH), 125.1 (C, aromatic C), 126.7 (CH, aromatic CH), 127.3 (C, aromatic C), 127.9 (CH, 2 × aromatic CH), 128.2 (CH, aromatic CH), 128.3 (CH, 2 × aromatic CH), 128.5 (CH, 2 × aromatic CH), 128.6 (CH, aromatic CH), 128.7 (CH, 2 × aromatic CH), 131.3 (C, aromatic C), 132.1 (C, aromatic

C), 134.6 (C, aromatic C), 139.9 (CH, aromatic CH), 140.5 (CH, aromatic CH), 141.1 (C, aromatic C), 144.3 (C, aromatic C), 144.5 (C, aromatic C), 152.0 (CH, aromatic CH), 162.2 (C, C=O); m/z (ESI+): 394 [(M+H)$^+$ 20%], 305 (20%), 108 (100%); HRMS (ESI+): Exact mass calculated for $[C_{25}H_{20}N_3O_2]^+$ 394.1556. Found 394.1560.

9-((Benzylamino)methyl)-5-methyl-6*H*-pyrido[4,3-*b*]carbazole-11-carboxylic acid 17. A solution of benzylammonium 9-((benzylimino) methyl)-5-methyl-6*H*-pyrido[4,3-*b*]carbazole-11-carboxylate **16** (88 mg, 0.224 mmol) in absolute ethanol (12 mL) was treated with sodium cyanoborohydride (21 mg, 0.338 mmol) and heated to reflux for 4.5 h. The solution was evaporated under reduced pressure and water (10 mL) was added. The mixture was stirred for 15 min, cooled and filtered. The orange solid was washed with water (5 mL) and diethyl ether (10 mL) and dried at 0.1 mbar for 24 h (56 mg, 62.9%). m.p. >300 °C (without melting); vmax/cm^{-1} (KBr): 3370 (NH), 3188 (OH, broad), 3056 (CH), 1596 (C=O), 1565 (C=C arom.), 1482, 1403, 1348, 1247 (C-O stretch); δH (600 MHz, DMSO-d_6): 2.73 [3H, s, C(5)CH_3], 3.89 [2H, s, one of CH_2], 4.04 [2H, s, one of CH_2], 7.21–7.26 [3H, m, *N*-benzyl-C(3)H, C(4)H, C(5)H], 7.39–7.40 [2H, m, N-benzyl-C(2)H, C(6)H], 7.46 [1H, d, *J* = 7.3, C(7)H], 7.53 [1H, d, *J* = 7.5, C(8)H], 7.82 [1H, d, *J* = 5.6, C(3)H], 8.29 [1H, d, *J* = 5.6, C(4)H], 8.42 [1H, s, C(10)H], 9.44 [1H, s, C(1)H], 11.39 [1H, s, N(6)H]; δC (150.9 MHz, DMSO-d_6): 12.0 [CH_3, C(5)CH_3], 50.3 (CH_2), 51.4 (CH_2), 108.3 (C, aromatic C), 110.4 [CH, C(7)H], 115.6 [CH, C(3)H], 119.1 (C, aromatic C), 119.3 (C, aromatic C), 122.4 (C, aromatic C), 124.5 [CH, C(10)H], 127.7 [CH, *N*-benzyl-C(4)H], 128.1 (CH, C(8)H], 128.3 [CH, *N*-benzyl-C(3)H, *N*-benzyl-C(5)H], 129.0 [CH, *N*-benzyl-C(2)H, *N*-benzyl-C(6)H], 129.1 (C, aromatic C), 132.0 (C, aromatic C), 133.7 (C, aromatic C), 136.0 (C, aromatic C), 140.2 [CH, C(4)H], 141.3 (C, aromatic C), 142.2 (C, aromatic C), 152.2 [CH, C(1)H], 170.8 (C, C=O); m/z (ESI+): 396 [(M+H)$^+$ 80%], 306 (100%); HRMS (ESI+): Exact mass calculated for $[C_{25}H_{22}N_3O_2]^+$ 396.1712. Found 396.1729.

Topoisomerase II decatenation assay. The decatenation assay kit was obtained from Inspiralis, Norwich Bioincubator, Norwich Research Park, Colney, Norwich, UK. The kit comprised of the following: assay buffer (supplied as 10× stock) containing 50 mM Tris.HCl (pH 7.5), 125 mM NaCl, 10 mM MgCl2, 5 mM DTT and 100 µg/mL albumin; dilution buffer containing 50 mM Tris. HCl (pH 7.5), 100 mM NaCl, 1 mM DTT, 0.5 mM EDTA, 50% (v/v) glycerol, 50 µg/mL albumin; ATP 30 mM; kDNA (100 ng/µl); 10 U/µL human topoisomerase II in dilution buffer; 5× stop buffer containing 2.5% SDS, 15% Ficoll-400, 0.05% bromophenol blue, 0.05% xylene cyanol and 25 mM EDTA. Tris-acetate-EDTA buffer (supplied as 10X buffer) and agarose were obtained from Sigma Life Sciences (Dublin, Ireland) and Safe View Stain was supplied by NBS Biologicals, Cambridgeshire, England.

The topo II decatenation assay protocol involved initial incubation of each inhibitor candidate (100 µM) along with a stock solution containing water, ATP, assay buffer, kDNA obtained from the mitochondrial DNA of Crithidia fasciculate, and topo II, at 37 °C for 1 h. Following addition of stop buffer, agarose DNA gel electrophoresis was run at 50 V for 2 h using a Consort EV243 power pack, to determine the relative amounts of decatenated DNA bands obtained in each compound lane. Positive (water), as well as negative controls (ellipticine) were incorporated in order to validate the results of each run. The resulting gels were viewed under UV light using a DNR Bio-Imaging System and photographed using GelCapture software.

NCI-60 Anti-cancer screening. Tested compounds were initially solubilised in DMSO, diluted into RPMI 1640 and 5% fetal bovine serum/L-glutamine, and added to 96-well plates containing cell lines previously cultured for 24 h. After 48-h incubation, the media were removed, and the cells were fixed and stained with sulforhodamine B to determine overall percent growth/total protein content. Unbound dye was removed with five washes of 1% acetic acid, and the plates were allowed to air dry. The dye was then resolubilised in Tris buffer, and the colorimetric absorbance was measured (515 nm). Growth inhibition was measured relative to the response generated from proliferating cells cultured under identical conditions for 48 h. In the five dose study, serial 5 × 10-fold dilution from an initial DMSO stock solution was performed, prior to incubation at each individual concentration (10 nM, 100 nM, 1 µM, 10 µM and 100 µM).

Using seven absorbance measurements (time zero (Tz), control growth (C), and test growth in the presence of drug at the five concentration levels (Ti)), the percentage growth was calculated at each of the drug concentrations levels. Percentage growth inhibition was calculated as:

$[(Ti-Tz)/(C-Tz)] \times 100$ for concentrations for which $Ti \geq Tz$

$[(Ti-Tz)/Tz] \times 100$ for concentrations for which $Ti < Tz$.

Three dose response parameters were calculated for each experimental agent. Growth inhibition of 50% (GI50) was calculated from $[(Ti-Tz)/(C-Tz)] \times 100 = 50$, which is the drug concentration resulting in a 50% reduction in the net protein increase (as measured by Sulforhodamine B staining) in control cells during the drug incubation. The drug concentration resulting in total growth inhibition (TGI) was calculated from $Ti = Tz$. The LC50 (concentration of drug resulting in a 50% reduction in the measured protein at the end of the drug treatment as compared to that at the beginning) indicating a net loss of cells following treatment was calculated from $[(Ti-Tz)/Tz] \times 100 = -50$. Values were calculated for each of these three parameters if the level of activity was reached; however, if the effect was not reached or was exceeded, the value for that parameter was expressed as greater or less than the maximum or minimum concentration tested [36,37]. Data from one dose experiments pertains to the percentage growth at 10 μM.

COMPARE analysis. COMPARE analysis was conducted using the private access system provided by the National Cancer Institute (https://dtp.cancer.gov/databases_tools/compare.htm). Seed compounds were analysed using a number of target sets: synthetic compounds, mechanistic set, standard agents, marketed drugs and diversity set. While the minimum correlation was set to 0.4, correlations of less than 0.5 were discounted. All other criteria were unchanged. Experiments that were carried out at different concentrations to the seed compound were ignored unless the concentration deviated by ±0.1, as was usual for older testing methods. COMPARE analysis was conducted solely on five dose data for compounds **11** and **13** [38].

4. Conclusions

Novel ellipticines substituted at the 11-position are described and their activity evaluated against topoisomerase II and cell growth in the National Cancer Institute's 60 cell line screening platform. Two of the novel compounds (**13** and **16**) show limited promise as topoisomerase II inhibitors at high concentrations (>10 μM). On evaluation of anticancer effect at the NCI, compounds **11** and **13** show real promise as future leads. Benzylamide **11** and unsaturated ketone **13** appear to have different modes of action in their cellular effects with broad cytotoxicity seen for compound **13** but some selectivity of cellular response seen for compound **11**. COMPARE analysis identified a potential target for compound **11** in Aurora kinase due to correlation of 0.6 with the known inhibitor SCH1473759. This will be investigated further in the future by synthesis of a series of ellipticine 11-amides to probe if this activity can be tuned further.

Supplementary Materials: The following are available online at http://www.mdpi.com/1424-8247/12/2/90/s1: Figures S1–S3, ^{1}H NMRs of relevant compounds; Figure S4, Three-fold dilution topoisomerase II inhibition assay of compounds **13** and **16**; Figures S5–S10, One dose NCI 60 cancer cell growth data (10 μM); Figures S11–S13, Five dose NCI 60 cancer cell growth data with GI50, TGI and LC50 data for compound **11**; Figures S14–S16, Five dose NCI 60 cancer cell growth data with GI50, TGI and LC50 data for compound **13**; Figure S17 COMPARE Analysis data for compound 13 in direct comparison with SCH1473759 (NSC761691), an Aurora kinase inhibitor.

Author Contributions: F.M.C. conceived and designed the experiments and wrote the manuscript; C.M.M. and E.O.S. performed the experiments, characterized the synthetic products and analysed the data.

Acknowledgments: The authors would like to acknowledge the Irish Research Council and the Higher Education Authority of Ireland under the PRTLI4 programme for funding. In addition, the authors would like to recognize the contribution from National Cancer Institute (NCI) screening program.

Conflicts of Interest: The authors declare no conflict of interest.

Abbreviations

The following abbreviations are used in this manuscript:

AKT	Protein Kinase B
CK2	Casein Kinase 2
GI50	Growth Inhibition 50%
LC50	Lethal concentration 50%
NCI	National Cancer Institute
NSC	numeric identifier for substances submitted to the National Cancer Institute (NCI)
Topo	Topoisomerase
SAR	Structure Activity Relationship

References

1. Hanahan, D.; Weinberg, R.A. Hallmarks of cancer: the next generation. *Cell* **2011**, *144*, 646–674. [CrossRef] [PubMed]
2. Goodwin, S.; Smith, A.F.; Horning, E.C. Alkaloids of Ochrosia elliptica Labill. *J. Am. Chem. Soc.* **1959**, *81*, 1903–1908. [CrossRef]
3. Miller, C.M.; McCarthy, F.O. Isolation, biological activity and synthesis of the natural product ellipticine and related pyridocarbazoles. *R. Soc. Chem. Adv.* **2012**, *2*, 8883–8918. [CrossRef]
4. O'Sullivan, E.C.; Miller, C.M.; Deane, F.M.; McCarthy, F.O. *Emerging Targets in the Bioactivity of Ellipticines and Derivatives. Studies in Natural Products Chemistry*; Elsevier: Amsterdam, The Netherlands, 2013; pp. 189–232.
5. Paoletti, C.; Le Pecq, J.B.; Dat-Xuong, N.; Juret, P.; Garnier, H.; Amiel, J.L.; Rouesse, J. Antitumor activity, pharmacology, and toxicity of ellipticines, ellipticinium, and 9-hydroxy derivatives: preliminary clinical trials of 2-methyl-9-hydroxy ellipticinium (NSC 264-137). *Recent Results Cancer Res.* **1980**, *74*, 107–123. [PubMed]
6. Ohashi, M.; Oki, T. Ellipticine and related anticancer agents. *Expert Opin. Ther. Pat.* **1996**, *6*, 1285–1294. [CrossRef]
7. Rouesse, J.; Spielmann, M.; Turpin, F.; Le Chevalier, T.; Azab, M.; Mondesir, J.M. Phase II study of elliptinium acetate salvage treatment of advanced breast cancer. *Eur. J. Cancer* **1993**, *6*, 856–859. [CrossRef]
8. Monnot, M.; Mauffret, O.; Simon, V.; Lescot, E.; Psaume, B.; Saucier, J.M.; Charra, M.; Belehradek, J., Jr.; Fermandjian, S. DNA-drug recognition and effects on topoisomerase II-mediated cytotoxicity. A three-mode binding model for ellipticine derivatives. *J. Biol. Chem.* **1991**, *266*, 1820–1829.
9. Froelich-Ammon, S.J.; Patchan, M.W.; Osheroff, N.; Thompson, R.B. Topoisomerase II binds to ellipticine in the absence or presence of DNA. Characterization of enzyme-drug interactions by fluorescence spectroscopy. *J. Biol. Chem.* **1995**, *270*, 14998–15004. [CrossRef]
10. Fossé, P.; René, B.; Charra, M.; Paoletti, C.; Saucier, J.M. Stimulation of topoisomerase II-mediated DNA cleavage by ellipticine derivatives: structure-activity relationship. *Mol. Pharmacol.* **1992**, *42*, 590–595.
11. Poljakova, J.; Eckschlager, T.; Hrabeta, J.; Hrebackova, J.; Smutny, S.; Frei, E.; Martinek, V.; Kizek, R.; Stiborova, M. The mechanism of cytotoxicity and DNA adduct formation by the anticancer drug ellipticine in human neuroblastoma cells. *Biochem. Pharmacol.* **2009**, *77*, 1466–1479. [CrossRef]
12. Vendôme, J.; Letard, S.; Martin, F.; Svinarchuk, F.; Dubreuil, P.; Auclair, C.; Le Bret, M. Molecular modelling of wild-type and D816V c-kit inhibition based on ATP-competitive binding of ellipticine derivatives to tyrosine kinases. *J. Med. Chem.* **2005**, *48*, 6194–6201. [CrossRef] [PubMed]
13. Prudent, R.; Vassal-Stermann, E.; Nguyen, C.-H.; Pillet, C.; Martinez, A.; Prunier, C.; Barette, C.; Soleilhac, E.; Filhol, O.; Beghin, A. Pharmacological inhibition of LIM kinase stabilizes microtubules and inhibits neoplastic growth. *Cancer Res.* **2012**, *72*, 4429–4439. [CrossRef] [PubMed]
14. Lu, C.; Wang, W.; El-Deiry, W.S. Non-genotoxic anti-neoplastic effects of ellipticine derivative NSC176327 in p53-deficient human colon carcinoma cells involve stimulation of p73. *Cancer Biol. Ther.* **2008**, *7*, 2039–2046. [CrossRef] [PubMed]
15. Andrews, W.J.; Panova, T.; Normand, C.; Gadal, O.; Tikhonova, I.G.; Panov, K.I. Old drug, new target: ellipticines selectively inhibit RNA polymerase I transcription. *J. Biol. Chem.* **2013**, *288*, 4567–4582. [CrossRef] [PubMed]

16. Brown, R.V.; Wang, T.; Chappeta, V.R.; Wu, G.; Onel, B.; Chawla, R.; Quijada, H.; Camp, S.M.; Chiang, E.T.; Lassiter, Q.R.; et al. The Consequences of Overlapping G-Quadruplexes and i-Motifs in the Platelet-Derived Growth Factor Receptor β Core Promoter Nuclease Hypersensitive Element Can Explain the Unexpected Effects of Mutations and Provide Opportunities for Selective Targeting of Both Structures by Small Molecules To Downregulate Gene Expression. *J. Am. Chem. Soc.* **2017**, *139*, 7456–7475. [PubMed]
17. Miller, C.M.; O'Sullivan, E.C.; Devine, K.J.; McCarthy, F.O. Synthesis and biological evaluation of novel isoellipticine derivatives and salts. *Org. Biomol. Chem.* **2012**, *10*, 7912–7921. [CrossRef]
18. Deane, F.M.; O'Sullivan, E.C.; Maguire, A.R.; Gilbert, J.; Sakoff, J.A.; McCluskey, A.; McCarthy, F.O. Synthesis and evaluation of novel ellipticines as potential anti-cancer agents. *Org. Biomol. Chem.* **2013**, *11*, 1334–1344. [CrossRef]
19. Russell, E.G.; O'Sullivan, E.C.; Miller, C.M.; Stanicka, J.; McCarthy, F.O.; Cotter, T.G. Ellipticine derivative induces potent cytostatic effect in acute myeloid leukaemia cells. *Investig. New Drugs* **2014**, *32*, 1113–1122. [CrossRef]
20. Russell, E.G.; Guo, J.; O'Sullivan, E.C.; O'Driscoll, C.M.; McCarthy, F.O.; Cotter, T.G. 7-formyl-10-methylisoellipticine, a novel ellipticine derivative, induces mitochondrial reactive oxygen species (ROS) and shows anti-leukaemic activity in mice. *Investig. New Drugs* **2016**, *34*, 15–23. [CrossRef]
21. Kutney, J.P.; Noda, M.; Lewis, N.G.; Monteiro, B.; Mostowicz, D.; Worth, B.R. Dihydropyridines in synthesis and biosynthesis. V. Synthesis of pyridocarbazole alkaloids: Olivacine and (±)-guantambuine. *Can. J. Chem.* **1982**, *60*, 2426–2430.
22. Mosher, C.W.; Crews, O.P.; Acton, E.M.; Goodman, L. Preparation and antitumor activity of olivacine and some new analogs. *J. Med. Chem.* **1966**, *9*, 237–241. [CrossRef] [PubMed]
23. Schmidt, U.; Theumer, G.; Jäger, A.; Kataeva, O.; Wan, B.; Franzblau, S.G.; Knölker, H.-J. Synthesis and Activity against Mycobacterium tuberculosis of Olivacine and Oxygenated Derivatives. *Molecules* **2018**, *23*, 1402. [CrossRef] [PubMed]
24. Awada, A.; Giacchetti, S.; Gerard, B.; Eftekhary, P.; Lucas, C.; de Valeriola, D.; Poullain, M.G.; Soudon, J.; Dosquet, C.; Brillanceau, M.-H. Clinical phase I and pharmacokinetic study of S 16020, a new olivacine derivative: report on three infusion schedules. *Ann. Oncol.* **2002**, *13*, 1925–1934. [CrossRef] [PubMed]
25. Thompson, D.; Miller, C.M.; McCarthy, F.O. Computer Simulations Reveal a Novel Nucleotide-type Binding Orientation for Ellipticine-based Anticancer c-kit Kinase Inhibitors. *Biochemistry* **2008**, *47*, 10333–10344. [CrossRef] [PubMed]
26. Gribble, G.W.; Saulnier, M.G.; Obaza-Nutaitis, J.A.; Ketcha, D.M. A versatile and efficient construction of the 6H-pyrido[4,3-b]carbazole ring system. Syntheses of the antitumor alkaloids ellipticine, 9-methoxyellipticine, and olivacine, and their analogs. *J. Org. Chem.* **1992**, *57*, 5891–5899. [CrossRef]
27. Saulnier, M.G.; Gribble, G.W. An efficient synthesis of ellipticine. *J. Org. Chem.* **1982**, *47*, 2810–2812. [CrossRef]
28. Saulnier, M.G.; Gribble, G.W. Efficient construction of the 10H-pyrido[3,4-b]carbazole ring system. Syntheses of isoellipticine and 7-methoxyisoellipticine. *J. Org. Chem.* **1983**, *48*, 2690–2695. [CrossRef]
29. Gribble, G.W.; Fletcher, G.L.; Ketcha, D.M.; Rajopadhye, M. Metalated heterocycles in the synthesis of ellipticine analogs. A new route to the 10H-pyrido[2,3-b]carbazole ring system. *J. Org. Chem.* **1989**, *54*, 3264–3269. [CrossRef]
30. Modi, S.P.; Carey, J.J.; Archer, S. Synthesis of 5-methyl-6h-pyrido[4,3-b]carbazole-11-methanol. *Tetrahedron Lett.* **1990**, *31*, 5845–5848. [CrossRef]
31. Modi, S.P.; Michael, M.A.; Archer, S.; Carey, J.J. An efficient synthesis of C-11 substituted 6H-pyrido[4,3-b] carbazoles. *Tetrahedron* **1991**, *47*, 6539–6548. [CrossRef]
32. Plug, J.P.M.; Koomen, G.-J.; Pandit, U.K. An Expedient Synthesis of 9-Hydroxyellipticine. *Synthesis* **1992**, *1992*, 1221–1222. [CrossRef]
33. Domcke, S.; Sinha, R.; Levine, D.A.; Sander, C.; Schultz, N. Evaluating cell lines as tumour models by comparison of genomic profiles. *Nat. Commun.* **2013**, *4*, 2126. [CrossRef] [PubMed]
34. Yu, T.; Tagat, J.R.; Kerekes, A.D.; Doll, R.J.; Zhang, Y.; Xiao, Y.; Esposite, S.; Belanger, D.B.; Curran, P.J.; Mandal, A.K.; et al. Discovery of a Potent, Injectable Inhibitor of Aurora Kinases Based on the Imidazo-[1,2-a]-Pyrazine Core. *ACS Med. Chem. Lett.* **2010**, *1*, 214–218. [CrossRef] [PubMed]
35. Pang, B.; Qiao, X.; Janssen, L.; Velds, A.; Groothuis, T.; Kerkhoven, R.; Nieuwland, M.; Ovaa, H.; Rottenberg, S.; van Tellingen, O.; et al. Drug-induced histone eviction from open chromatin contributes to the chemotherapeutic effects of doxorubicin. *Nat. Commun.* **2013**, *4*, 1908. [CrossRef] [PubMed]

36. National Cancer Institute. Developmental Therapeutics Program. NCI-60 Human Tumour Cell Lines Screen. Available online: https://dtp.cancer.gov/discovery_development/nci-60/default.htm (accessed on 14 May 2019).
37. Shoemaker, R.H. The NCI60 human tumour cell line anticancer drug screen. *Nat. Rev. Cancer* **2006**, *6*, 813–823. [CrossRef]
38. Paull, K.D.; Shoemaker, R.H.; Hodes, L.; Monks, A.; Scudiero, D.A.; Rubinstein, L.; Plowman, J.; Boyd, M.R. Display and Analysis of Patterns of Differential Activity of Drugs Against Human Tumor Cell Lines: Development of Mean Graph and COMPARE Algorithm. *J. Natl. Cancer Inst.* **1989**, *81*, 1088–1092. [CrossRef]

pharmaceuticals

Article

Protective Effect of Cashew Gum (*Anacardium occidentale* L.) on 5-Fluorouracil-Induced Intestinal Mucositis

João Antônio Leal de Miranda [1,2,*], João Erivan Façanha Barreto [1], Dainesy Santos Martins [1], Paulo Vitor de Souza Pimentel [1], Deiziane Viana da Silva Costa [1], Reyca Rodrigues e Silva [2], Luan Kelves Miranda de Souza [2], Camila Nayane de Carvalho Lima [3], Jefferson Almeida Rocha [4], Ana Paula Fragoso de Freitas [1], Durcilene Alves da Silva [2], Ariel Gustavo Scafuri [1], Renata Ferreira de Carvalho Leitão [1], Gerly Anne de Castro Brito [1], Jand Venes Rolim Medeiros [2] and Gilberto Santos Cerqueira [1,2]

1 Department of Morphology, Faculty of Medicine, Federal University of Ceará, s/n Delmiro de Farias Street, Porangabuçu Campus, Fortaleza 60416-030, Brazil; erivanfacanha@yahoo.com.br (J.E.F.B.); dainy.santos@gmail.com (D.S.M.); paulo_vitordesouza@hotmail.com (P.V.d.S.P.); deiziane2009@gmail.com (D.V.d.S.C.); paulinhaff2@hotmail.com (A.P.F.d.F.); urologia@gmail.com (A.G.S.); leitao_renata@yahoo.com.br (R.F.d.C.L.); gerlybrito@hotmail.com (G.A.d.C.B.); giufarmacia@hotmail.com (G.S.C.)

2 Biotechnology and Biodiversity Center Research, BIOTEC, Federal University of Piauí, Parnaíba, Piauí 64202-020, Brazil; reyca_14@hotmail.com (R.R.e.S.); luankelves11@gmail.com (L.K.M.d.S.); durcileneas@yahoo.com.br (D.A.d.S.); jandvenes@ufpi.edu.br (J.V.R.M.)

3 Nucleus of Research and Development of Medications (NPDM), Federal University of Ceará, Coronel Nunes de Melo Street, 100, Fortaleza 60430-275, Brazil; camilacarvalhoenf@yahoo.com.br

4 Research Group in Natural Sciences and Biotechnology, Federal University of Maranhão, s/n Avenue Aurila Maria Santos Barros de Sousa, Frei Alberto Beretta, Grajaú-MA 65940-000, Brazil; jeffersonkalel@hotmail.com

* Correspondence: joaoantonio@ufpi.edu.br; Tel.: +55-85-3366-8492

Received: 31 December 2018; Accepted: 15 March 2019; Published: 3 April 2019

Abstract: Intestinal mucositis is a common complication associated with 5-fluorouracil (5-FU), a chemotherapeutic agent used for cancer treatment. Cashew gum (CG) has been reported as a potent anti-inflammatory agent. In the present study, we aimed to evaluate the effect of CG extracted from the exudate of *Anacardium occidentale* L. on experimental intestinal mucositis induced by 5-FU. Swiss mice were randomly divided into seven groups: Saline, 5-FU, CG 30, CG 60, CG 90, Celecoxib (CLX), and CLX + CG 90 groups. The weight of mice was measured daily. After treatment, the animals were euthanized and segments of the small intestine were collected to evaluate histopathological alterations (morphometric analysis), levels of malondialdehyde (MDA), myeloperoxidase (MPO), and glutathione (GSH), and immunohistochemical analysis of interleukin 1 beta (IL-1β) and cyclooxygenase-2 (COX-2). 5-FU induced intense weight loss and reduction in villus height compared to the saline group. CG 90 prevented 5-FU-induced histopathological changes and decreased oxidative stress through decrease of MDA levels and increase of GSH concentration. CG attenuated inflammatory process by decreasing MPO activity, intestinal mastocytosis, and COX-2 expression. Our findings suggest that CG at a concentration of 90 mg/kg reverses the effects of 5-FU-induced intestinal mucositis.

Keywords: intestinal mucositis; heteropolysaccharide; 5-fluorouracil; inflammation

1. Introduction

Cancer, a complex disease characterized by uncontrolled cell growth, is one of the main causes of morbidity and mortality in both developed and developing countries [1–3]. Chemotherapeutic agents can controlled the dissemination of several tumors and improve the quality of life in most patients with cancer. Currently, 5-fluorouracil (5-FU) is one of the major chemotherapeutic agents used for the treatment of cancer. 5-FU is a fluorinated pyrimidine with antimetabolite activity. However, it can cause side effects such as nausea, vomiting, diarrhea, myelosuppression, and intestinal mucositis [4–9].

Mucositis is initiated by basal cell lesions in the gastrointestinal tract, resulting in mucosal damage, intense inflammatory reaction, and consequent ulceration. It affects around 40% of patients treated with chemotherapeutic agents [10,11]. Intestinal mucositis can increase the risk of bacterial translocation and sepsis, thus impairing the continuity of anticancer treatment.

Owing to the lack of efficacious therapeutic tools for the treatment of intestinal mucositis, new alternative therapeutics that can reduce the side effects of 5-FU, without impairing cancer treatment, have been investigated.

Cashew gum (CG), a high-molecular weight complex heteropolysaccharide, is obtained from the exudate of cashew tree (*Anacardium occidentale* L.) through condensation of a large number of aldose and ketose molecules [12,13]. Its anti-inflammatory, antiulcerogenic, and antidiarrheal activity have been reported in previous studies [14–17]. In this study, we investigated the effect of CG on 5-FU-induced experimental intestinal mucositis. In addition, we evaluated its effect on inflammatory process and oxidative stress, as well as the involvement of cyclooxygenase 2 (COX-2).

2. Results

2.1. Weight Analysis

As expected, from the second day, all mice subjected to 5-FU-induced intestinal mucositis presented progressive weight loss, which was significant compared to the saline group ($p < 0.05$). Notably, only CG 60 pretreatment prevented weight loss induced by 5-FU ($p < 0.05$). CG 30 and CG 90 were unable to reverse 5-FU-induced weight loss (Figure 1).

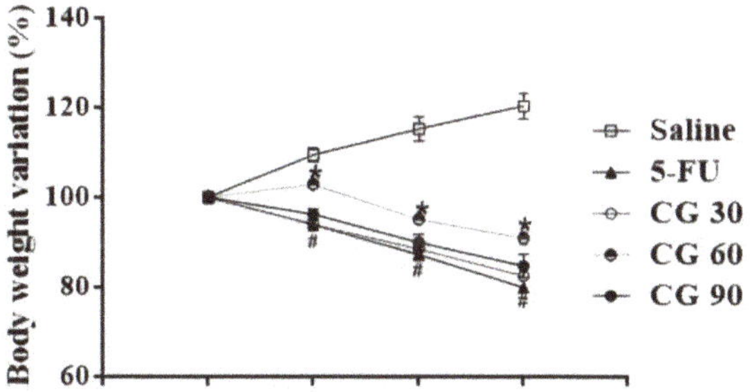

Figure 1. Body weight variation in mice subjected to intestinal mucositis (5-FU, 450 mg/kg, ip, single dose) and treated with CG (30, 60 and 90 mg/kg for 4 days). The results are expressed as the mean ± SEM of the weight evaluation percentage of the initial weight, of a minimum of 6 animals per group. Two-way ANOVA followed by the Tukey's test were used for the statistical analysis, where # $p < 0.05$ vs. saline and * $p < 0.05$ vs. 5-FU.

2.2. Histopathological and Morphometric Analysis

The 5-FU group showed intense inflammatory cell infiltration, disruption of intestinal mucosal architecture, and a significant reduction in villus height, crypt depth, and villus/crypt ratio compared to saline group ($p < 0.05$) (Figure 2B). Notably, all doses of CG attenuated the effects induced by 5-FU ($p < 0.05$) (Figure 2C–H). Moreover, a significant increase in histopathological scores was found in 5-FU group ($p < 0.05$) compared to the saline group (Table 1). CG 90 pretreatment decreased the histopathological scores compared to the 5-FU group ($p < 0.05$). However, CG 30 and CG 60 pretreatment did not reduce histopathological scores.

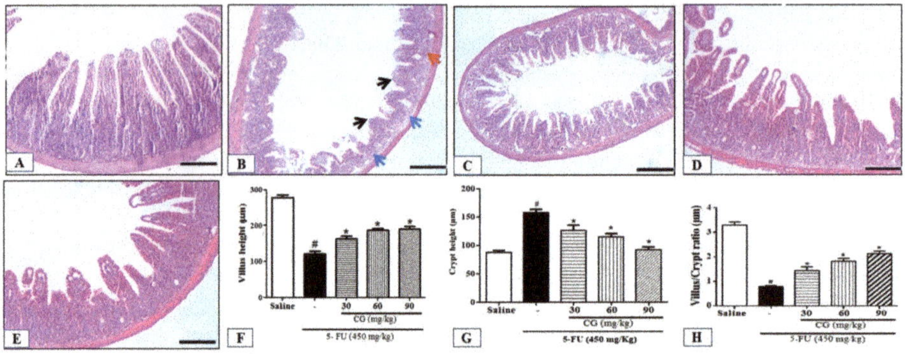

Figure 2. Histopathological analysis. (**A**) Saline; (**B**) 5-FU; (**C**) CG 30; (**D**) CG 60; (**E**) CG 90. 5 FU induced inflammatory cell infiltrate (red arrow), decreased intestinal villi (black arrow), loss of intestinal crypt architecture (blue arrow). Pretreatment with CG (30, 60 and 90 mg/kg) decreased the inflammatory infiltrate and prevented the shortening of the villi (**F**), increased crypt depth (**G**) and decreased villus/crypt ratio (**H**), with greater reversion of the 5-FU effect in the CG 90 + 5-FU group. All panels were obtained on the 100 µm scale (×200). Values were expressed as mean ± SEM. One-way ANOVA followed by the Tukey's test were used for the statistical analysis was used, where # $p < 0.05$ vs. saline group and * $p < 0.05$ vs. group 5-FU.

Table 1. Histopathological scores of mice subjected to 5-FU-induced intestinal mucositis and pretreated with CG.

Groups	Scores
Saline	0 (0-0)
5-FU	2 (1-3) #
CG 30	3 (3-3)
CG 60	1 (1-2)
CG 90	1 (0-1) *

Values were expressed as median, where # $p < 0.05$ vs. saline and * $p < 0.05$ vs. 5-FU (n = 6/group). The data was analyzed by the Kruskal-Wallis test followed by the Dunns multiple comparisons test.

2.3. Leukocyte Count

Analysis of leukocyte count in blood showed a significant decrease ($p < 0.05$) in the number of total leukocytes in 5-FU group compared to that in the saline group. In contrast, CG pretreatment reduced 5-FU-induced leukopenia ($p < 0.05$) (Figure 3A).

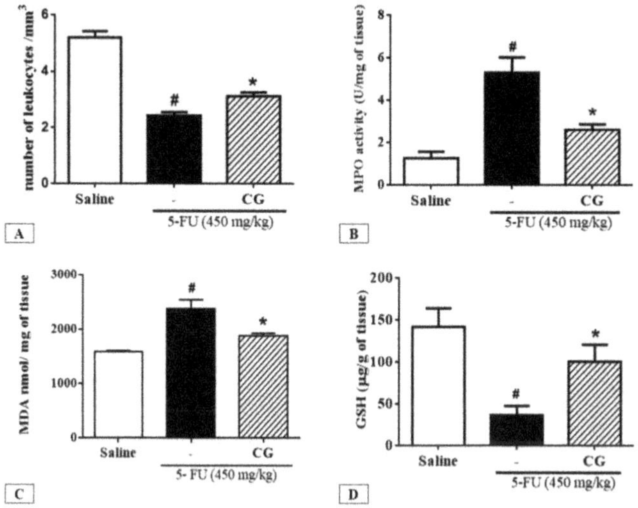

Figure 3. (**A**) Total leukocyte count; (**B**) Activity of myeloperoxidase (MPO); (**C**) Level of malondialdehyde (MDA); (**D**) concentration of glutathione (GSH). Values were presented as mean ± SEM. For the statistical analysis, one-way ANOVA followed by Tukey's test was used, where # $p < 0.05$ vs. saline group and * $p < 0.05$ vs. group 5-FU.

2.4. Myeloperoxidase Assay (MPO)

To investigate the effects of CG pretreatment on neutrophil recruitment in 5-FU-induced intestinal mucositis, we determined the activity of myeloperoxidase (MPO), a neutrophil marker. The 5-FU group presented a significant increase in MPO levels in the duodenum compared to the saline group ($p < 0.05$). CG (90 mg/kg) pretreatment decreased MPO levels in the duodenum of mice subjected to 5-FU-induced intestinal mucositis ($p < 0.05$), which in turn decreased polymorphonuclear leukocyte infiltration (Figure 3B).

2.5. Malondialdehyde (MDA) and Glutathione (GSH) Levels

To investigate the effect of CG pretreatment on 5-FU-induced oxidative stress in the duodenum, MDA and GSH levels (end products of oxidative stress) were evaluated. We found that 5-FU elevated MDA levels in the duodenum compared to the saline group (Figure 3C). CG (90 mg/kg) pretreatment reduced MDA levels compared to the 5-FU group ($p < 0.05$), thereby reducing 5-FU-induced oxidative stress (Figure 3C). Animals treated with 5-FU showed a significant ($p < 0.05$) decrease in GSH levels compared to the saline group. In contrast, CG (90 mg/kg) increased GSH levels compared to the 5- FU group ($p < 0.05$) (Figure 3D).

2.6. Mast Cell Concentration Analysis

To evaluate the effect of CG pretreatment on 5-FU-induced mastocytosis, the number of mast cells in the duodenum was measured. 5-FU (Figure 4B) increased the number of mast cells per field in the duodenum compared to the saline group (Figure 4A) ($p < 0.05$). CG (90 mg/kg) pretreatment (Figure 4C) decreased the number of mast cells compared to the 5-FU group ($p < 0.05$) (Figure 4D).

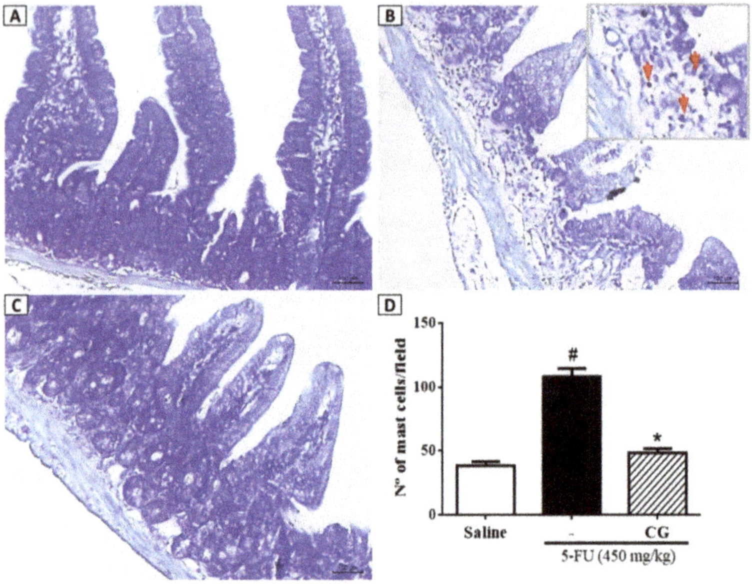

Figure 4. Mast cell counts in the duodenum samples. In (**B**) demonstrates that 5-FU promoted increased mast cell counts (red arrows) when compared to saline group (**A**). CG 90 (**C**) reversed the 5-FU-induced mastocytosis. All the panels were obtained at ×400 magnification. (**D**) Values were presented as mean ± SEM of the number of mast cells per field. For the statistical analysis, tone-way ANOVA followed by Tukey's test was used, where # $p < 0.05$ vs. saline group and * $p < 0.05$ vs. group 5-FU.

2.7. *Effect of CG on Cyclooxygenase-2 Pathway in Histopathological and Morphometric Analyses*

To investigate whether the effects of CG on reduction of 5-FU-induced intestinal injury, oxidative stress, and inflammation are mediated by cyclooxygenase-2 (COX-2) pathway, we blocked COX-2 by injecting celecoxib (CLX) in the presence or absence of CG in mice subjected to 5-FU-induced intestinal mucositis. Pretreatment with COX-2 blocker (CLX) (Figure 5D), as well as pretreatment with the combination of CLX and CG (90 mg/kg) (Figure 5E) prevented 5-FU-induced shortening of villus, cellular vacuolization, infiltration of inflammatory cells, edema, and loss of cellular architecture (Figure 5B).

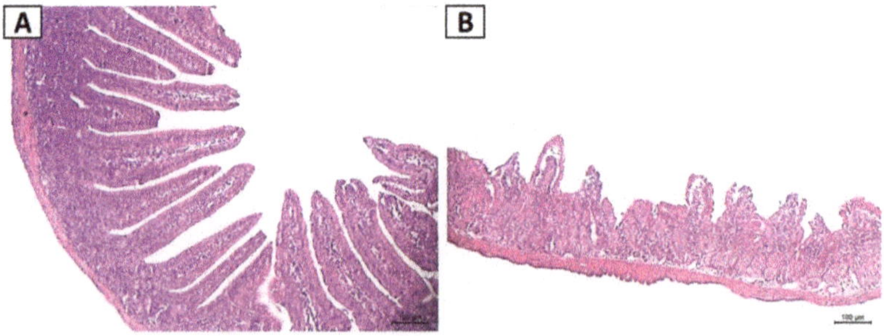

Figure 5. *Cont.*

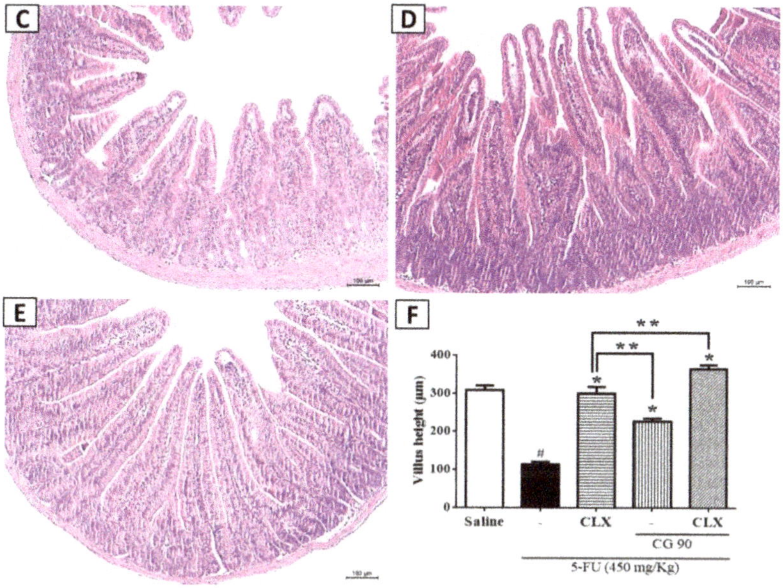

Figure 5. Effect of GC on the cyclooxygenase-2 pathway (COX-2) in histopathological and morphometric. The histopathological analysis represented by the groups (**A**) Saline; (**B**) 5-FU; (**C**) CG 90; (**D**) Celecoxib (CLX); (**E**) CLX and CG 90, as well as morphometric analysis of villus height (**F**) showed that 5-FU caused a decrease in villi and loss of cellular architecture when compared to the saline group. C, D, and E reversed the effect of 5-FU. All panels were obtained at ×200 magnification. Values were expressed as mean ± SEM for villi height in µm. For statistical analysis, one-way ANOVA followed by Tukey's test was used, where # $p < 0.05$ vs. saline group, * $p < 0.05$ vs. group 5-FU, ** $p < 0.05$ vs. group CLX.

CLX pretreatment decreased 5-FU-induced villus shortening ($p < 0.05$). In addition, pretreatment with the combination of CLX and CG (90 mg/kg) reverted villus shortening induced by 5-FU ($p < 0.05$). Moreover, the combination of CLX and CG (90 mg/kg) (Figure 5F) showed a greater effect on the recovery of duodenal villus in mice subjected to 5-FU-induced intestinal mucositis than pretreatment with CG 90 (Figure 5C) or CLX alone (Figure 5C) ($p < 0.05$).

2.8. Immunohistochemistry for the Detection of COX-2 and IL-1β

We investigated the effects of CG (90 mg/kg) in the presence or absence of CLX on COX-2 and IL-1β expression during 5-FU-induced intestinal mucositis through immunohistochemical analysis. 5-FU promoted intense immunostaining of COX-2 (Figure 6C) and IL-1β (Figure 6D) in the duodenal mucosa compared to the saline group (Figure 6A,B,K,L, $p < 0.05$). As shown in Figure 6E,F CG (90 mg/kg) pretreatment decreased immunostaining for COX-2 and IL-1β, respectively, compared to 5-FU group (Figure 6K,L, $p < 0.05$). Similarly, CLX alone (Figure 6G,H) or the combination of CLX and CG (90 mg/kg) (Figure 6I,J) decreased cell immunostaining forproinflammatory molecules in mice subjected to 5-FU-induced intestinal mucositis compared to the 5-FU group (Figure 6K,L, $p < 0.05$). Intense immunostaining was evidenced for the 5-FU lesion group, on the lamina followed by mild mucosal immunostaining, also was observed an absence of labeling in the epithelial cells.

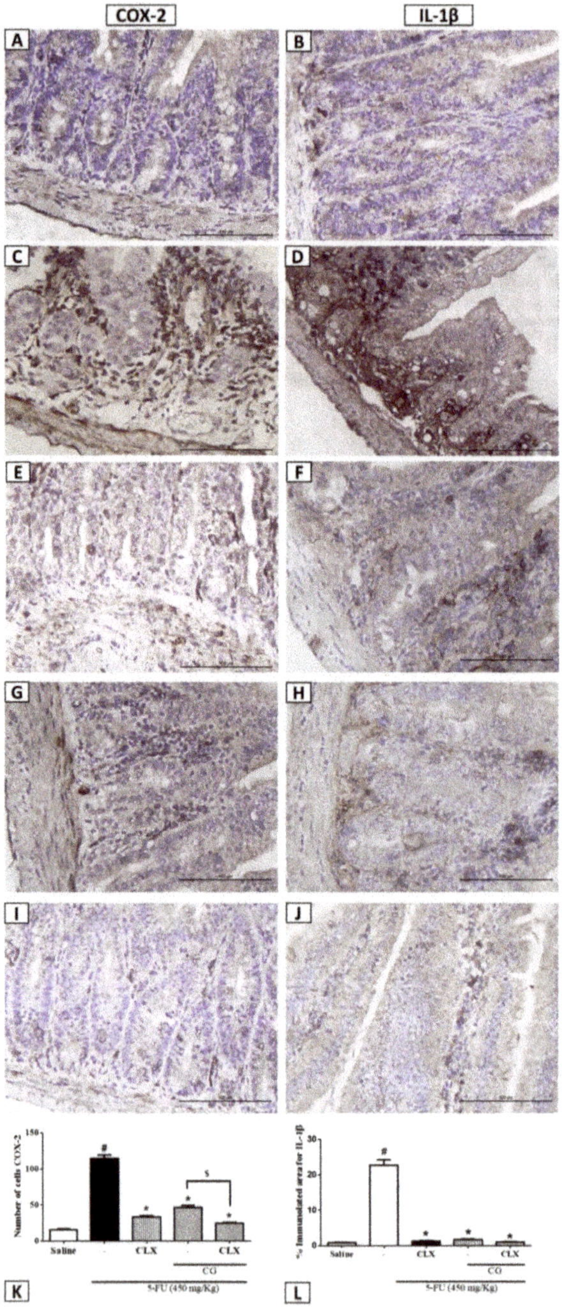

Figure 6. Immunohistochemistry analysis for COX-2 and IL-1β. (**A**,**B**) Saline; (**C**,**D**) 5-FU; (**E**,**F**) CLX; (**G**,**H**) CG 90; (**I**,**J**) CLX + CG 90. (**K**) a number of cells immunolabelled for cox-2. (**L**) % immunolabelled for IL-1β. Values were expressed as mean ± SEM. For statistical analysis, one-way ANOVA followed by Tukey´s test was used, where # $p < 0.05$ vs. saline group, * $p < 0.05$ vs. group 5-FU, $ $p < 0.05$ vs. group CLX.

3. Discussion

In the present study, we evaluated the effects of CG on intestinal mucositis induced by 5-FU and found that CG reversed the effects of 5-FU-induced intestinal mucositis at a concentration of 90 mg/kg. With the continuous expanded use of medicinal plants for the prevention and treatment of different pathologies worldwide, there has been increasing interest in the discovery of natural products with pharmacological effects. In Brazil, many herbal extracts are used in folk medicine to treat various digestive disorders, and several studies have documented the benefits of Brazilian plants in the prevention of gastrointestinal lesions [18,19].

A previous study reported that the extract of *Spondias pinnata*, belonging to the family Anacardiaceae, decreased histological severity scores and intestinal inflammation, and altered the mucosal architecture after chemotherapy. This indicated that *S. pinnata* extract could be an important pharmacological agent in promoting healing of damaged intestine after chemotherapy [20]. *A. occidentale* L. has been reported to possess diverse pharmacological properties. Its bark, leaves, and bark oil are used in anti-inflammatory and astringent preparations for the treatment of diarrhea [21]. Previous studies using the extracts of cashew tree bark have reported hypoglycemic [22,23], antioxidant and anti-inflammatory [24], antimicrobial [25], antihypertensive [26], and anticancer effects. It also showed beneficial effects in the treatment of gastritis, diarrhea, and wounds [22,27]. The anti-inflammatory activities and wound healing potential of cashew nuts have also been reported [28].

Weight loss is considered one of the common side effects of 5-FU chemotherapy. Therefore, body mass measure is one of the daily evaluated parameters to confirm the model of intestinal mucositis induced by 5-FU. Similar to our results, previous studies showed a decrease in body weight of animals after 5-FU-induced intestinal mucositis [29–31]. In this study, we showed that CG 60mg/kg decreased 5-FU-induced weight loss in mice, instead of the other CG doses which the loss weight was irreversible. Studies with probiotics and olmesartan showed that doses of these drugs were considered effective in reversing the harmful effects promoted by chemotherapy in mucositis model, after evaluation of histopathological parameters and inflammatory markers, however they were not effective in reverse weight loss as presented in ours studies [32,33].

Previous studies reported that 5-FU promoted decrease and vacuolization of intestinal villi, cryptic necrosis, infiltration of inflammatory cells, loss of cell architecture, and a decrease in villus/crypt ratio [34–37]. These findings are consistent with those of the present study. In addition, we found that CG at a concentration of 90 mg/kg was able to reduce the harmful effects of 5-FU on the duodenal mucosa. The anti-inflammatory effect of CG has been reported in skin lesions [15]. Araújo et al. [17] reported that 90 and 60 mg/kg of CG were effective in the treatment of acute inflammatory diarrhea. Similarly, 90 mg/kg was the best treatment concentration to prevent histopathological changes in 5-FU-induced intestinal mucositis.

Mucositis and myelosuppression are the main adverse effects related to 5-FU treatment [7,9,38]. In the present study, we showed that CG (90 mg/kg) attenuated leukopenia, the decrease in a number of total leukocytes, induced by 5-FU. Soares et al. [39] and Quaresma [40] demonstrated leukopenia in mice following a single administration of 5-FU (450 mg/kg).

The ulcerative phase of mucositis is characterized by loss of epithelial integrity of the mucosa, which facilitates a propitious environment for the invasion of bacteria. In addition, leucopenia may potentialize this process, resulting in bacteremia or sepsis [11,41,42]. We suggested that CG can be fundamental in preventing potential generalized bacterial infections during 5-FU treatment because it attenuated 5-FU-induced leukopenia. However, further investigations are needed to confirm this.

CG 90 prevented a 5-FU-induced increase in MPO levels in the duodenum. Similar to the present study, Bastos et al. [43], Justino et al. [44], Ávila et al. [45], Al-Asmari et al. [46], and Carvalho et al. [30] showed an increase in MPO activity after induction of intestinal mucositis by 5-FU. MPO has been used as a quantitative marker of neutrophil infiltration into various organs, including the gastrointestinal tract.

We showed that CG exerted antioxidant effects against intestinal mucositis by increasing GSH levels and decreasing MDA levels in the duodenum of mice subjected to 5-FU-induced intestinal mucositis. This finding is in agreement with the result of a previous study demonstrating that CG formulations exerted an antioxidant effect by decreasing MDA levels [47].

Our findings showed that CG reversed 5-FU-induced mastocytosis (increase in a number of mast cells) in the duodenum, indicating potent anti-inflammatory effects of CG in mice with 5-FU-induced intestinal mucositis. Previous studies have shown intense mastocytosis during intestinal mucositis induced by chemotherapeutics in mice [46,48]. The role of mast cells in the gastrointestinal tract is paradoxical, as their function depends on the mediators released and receptors activated. Mast cells contribute to intestinal homeostasis through immune protection, regulation of architecture and permeability of the epithelial barrier, and mucosal tissue remodeling through stimulation of fibroblast growth [49]. However, they are considered critical in the pathogenesis of inflammatory processes such as mucositis, because their overexpression consequently leads to amplification of inflammatory response caused by the selective release of mediators [50,51]. Besides exacerbation of inflammation, mastocytosis in the gastrointestinal tract has been reported to culminate in alteration of architecture and impairment of the gastrointestinal barrier, such as villus enlargement and changes in crypt size in the small intestine [52,53].

In the present study, we evaluated the effect of CG on COX-2 pathway by pretreating mice subjected to intestinal mucositis with a combination of CLX (a COX-2 blocker) and CG (90 mg/kg). In addition, we investigated whether the protective effect of CG on morphometric and histopathological changes induced by 5-FU was related to COX-2 inhibition. We found that the combination of CLX and CG (90 mg/kg) completely reverted 5-FU-induced decrease in villi, cryptic necrosis, inflammatory cell infiltration, and loss of cellular architecture in the duodenum. Our findings demonstrated that pretreatment with the combination of CG and CLX during 5-FU-induced intestinal mucositis was more effective in reversing histopathological effects than treatment with CLX alone, a commercially available nonsteroidal anti-inflammatory drug that acts as a selective inhibitor of COX-2. Short et al. [54] suggested that low doses of CLX can be used therapeutically for the protection of the intestinal barrier in patients with inflammatory bowel disorders, because of its ability to reduce COX-2 expression. Javle et al. [55] found that the combination of irinotecan (CPT-11) and CLX resulted in antitumor effects, with improvement in irinotecan-induced diarrhea and lethality. Furthermore, CG (90 mg/kg) alone or in combination with CLX was able to decrease 5-FU-induced COX-2 and IL-1β immunostaining in the duodenum. It is known that IL-1β is produced by macrophages, monocytes, and glial cells. This proinflammatory cytokine induces the expression of inflammatory mediators, such as COX-2 with subsequent release of prostaglandins, and the onset of primary tissue damage and progression [56–58]. The gene expression and tissue levels of IL-1β are correlated with intestinal mucosal injury induced by chemotherapy [59].

The study and use of natural polysaccharides in inflammatory bowel diseases, especially mucositis, is a current reality and future promise for the development of effective drugs in the treatment of 5-FU-induced intestinal mucositis. The present study has however a limitation. As intestinal inflammation is a complex process involving multiple mechanisms of activation and maintenance of the inflammatory process, the hypothetical model of action of CG on 5-FU-induced intestinal mucositis in mice proposed using the results of the present study (Figure 7) may be inadequate. Further studies are needed to elucidate the other possible mechanisms of CG action in intestinal mucositis.

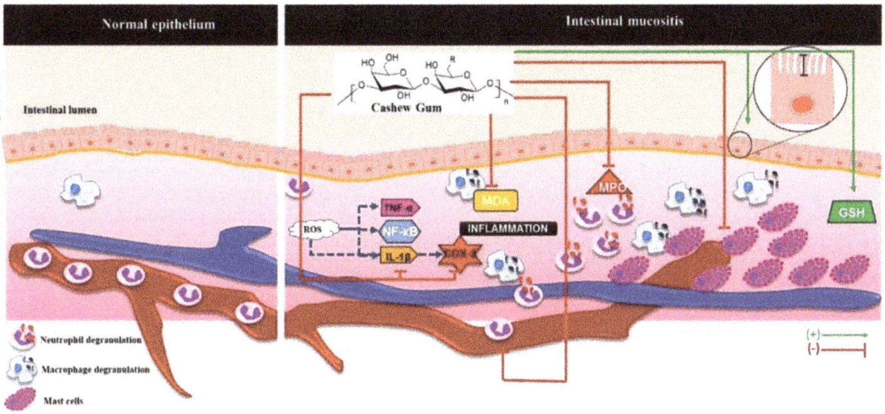

Figure 7. Hypothetical model of action of CG in intestinal mucositis induced by 5-FU. CG prevented the 5-FU-induced injury intestinal through inhibition of MDA formation, neutrophil recruitment (decreasing MPO levels), mast cells activation and IL-1β and COX-2 immunostaining marker and inhibited leucopenia. CG also stimulate villus enlargement and increase levels of GSH, an antioxidant. ROS: Reactive Oxygen Species; TNF-α: Tumor Necrosis Factor-alpha; NF-κB: transcription factor nuclear kappa b; IL-1β: Interleukin 1 beta; COX-2: Cyclooxygenase 2; MDA: Malondialdehyde; MPO: Myeloperoxidase; GSH: Reduced glutathione. Arrows green (stimulate / increase), red arrows (inhibit).

4. Materials and Methods

4.1. Animals

The animals were obtained from the Department of Surgery of the Federal University of Ceara (UFC) were used. The male Swiss mice (25–30 g) were housed in polypropylene cages, lined with wood, in a controlled environment with a temperature of 23 ± 2 °C, in a cycle of 12 h light/12 h dark, with free access to water and standard feed. The procedures and experimental protocols were approved by the Ethics Committee on Animal Use (n° 208/16) from the Federal University of Piaui (CEUA/UFPI).

4.2. Drugs and Plant Materials

Two drug drugs were used for mucositis induction and treatment, respectively: 5-FU (FauldFluor®, Libbs, Sao Paulo, Brazil) celecoxib (CLX- Celebra®, Pfizer, Sao Paulo, Brazil). Raw samples of CG were collected in 2013 by the Biotechnology and Biodiversity Center Research–BIOTEC, Parnaíba, Brazil, from the trunk of native cashew trees (*A. occidentale* L.) in Ilha Grande de Santa Isabel, Piauí, Brazil (Latitude, decimal degrees S-2.8242; Longitude, decimal degrees W-41.7331). The tree was identified and a voucher specimen, voucher number 52, was deposited at the HDELTA herbarium (Federal University of Piauí, Parnaíba, Piauí, Brazil).

4.3. Extraction and Purification of Cashew Gum

The CG was purified with sodium salt, as previously described [60]. Bark free nodules were selected and dissolved at a final concentration of 5% (*w*/*v*) in distilled water. The pH of the solution was adjusted to approximately 7.0. The clear solution was successively filtered through sintered glass and the heteropolysaccharide was precipitated with ethanol [61,62].

4.4. Induction of Experimental Intestinal Mucositis

The experimental intestinal mucositis model in Swiss Mice was induced as described by Soares et al. [39]. The 5-FU (450 mg/kg) was given intraperitoneally (i.p) in a single dose on the first day of the experimental protocol. Three days of treatment with CG were performed. The mice were pretreated daily with oral CG (30, 60, 90 mg/kg), 1h before the injection of 5- FU, after then the same oral doses were performed once a day. After four days of treatment, the animals were euthanized by ketamine (270 mg/kg) and xylazine (15 mg/kg) and the intestinal samples were collected. The body weight of mice was measured daily before the treatment administered to confirm the experimental model of intestinal mucositis induced by 5-FU. In this study, the mice was randomly allocated in seven groups ($n = 6$): Saline (NaCl 0.9%), 5-FU (5-FU + NaCl 0.9%), CG 30 (5-FU + CG 30 mg/kg), CG 60 (5-FU + CG 60 mg/kg), CG 90 (5-FU + CG 90 mg/kg), CLX (5-FU + celecoxib 7.5 mg/kg, i.p), CLX + CG 90 (5-FU + celecoxib 7.5 mg/kg, i.p + CG 90 mg/kg). To investigate the participation of COX-2 on the effects of treatment with CG during intestinal mucositis induced by 5-FU, COX-2 was blocked by celecoxib in an independent experiment. The mice were treated with celecoxib and CG 90 in combination or alone for three days.

4.5. Histopathological and Morphometric Analysis

After euthanasia, duodenum samples were obtained and fixed in 10% formaldehyde for performing the histopathological and morphometric analysis [63,64]. These samples were embedded in paraffin, sectioned at 4 μm and stained with hematoxylin and eosin (H&E). A blinded and randomized histopathological analysis was performed by an experienced histopathologist to assess the severity of mucositis using a scores system [65], the tissues were ranging from 0 (absence of lesion/normal histological findings) to 3 (maximum lesion degree), indicating shortened villi with vacuolized cells, necrosis of crypts, intense infiltration of inflammatory cells, vacuolization and edema in the mucosal layer and muscular layer with edema, vacuolization and neutrophil infiltrate. The effective concentration of CG in the treatment of mucositis was determined following the histological analysis.

4.6. Leukocyte Count

Mice were anesthetized with a combination of anesthetics (xylazine 10m/kg and ketamine 80 mg/kg) and, a peripheral blood sample was collected from the ocular artery, and was diluted in the liquid of Turk at a ratio of 20 μL of blood to 380 μL of solution. The total leukocytes were counted using a Neubauer chamber [66], and the results were expressed as a total number of leukocytes per mm3 of blood.

4.7. Dosage of Malondialdehyde (MDA)

The MDA is a product of lipid peroxidation frequently used as a marker of oxidative stress. Briefly, the intestinal samples were homogenized (10%) with potassium phosphate buffer (1.15%). Then, were added phosphoric acid (1%) and thiobarbituric acid (0.6%) to the homogenates and incubated at (100 °C, for 45 min) followed by the addition of 1.5 mL *n*-butanol. The supernatant was obtained and measured after centrifugation (5000 rpm, for 10 min). The results were expressed as nMol of MDA/mg of tissue by 535 nm absorbance measure [67,68].

4.8. Concentration of Glutathione (GSH)

The concentration of GSH in the duodenal samples was performed according to the method described by Sedlak and Lindsay [69]. The levels of nonprotein sulfhydryl groups (NPSH) were determined from 50 to 100 mg of the intestinal mucosa of each animal. The tissues were homogenized in 1 mL of 0.02M EDTA for each sample. Aliquots of 100 μL of the homogenate were mixed with 80 μL of distilled water and 20 μL of 50% trichloroacetic acid (TCA) for precipitation of proteins. The tubes were centrifuged for 15 min at 3000 rpm at 4 °C. A total of 100 μL of the supernatant was added to 200 μL of 0.4 M Tris buffer (pH 8.9) and 5 μL of 0.01 M 5,5-dithiobis-(2-nitrobenzoic acid) (DTNB, Sigma Aldrich, St. Louis, Missouri, USA). The mixture was then homogenate for 3 min and the absorbance was read at 412 nm. Results were expressed as micrograms of NPSH groups per milliliter of homogenate (μg/mL).

4.9. Myeloperoxidase Assay (MPO)

MPO activity was determined by the technique described by Bradley et al [70]. Briefly, the duodenum segments (50–100 mg) were homogenized in 1 mL of potassium buffer containing 0.5% hexadecyltrimethylammonium bromide (HTAB), then centrifuged (4000 rpm, 7 min, 4 °C). The MPO activity was analyzed by measuring the absorbance at 450 nm using diisocyanate dihydrochloride and 1% hydrogen peroxide in the resuspended pellet. The results were recorded as MPO units per mg tissue.

4.10. Mast Cell Analysis

The paraffin blocks with duodenum samples were processed for toluidine blue staining to identified mast cells, according to Michalany [71]. The slides were deparaffinized with xylene, incubated for 3 min with toluidine blue solution (1 g of toluidine blue dissolved in 70% ethanol), washed three times in distilled water, dehydrated, and mounted. The total number of mast cells were counted manually, considering four specimens per group and ten fields per slide. The results were expressed as the mean of 10 fields in each group.

4.11. Immunohistochemistry for the Detection of COX-2 and IL-1β

Duodenal sections were deparaffinized with oven insertion (60 °C) and three cycles of xylol immersion for 5 min each. Then, the sections were rehydrated in decreasing alcohol concentrations (100, 90, 80 and 70%). The histological sections were then washed with distilled water for 10 min and the antigenic recovery in citrate buffer (pH 7.0, DAKO®, Sao Paulo, Brazil) was carried out for 20 min in the water bath (95 °C). The slides were then washed with phosphate-buffered saline solution (PBS) for 5 min at room temperature. Following, endogenous peroxidase blockade with 3% hydrogen peroxide solution (H_2O_2) was performed for 30 min. The sections were then incubated overnight with goat anti-COX-2 primary antibody (SantaCruz®, Dallas, TX, USA), and rabbit anti-IL-1β (SantaCruz®, Dallas, TX, USA) diluted in antibody diluent (1:100) for 60 min, respectively. After the slides were washed with PBS and incubated with rabbit IgG (GBI Labs®, Bothell, WA, USA) secondary antibody diluted (1:400) for 30 min. For revelation, the sections were incubated with the streptavidin conjugated peroxidase complex (ABC complex) for 30 min and chromogen 3,3′diaminobenzidine peroxide, DAB (DAKO®, Sao Paulo, Brazil), followed by counterstaining with hematoxylin (DAKO®, Sao Paulo, Brazil), for 10 min. Negative controls were processed simultaneously as described above, with the primary antibody being replaced for antibody diluent. The procedures were performed in an automated manner using Autostainer Plus (DAKO®, Sao Paulo, Brazil). To assess COX-2 immunostaining, quantification was performed by immunolabelled cells with the aid of Image J software. For IL-1β immunostaining images, quantification was performed by measuring the % immunolabelled area with the aid of Adobe Photoshop 10. All images were captured with the aid of an optical microscope to the image acquisition system (LEICA, Wetzlar, HE, Germany).

4.12. Statistical Analysis

Quantitative results were expressed as mean ± standard error of the mean (SEM) and the qualitative data (histological scores) were pointed scores and expressed by the median ± minimum and maximum. The results with a parametric distribution were analyzed by Analysis of Variance (ANOVA) followed by post hoc test Tuckey through the program GraphPad Prism version 6.0 (GraphPad Software Inc., La Jolla, CA, USA). The data obtained from non-parametric distribution were analyzed using Kruskal-Wallis test followed by Dunn's (multiple comparisons). Values of p-value < 0.05 were considered statistically significant.

5. Conclusions

In summary, CG decreased inflammation, oxidative stress, and intestinal injury induced by 5-FU in the duodenum. The effects of CG were found to be related to COX-2 pathway. The concomitant administration of CG and CLX completely reverted COX-2 and IL-1β immunostaining markers and intestinal injury induced by 5-FU. Thus, we suggest that CG has potential application in the development of novel drugs against intestinal mucositis due to antineoplastic agents. Additionally, we recommend further studies to elucidate the molecular mechanisms related to the effects of GC under pro-inflammatory cytokines expression as well as other possible mechanisms of action involved in the protective effect of CG on chemotherapy-induced intestinal mucositis.

Author Contributions: J.A.L.M., L.K.M.S., J.A.R., A.P.F.F., and G.S.C. conceived and designed the experiments; J.A.L.M., J.E.F.B., D.S.M., P.V.S.P., D.V.S.C., R.R.S., C.N.C.L., A.G.S., R.F.C.L., and D.A.S. performed the experiments; J.A.L.M., D.S.M., D.V.S.C., G.A.C.B., J.V.R.M. and G.S.C. analyzed the data; J.A.L.M., R.R.S., D.V.S.C. and G.S.C. wrote the paper.

Acknowledgments: This research was supported by Conselho Nacional de Desenvolvimento Científico e Tecnológico–CNPq, Coordenação de Aperfeiçoamento de Pessoal de Nıvel Superior–CAPES, Fundação Cearense de Apoio ao Desenvolvimento Científico e Tecnológico–FUNCAP. We thank Microscopy and Image Processing Core (NEMPI) at Federal University of Ceará.

Conflicts of Interest: The authors declare no conflict of interest.

References

1. Kumar, V.; Abbas, A.K.; Aster, J.C. *Robbins Basic Pathology E-Book*, 9th ed.; Elsevier Health Sciences: Rio de Janeiro, Brazil, 2013.
2. Ferreira, J.E.V.; de Figueiredo, A.F.; Barbosa, J.P.; Pinheiro, J.C. Chemometric study on molecules with anticancer properties. In *Chemometrics in Practical Applications*; IntechOpen: London, UK, 2012; pp. 185–186.
3. Organization, W.H. Cancer. Available online: http://www.who.int/cancer/en/ (accessed on 17 August 2018).
4. Chang, C.-T.; Ho, T.-Y.; Lin, H.; Liang, J.-A.; Huang, H.-C.; Li, C.-C.; Lo, H.-Y.; Wu, S.-L.; Huang, Y.-F.; Hsiang, C.-Y. 5-Fluorouracil induced intestinal mucositis via nuclear factor-κB activation by transcriptomic analysis and in vivo bioluminescence imaging. *PLoS ONE* **2012**, *7*, e31808. [CrossRef]
5. Udofot, O.; Affram, K.; Bridg'ette Israel, E.A. Cytotoxicity of 5-fluorouracil-loaded pH-sensitive liposomal nanoparticles in colorectal cancer cell lines. *Integr. Cancer Sci. Ther.* **2015**, *2*, 245–252. [CrossRef] [PubMed]
6. Wilhelm, M.; Mueller, L.; Miller, M.C.; Link, K.; Holdenrieder, S.; Bertsch, T.; Kunzmann, V.; Stoetzer, O.J.; Suttmann, I.; Braess, J. Prospective, multicenter study of 5-fluorouracil therapeutic drug monitoring in metastatic colorectal cancer treated in routine clinical practice. *Clin. Colorectal Cancer* **2016**, *15*, 381–388. [CrossRef] [PubMed]
7. Kawashima, R.; Fujimaki, M.; Ikenoue, Y.; Danjo, K.; Koizumi, W.; Ichikawa, T. Influence of an elemental diet on 5-fluorouracil-induced morphological changes in the mouse salivary gland and colon. *Support. Care Cancer* **2016**, *24*, 1609–1616. [CrossRef] [PubMed]
8. Kawashima, R.; Kawakami, F.; Maekawa, T.; Yamamoto, H.; Koizumi, W.; Ichikawa, T. Elemental diet moderates 5-fluorouracil-induced gastrointestinal mucositis through mucus barrier alteration. *Cancer Chemother. Pharmacol.* **2015**, *76*, 269–277. [CrossRef]
9. Kobuchi, S.; Ito, Y.; Sakaeda, T. Population Pharmacokinetic–Pharmacodynamic Modeling of 5-Fluorouracil for Toxicities in Rats. *Eur. J. Drug Metab. Pharmacokinet.* **2017**, *42*, 707–718. [CrossRef]
10. Peterson, D.; Bensadoun, R.-J.; Roila, F.; Group, E.G.W. Management of oral and gastrointestinal mucositis: ESMO Clinical Practice Guidelines. *Ann. Oncol.* **2011**, *22*, 78–84. [CrossRef]
11. Kim, H.J.; Kim, J.H.; Moon, W.; Park, J.; Park, S.J.; Am Song, G.; Han, S.H.; Lee, J.H. Rebamipide attenuates 5-fluorouracil-induced small intestinal mucositis in a mouse model. *Biol. Pharm. Bull.* **2015**, *38*, 179–183. [CrossRef]
12. Ofori-Kwakye, K.; Amekyeh, H.; El-Duah, M.; Kipo, S.L. Mechanical and tablet coating properties of cashew tree (Anacardium occidentale l) gum-based films. *Asian J. Pharm. Clin. Res.* **2012**, *5*, 62–68.
13. Olusola, A.; Toluwalope, G.; Olutayo, O. Carboxymethylation of Anacardium occidentale L. exudate gum: Synthesis and characterization. *Sch. Acad. J. Pharm.* **2014**, *3*, 213–216.

14. Schirato, G.V.; Monteiro, F.M.F.; Silva, F.d.O.; Luís, d.L.F.J.; Leão, A.M.d.A.C.; Porto, A.L.F. O polissacarídeo do Anacardium occidentale L. na fase inflamatória do processo cicatricial de lesões cutâneas. *Ciência Rural* **2006**, *36*, 149–154. [CrossRef]
15. Kumar, A.; Moin, A.; Ahmed, A.; Shivakumar, H.G. Cashew gum a versatile hydrophyllic polymer: A review. *Curr. Drug Ther.* **2012**, *7*, 2–12. [CrossRef]
16. Quelemes, P.V.; Araruna, F.B.; de Faria, B.E.; Kuckelhaus, S.A.; da Silva, D.A.; Mendonça, R.Z.; Eiras, C.; dos S Soares, M.J.; Leite, J.R.S. Development and antibacterial activity of cashew gum-based silver nanoparticles. *Int. J. Mol. Sci.* **2013**, *14*, 4969–4981. [CrossRef]
17. Araújo, T.S.; Costa, D.S.; Sousa, N.A.; Souza, L.K.; de Araújo, S.; Oliveira, A.P.; Sousa, F.B.M.; Silva, D.A.; Barbosa, A.L.; Leite, J.R.S. Antidiarrheal activity of cashew GUM, a complex heteropolysaccharide extracted from exudate of Anacardium occidentale L. in rodents. *J. Ethnopharmacol.* **2015**, *174*, 299–307. [CrossRef] [PubMed]
18. AlRashdi, A.S.; Salama, S.M.; Alkiyumi, S.S.; Abdulla, M.A.; Hadi, A.H.A.; Abdelwahab, S.I.; Taha, M.M.; Hussiani, J.; Asykin, N. Mechanisms of gastroprotective effects of ethanolic leaf extract of Jasminum sambac against HCl/ethanol-induced gastric mucosal injury in rats. *Evid.Based Complement. Altern. Med.* **2012**, *2012*, 786426. [CrossRef]
19. Bonacorsi, C.; Da Fonseca, L.M.; Raddi, M.S.G.; Kitagawa, R.R.; Vilegas, W. Comparison of Brazilian plants used to treat gastritis on the oxidative burst of Helicobacter pylori-stimulated neutrophil. *Evid. Based Complement. Altern. Med.* **2013**, *2013*, 851621. [CrossRef] [PubMed]
20. Reddy, S.C.; Shetty, B.V.; Rao, G.M. Oral Ingestion of Spondias pinnata Bark Extract Trim Down Severity of Small Intestinal Mucositis in Etoposide Treated Rats. *Cancer Sci. Ther.* **2015**, *7*, 030–033. [CrossRef]
21. Chikezie, P.C. Sodium metabisulfite–induced polymerization of sickle cell hemoglobin incubated in the extracts of three medicinal plants (Anacardium occidentale, Psidium guajava, and Terminalia catappa). *Pharmacogn. Mag.* **2011**, *7*, 126–132. [CrossRef]
22. Okpashi, V.E.; Bayim, B.P.-R.; Obi-Abang, M. Comparative effects of some medicinal plants: Anacardium occidentale, Eucalyptus globulus, Psidium guajava, and Xylopia aethiopica extracts in alloxan-induced diabetic male Wistar albino rats. *Biochem. Res. Int.* **2014**, *2014*. [CrossRef]
23. Jaiswal, Y.; Tatke, P.; Gabhe, S.; Vaidya, A. Antidiabetic activity of extracts of Anacardium occidentale Linn. leaves on n-streptozotocin diabetic rats. *J. Tradit. Complement. Med.* **2017**, *7*, 421–427. [CrossRef]
24. Souza, N.C.; de Oliveira, J.M.; Morrone, M.d.S.; Albanus, R.D.O.; Amarante, M.d.S.M.; Camillo, C.d.S.; Langassner, S.M.Z.; Gelain, D.P.; Moreira, J.C.F.; Dalmolin, R.J.S. Antioxidant and anti-inflammatory properties of Anacardium occidentale leaf extract. *Evid. Based Complement. Altern. Med.* **2017**, *2017*, 2787308. [CrossRef] [PubMed]
25. Silva, J.G.d.; Souza, I.A.; Higino, J.S.; Siqueira-Junior, J.P.; Pereira, J.V.; Pereira, M.d.S.V. Atividade antimicrobiana do extrato de Anacardium occidentale Linn. em amostras multiresistentes de Staphylococcus aureus. *Rev. Bras. Farmacogn.* **2007**, *17*, 572–577. [CrossRef]
26. Tchikaya, F.O.; Bantsielé, G.B.; Kouakou-Siransy, G.; Datté, J.Y.; Datté, P.; Zirihi, N.G.; Offoumou, M.A. Anacardium occidentale Linn.(Anacardiaceae) stem bark extract induces hypotensive and cardio-inhibitory effects in experimental animal models. *Afr. J. Tradit. Complement. Altern. Med.* **2011**, *8*, 452–461. [CrossRef]
27. Cardoso Palheta, I.; Caldeira Tavares-Martins, A.C.; Araujo Lucas, F.C.; Goncalves Jardim, M.A. Ethnobotanical study of medicinal plants in urban home gardens in the city of Abaetetuba, Pará state, Brazil. *Boletín Latinoamericano y del Caribe de Plantas Medicinales y Aromáticas* **2017**, *16*, 206–262.
28. Vasconcelos, M.d.S.; Rochette, N.F.G.; de Oliveira, M.L.M.; Nunes-Pinheiro, D.C.S.; Tomé, A.R.; Maia de Sousa, F.Y.; Pinheiro, F.G.M.; Moura, C.F.H.; Miranda, M.R.A.; Mota, E.F. Anti-inflammatory and wound healing potential of cashew apple juice (Anacardium occidentale L.) in mice. *Exp. Biol. Med.* **2015**, *240*, 1648–1655. [CrossRef]
29. Yeung, C.-Y.; Chan, W.-T.; Jiang, C.-B.; Cheng, M.-L.; Liu, C.-Y.; Chang, S.-W.; Chiau, J.-S.C.; Lee, H.-C. Amelioration of chemotherapy-induced intestinal mucositis by orally administered probiotics in a mouse model. *PLoS ONE* **2015**, *10*, e0138746. [CrossRef]
30. Carvalho, R.D.; Breyner, N.; Menezes-Garcia, Z.; Rodrigues, N.M.; Lemos, L.; Maioli, T.U.; Souza, D.G.; Carmona, D.; Faria, A.M.; Langella, P. Secretion of biologically active pancreatitis-associated protein I (PAP) by genetically modified dairy Lactococcus lactis NZ9000 in the prevention of intestinal mucositis. *Microb. Cell Factories* **2017**, *16*, 27. [CrossRef]

31. Li, Y.; Liu, M.; Zuo, Z.; Liu, J.; Yu, X.; Guan, Y.; Zhan, R.; Han, Q.; Zhang, J.; Zhou, R. TLR9 Regulates the NF-κB–NLRP3–IL-1β Pathway Negatively in Salmonella-Induced NKG2D-Mediated Intestinal Inflammation. *J. Immunol.* **2017**, *199*, 761–773. [CrossRef]
32. Gerhard, D.; Sousa, F.J.D.S.S.; Andraus, R.A.C.; Pardo, P.E.; Nai, G.A.; Neto, H.B.; Messora, M.R.; Maia, L.P. Probiotic therapy reduces inflammation and improves intestinal morphology in rats with induced oral mucositis. *Braz. Oral Res.* **2017**, *31*, 1–11. [CrossRef]
33. De Araújo, A.A.; Borba, P.B.; de Souza, F.H.D.; Nogueira, A.C.; Saldanha, T.S.; Araújo, T.E.F.; Silva, A.I.; de Araújo Júnior, R.F. In a methotrexate-induced model of intestinal mucositis, olmesartan reduced inflammation and induced enteropathy characterized by severe diarrhea, weight loss, and reduced sucrose activity. *Biol. Pharm. Bull.* **2015**, *38*, 746–752. [CrossRef]
34. De Barros, P.A.V.; Andrade, M.E.R.; de Vasconcelos Generoso, S.; Miranda, S.E.M.; dos Reis, D.C.; Leocádio, P.C.L.; e Souza, É.L.d.S.; dos Santos Martins, F.; da Gama, M.A.S.; Cassali, G.D. Conjugated linoleic acid prevents damage caused by intestinal mucositis induced by 5-fluorouracil in an experimental model. *Biomed. Pharmacother.* **2018**, *103*, 1567–1576. [CrossRef] [PubMed]
35. Al-Asmari, A.K.; Khan, A.Q.; Al-Asmari, S.A.; Al-Rawi, A.; Al-Omani, S. Alleviation of 5-fluorouracil-induced intestinal mucositis in rats by vitamin E via targeting oxidative stress and inflammatory markers. *J. Complement. Integr. Med.* **2016**, *13*, 377–385. [CrossRef] [PubMed]
36. Han, X.; Wu, Z.; Di, J.; Pan, Y.; Zhang, H.; Du, Y.; Cheng, Z.; Jin, Z.; Wang, Z.; Zheng, Q. CXCL9 attenuated chemotherapy-induced intestinal mucositis by inhibiting proliferation and reducing apoptosis. *Biomed. Pharmacother.* **2011**, *65*, 547–554. [CrossRef]
37. Zhang, S.; Liu, Y.; Xiang, D.; Yang, J.; Liu, D.; Ren, X.; Zhang, C. Assessment of dose-response relationship of 5-fluorouracil to murine intestinal injury. *Biomed. Pharmacother.* **2018**, *106*, 910–916. [CrossRef] [PubMed]
38. Kumar, S.; Aninat, C.; Michaux, G.; Morel, F. Anticancer drug 5-fluorouracil induces reproductive and developmental defects in Caenorhabditis elegans. *Reprod. Toxicol.* **2010**, *29*, 415–420. [CrossRef] [PubMed]
39. Soares, P.M.; Mota, J.M.S.; Gomes, A.S.; Oliveira, R.B.; Assreuy, A.M.S.; Brito, G.A.C.; Santos, A.A.; Ribeiro, R.A.; Souza, M.H. Gastrointestinal dysmotility in 5-fluorouracil-induced intestinal mucositis outlasts inflammatory process resolution. *Cancer Chemother. Pharmacol.* **2008**, *63*, 91–98. [CrossRef]
40. Quaresma, M.P. *Lactobacillus spp. e Bifidobacterium sp. Attenuate Experimental Intestinal Mucositis Induced by 5-Fluorouracil in Mice*; Federal University of Ceará: Fortaleza, Brazil, 2016.
41. Sonis, S.T. A biological approach to mucositis. *J. Support. Oncol.* **2004**, *2*, 21–32.
42. Guabiraba, R.; Besnard, A.; Menezes, G.; Secher, T.; Jabir, M.; Amaral, S.; Braun, H.; Lima-Junior, R.C.; Ribeiro, R.; Cunha, F. IL-33 targeting attenuates intestinal mucositis and enhances effective tumor chemotherapy in mice. *Mucosal Immunol.* **2014**, *7*, 1079–1093. [CrossRef]
43. Bastos, C.C.C.; de Ávila, P.H.M.; dos Santos Filho, E.X.; de Ávila, R.I.; Batista, A.C.; Fonseca, S.G.; Lima, E.M.; Marreto, R.N.; de Mendonca, E.F.; Valadares, M.C. Use of Bidens pilosa L.(Asteraceae) and Curcuma longa L.(Zingiberaceae) to treat intestinal mucositis in mice: Toxico-pharmacological evaluations. *Toxicol. Rep.* **2016**, *3*, 279–287. [CrossRef] [PubMed]
44. Justino, P.F.; Melo, L.F.; Nogueira, A.F.; Costa, J.V.; Silva, L.M.; Santos, C.M.; Mendes, W.O.; Costa, M.R.; Franco, A.X.; Lima, A.A.; et al. Treatment with Saccharomyces boulardii reduces the inflammation and dysfunction of the gastrointestinal tract in 5-fluorouracil-induced intestinal mucositis in mice. *Br. J. Nutr.* **2014**, *111*, 1611–1621. [CrossRef] [PubMed]
45. De Ávila, P.H.M.; de Ávila, R.I.; dos Santos Filho, E.X.; Bastos, C.C.C.; Batista, A.C.; Mendonca, E.F.; Serpa, R.C.; Marreto, R.N.; da Cruz, A.F.; Lima, E.M. Mucoadhesive formulation of Bidens pilosa L.(Asteraceae) reduces intestinal injury from 5-fluorouracil-induced mucositis in mice. *Toxicol. Rep.* **2015**, *2*, 563–573. [CrossRef]
46. Al-Asmari, A.; Al-Zahrani, A.; Khan, A.; Al-Shahrani, H.; Ali Al Amri, M. Taurine ameliorates 5-flourouracil-induced intestinal mucositis, hepatorenal and reproductive organ damage in Wistar rats: A biochemical and histological study. *Hum. Exp. Toxicol.* **2016**, *35*, 10–20. [CrossRef] [PubMed]
47. Heber, D. Oxidative Stress Markers and Inflammation: The Role of Spices and Herbs. *Nutr. Today* **2014**, *49*, S4–S5. [CrossRef]
48. Nogueira, L.T.; Costa, D.V.; Gomes, A.S.; Martins, C.S.; Silva, A.M.; Coelho-Aguiar, J.M.; Castelucci, P.; Lima-Júnior, R.C.; Leitão, R.F.; Moura-Neto, V.; et al. The involvement of mast cells in the irinotecan-induced enteric neurons loss and reactive gliosis. *J. Neuroinflamm.* **2017**, *14*, 79. [CrossRef]

49. Hamilton, M.J.; Frei, S.M.; Stevens, R.L. The multifaceted mast cell in inflammatory bowel disease. *Inflamm. Bowel Dis.* **2014**, *20*, 2364–2378. [CrossRef] [PubMed]
50. De Winter, B.Y.; van den Wijngaard, R.M.; de Jonge, W.J. Intestinal mast cells in gut inflammation and motility disturbances. *Biochim. Biophys. Acta Mol. Basis Dis.* **2012**, *1822*, 66–73. [CrossRef]
51. Theoharides, T.C.; Alysandratos, K.-D.; Angelidou, A.; Delivanis, D.-A.; Sismanopoulos, N.; Zhang, B.; Asadi, S.; Vasiadi, M.; Weng, Z.; Miniati, A.; et al. Mast cells and inflammation. *Biochim. Biophys. Acta Mol. Basis Dis.* **2012**, *1822*, 21–33. [CrossRef]
52. Ramsay, D.B.; Stephen, S.; Borum, M.; Voltaggio, L.; Doman, D.B. Mast cells in gastrointestinal disease. *Gastroenterol. Hepatol.* **2010**, *6*, 772–777.
53. Bischoff, S.C. Mast cells in gastrointestinal disorders. *Eur. J. Pharmacol.* **2016**, *778*, 139–145. [CrossRef]
54. Short, S.S.; Wang, J.; Castle, S.L.; Fernandez, G.E.; Smiley, N.; Zobel, M.; Pontarelli, E.M.; Papillon, S.C.; Grishin, A.V.; Ford, H.R. Low doses of celecoxib attenuate gut barrier failure during experimental peritonitis. *Lab. Investig.* **2013**, *93*, 1265–1275. [CrossRef] [PubMed]
55. Javle, M.M.; Cao, S.; Durrani, F.A.; Pendyala, L.; Lawrence, D.D.; Smith, P.F.; Creaven, P.J.; Noel, D.C.; Iyer, R.V.; Rustum, Y.M. Celecoxib and mucosal protection: Translation from an animal model to a phase I clinical trial of celecoxib, irinotecan, and 5-fluorouracil. *Clin. Cancer Res.* **2007**, *13*, 965–971. [CrossRef] [PubMed]
56. Verri Jr, W.A.; Cunha, T.M.; Parada, C.A.; Poole, S.; Cunha, F.Q.; Ferreira, S.H. Hypernociceptive role of cytokines and chemokines: Targets for analgesic drug development? *Pharmacol. Ther.* **2006**, *112*, 116–138. [CrossRef] [PubMed]
57. Al-Azri, A.R.; Gibson, R.J.; Bowen, J.M.; Stringer, A.M.; Keefe, D.M.; Logan, R.M. Involvement of matrix metalloproteinases (MMP-3 and MMP-9) in the pathogenesis of irinotecan-induced oral mucositis. *J. Oral Pathol. Med.* **2015**, *44*, 459–467. [CrossRef]
58. Ribeiro, R.A.; Wanderley, C.W.; Wong, D.V.; Mota, J.M.S.; Leite, C.A.; Souza, M.H.; Cunha, F.Q.; Lima-Junior, R.C. Irinotecan-and 5-fluorouracil-induced intestinal mucositis: Insights into pathogenesis and therapeutic perspectives. *Cancer Chemother. Pharmacol.* **2016**, *78*, 881–893. [CrossRef]
59. Al-Dasooqi, N.; Sonis, S.T.; Bowen, J.M.; Bateman, E.; Blijlevens, N.; Gibson, R.J.; Logan, R.M.; Nair, R.G.; Stringer, A.M.; Yazbeck, R.; et al. Emerging evidence on the pathobiology of mucositis. *Support. Care Cancer* **2013**, *21*, 2075–2083. [CrossRef]
60. De Paula, R.; Santana, S.; Rodrigues, J. Composition and rheological properties of Albizia lebbeck gum exudate. *Carbohydr. Polym.* **2001**, *44*, 133–139. [CrossRef]
61. Silva, D.A.; Feitosa, J.P.; Maciel, J.S.; Paula, H.C.; de Paula, R.C. Characterization of crosslinked cashew gum derivatives. *Carbohydr. Polym.* **2006**, *66*, 16–26. [CrossRef]
62. Da Silva, D.A.; Feitosa, J.P.; Paula, H.C.; de Paula, R.C. Synthesis and characterization of cashew gum/acrylic acid nanoparticles. *Mater. Sci. Eng. C* **2009**, *29*, 437–441. [CrossRef]
63. Soares, P.M.; Mota, J.M.S.; Souza, E.P.; Justino, P.F.; Franco, A.X.; Cunha, F.Q.; Ribeiro, R.A.; Souza, M.H. Inflammatory intestinal damage induced by 5-fluorouracil requires IL-4. *Cytokine* **2013**, *61*, 46–49. [CrossRef]
64. Dos Santos Filho, E.X.; Ávila, P.H.M.; Bastos, C.C.C.; Batista, A.C.; Naves, L.N.; Marreto, R.N.; Lima, E.M.; Mendonca, E.F.; Valadares, M.C. Curcuminoids from Curcuma longaL. reduced intestinal mucositis induced by 5-fluorouracil in mice: Bioadhesive, proliferative, anti-inflammatory and antioxidant effects. *Toxicol. Rep.* **2016**, *3*, 55–62. [CrossRef]
65. MacPherson, B.; Pfeiffer, C. Experimental production of diffuse colitis in rats. *Digestion* **1978**, *17*, 135–150. [CrossRef] [PubMed]
66. Moura, R.; Wada, C.; Purchio, A.; Almeida, T. *Studies of the Figurative Elements of Blood*, 3rd ed.; Atheneu: São Paulo, Brazil, 1998.
67. Bradford, M.M. A rapid and sensitive method for the quantitation of microgram quantities of protein utilizing the principle of protein-dye binding. *Anal. Biochem.* **1976**, *72*, 248–254. [CrossRef]
68. Ohkawa, H.; Ohishi, N.; Yagi, K. Assay for lipid peroxides in animal tissues by thiobarbituric acid reaction. *Anal. Biochem.* **1979**, *95*, 351–358. [CrossRef]
69. Sedlak, J.; Lindsay, R.H. Estimation of total, protein-bound, and nonprotein sulfhydryl groups in tissue with Ellman's reagent. *Anal. Biochem.* **1968**, *25*, 192–205. [CrossRef]

70. Bradley, P.P.; Priebat, D.A.; Christensen, R.D.; Rothstein, G. Measurement of cutaneous inflammation: Estimation of neutrophil content with an enzyme marker. *J. Investig. Dermatol.* **1982**, *78*, 206–209. [CrossRef] [PubMed]
71. Michalany, J. *Histological Technique Pathological Anatomy: With Instructions for the Surgeon, Nurse, Cytotechnician*, 3rd ed.; Michalany: São Paulo, Brazil, 2008.

pharmaceuticals

MDPI

Article

Mechanism of the Dual Activities of Human CYP17A1 and Binding to Anti-Prostate Cancer Drug Abiraterone Revealed by a Novel V366M Mutation Causing 17,20 Lyase Deficiency

Mónica Fernández-Cancio [1,†], Núria Camats [1,2,3,†], Christa E. Flück [2,3,†], Adam Zalewski [2,3,†], Bernhard Dick [4], Brigitte M. Frey [4], Raquel Monné [5], Núria Torán [6], Laura Audí [1] and Amit V. Pandey [2,3,*]

1 Growth and Development Research Unit, Vall d'Hebron Research Institute (VHIR), Center for Biomedical Research on Rare Diseases (CIBERER), Instituto de Salud Carlos III, Autonomous University of Barcelona, Barcelona 08035, Spain; monica.fernandez.cancio@vhir.org (M.F.-C.); nuria.camats@vhir.org (N.C.); laura.audi@vhir.org (L.A.)

2 Pediatric Endocrinology Unit, Department of Paediatrics, University Children's Hospital Bern, Bern 3010, Switzerland; christa.flueck@dbmr.unibe.ch (C.E.F.); adam.zalewski@mail.com (A.Z.)

3 Department of Biomedical Research, University of Bern, Bern 3010, Switzerland

4 Department of Nephrology and Hypertension, University of Bern, Bern 3010, Switzerland; Bernhard.dick@gmx.ch (B.D.); brigitte.frey@dbmr.unibe.ch (B.M.F.)

5 Pediatric Service, Hospital Joan XXIII, Tarragona 43005, Spain; raquel.monne@urv.cat

6 Pathology Department, Hospital Universitari Vall d'Hebron, CIBERER, Barcelona 08035, Spain; toranfuentesn@gmail.com

* Correspondence: amit@pandeylab.org; Tel.: +41-31-632-9637

† These authors contributed equally.

Received: 4 April 2018; Accepted: 25 April 2018; Published: 29 April 2018

Abstract: The *CYP17A1* gene regulates sex steroid biosynthesis in humans through 17α-hydroxylase/17,20 lyase activities and is a target of anti-prostate cancer drug abiraterone. In a 46, XY patient with female external genitalia, together with a loss of function mutation S441P, we identified a novel missense mutation V366M at the catalytic center of CYP17A1 which preferentially impaired 17,20 lyase activity. Kinetic experiments with bacterially expressed proteins revealed that V366M mutant enzyme can bind and metabolize pregnenolone to 17OH-pregnenolone, but 17OH-pregnenolone binding and conversion to dehydroepiandrosterone (DHEA) was impaired, explaining the patient's steroid profile. Abiraterone could not bind and inhibit the 17α-hydroxylase activity of the CYP17A1-V366M mutant. Molecular dynamics (MD) simulations showed that V366M creates a "one-way valve" and suggests a mechanism for dual activities of human CYP17A1 where, after the conversion of pregnenolone to 17OH-pregnenolone, the product exits the active site and re-enters for conversion to dehydroepiandrosterone. The V366M mutant also explained the effectiveness of the anti-prostate cancer drug abiraterone as a potent inhibitor of CYP17A1 by binding tightly at the active site in the WT enzyme. The V366M is the first human mutation to be described at the active site of CYP17A1 that causes isolated 17,20 lyase deficiency. Knowledge about the specificity of CYP17A1 activities is of importance for the development of treatments for polycystic ovary syndrome and inhibitors for prostate cancer therapy.

Keywords: P450c17; prostate cancer; abiraterone; steroidogenesis; androgens; dehydroepiandrosterone; *CYP17A1*; cytochrome P450; anti-cancer drugs; DSD

1. Introduction

The Cytochrome P450 proteins that are located in the endoplasmic reticulum are responsible for the metabolism of xenobiotics, drugs and steroid hormones (Figure 1) and are part of the microsomal mixed oxidase system [1–3]. Cytochrome P450c17 (CYP17A1) is required for the biosynthesis of steroid hormones in all vertebrates. The CYP17A1 is the qualitative regulator of the biosynthesis of sex steroid in humans (Figure 2) [4]. CYP17A1 catalyses multiple reactions in the steroid pathway [5–7]; chiefly among them, its 17α-hydroxylase activity is essential for the production of 17OH-pregnenolone (17OH-PREG) and 17OH-progesterone (17OH-PROG) which are precursors of cortisol, and its 17,20 lyase activity is required for the generation of the precursor of sex steroids, dehydroepiandrosterone (DHEA) (Figure 2). These two activities of the CYP17A1 determine the type of steroid hormone synthesized in different cells and tissues; if the CYP17A1 is absent, mineralocorticoids are produced, if only the 17α-hydroxylase activity of the CYP17A1 is present, glucocorticoids are made; and if both the 17α-hydroxylase and the 17,20 lyase activities of the CYP17A1 are present, sex steroid precursors are generated [4]. Overproduction of androgens by the specific activation of CYP17A1-17,20 lyase activity has been implicated in the pathogenesis of the polycystic ovary syndrome [4]. CYP17A1 is a target for prostate cancer therapy by inhibitor abiraterone (Zytiga by Johnson & Johnson, New Brunswick, USA) [8–12].

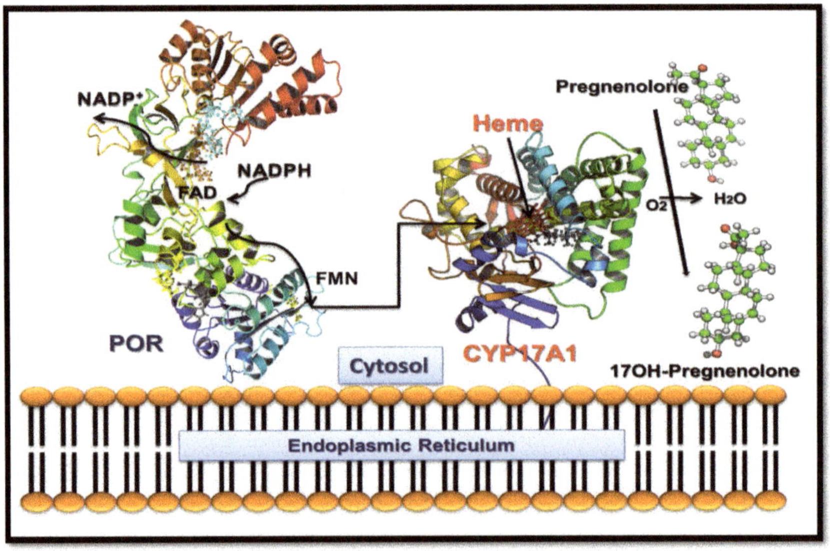

Figure 1. Schematic diagram of CYP17A1 and P450 oxidoreductase (POR) interaction in the membranes. The nicotinamide adenine dinucleotide phosphate (NADPH) molecules bind to POR, which is embedded into the membranes of endoplasmic reticulum and donate a pair of electrons, one at a time, which are received by the FAD. Transfer of electrons to FAD creates a change in conformation of POR, allowing the FAD and FMN groups to move towards each other, which facilitates the transfer of electrons from FAD to FMN. The FMN domain of POR interacts with the CYP17A1 and transfers electrons for catalytic activities.

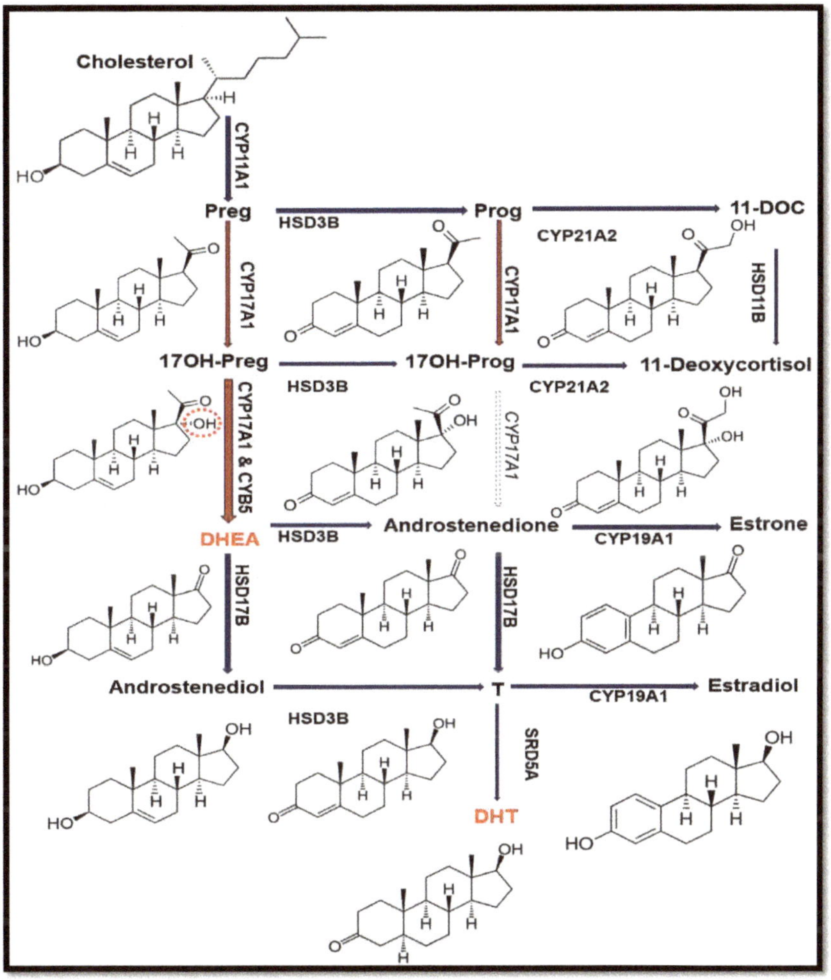

Figure 2. Steroid biosynthetic pathway. In humans, 17,20 lyase activity of *CYP17A1* converts 17α-hydroxypregnenolone (17OH-PREG) to dehydroepiandrosterone (DHEA) but does not effectively convert 17α-hydroxyprogesterone (17OH-PROG) to androstenedione. The DHEA is the precursor for androgen production and (dihydrotestosterone) DHT is the potent form of androgen with higher affinity towards androgen receptor (AR) than testosterone (T). The 17α-hydroxy position of 17OH-PREG is highlighted in red to show the difference from PREG.

Similar to other microsomal P450 proteins, CYP17A1 also requires electrons supplied from reduced nicotinamide adenine dinucleotide phosphate (NADPH) through cytochrome P450 oxidoreductase (POR) (Figure 1) [2,13–16]. The 17,20 lyase activity of CYP17A1 is influenced by the presence of cytochrome b_5 (CYB5A) in specific locations in different cells and tissues and guides the steroid hormone pathway in different directions [4] (Figure 2).

Along with CYB5A, higher molecular ratios of POR and phosphorylation of CYP17A1 also influence 17,20 lyase activity [17–21]. Recently several X-ray crystal structures of solubilized human CYP17A1 have been reported, but the structural basis of 17α-hydroxylase and 17,20, lyase activities remains unknown [22–26]. Generally, the mutations that affect the steroid-binding domain of CYP17A1 or disturb the interaction with P450 oxidoreductase (POR) for electron transfer, cause combined 17α-hydroxylase and 17,20 lyase deficiency, and are those more frequently found in humans [4,25]. Very few point mutations in CYP17A1 (R347C/H, R358Q) have been reported to cause isolated 17,20 lyase deficiency [27–30] (Table 1). These mutations are thought to interfere with CYB5A binding and/or electron transfer from POR to CYP17A1 during the 17,20 lyase reaction.

Table 1. Reported cases of *CYP17A1* mutations causing isolated 17,20 lyase deficiency [27–30]. The mutation E305G which was initially reported by Sherbet et al. [28] to cause isolated 17,20 lyase deficiency, was later reported by Tiosano et al. [30] to also result in combined 17α-hydroxylase/17,20 lyase deficiency, similar to other common mutations in *CYP17A1* [30].

17OH Steroids Basal	17OH Steroids Stimulated	Cortisol Basal	Cortisol Stimulated	Activities (% of WT)		Ref
				17OHase	17,20 lyase	
Normal	Hyperresponsive	Normal	Areactive	65	5	Geller 1997 [27]
Elevated	Hyperresponsive	Normal	Areactive	65	5	Geller 1997 [27]
Slightly elevated	Not reactive	Low normal	Areactive			van den Akker 2002 [29]
Normal	Normal	Low normal	Areactive			van den Akker 2002 [29]
Normal/Elevated	Reactive	Low normal	Hyporeactive	60	0	van den Akker 2002 [29]
Normal/Elevated	Reactive	Low normal	Hyporeactive	60	0	van den Akker 2002 [29]
Normal/Elevated	Reactive	Low	Hyporeactive	100	0	Sherbet 2003 [28]
Normal/Elevated	Normal	Low normal	Hyporeactive			Tiosano 2008 [30]
Normal/Elevated	Normal	Low normal	Hyporeactive			Tiosano 2008 [30]
Normal/Elevated	Normal	Low normal	Hyporeactive			Tiosano 2008 [30]
Normal/Elevated	Normal	Low normal	Hyporeactive			Tiosano 2008 [30]
Normal/Elevated	Normal	Low normal	Hyporeactive			Tiosano 2008 [30]
Normal/Elevated	Normal	Low normal	Hyporeactive			Tiosano 2008 [30]
Normal/low	Hyporeactive	Low normal	Areactive	43	0/0	This report

Lack of 17α-hydroxylase activity of CYP17A1 results in a compensatory overproduction of corticosterone and deoxycorticosterone with a weak glucocorticoid and significant mineralocorticoid action, which results in severe hypertension and hypokalemia. On the other hand, the 17,20 lyase deficiency results in a lack of sex steroids, leading to the 46, XY disorder of sexual development (DSD) with severe undervirilization in the "male" newborn, and deficient pubertal development and fertility in both sexes [4]. Previously, we have reported that disturbing the interaction of CYP17A1 with P450 oxidoreductase (POR) for electron transfer causes combined 17α-hydroxylase and 17,20 lyase deficiency [2,14,16,31–34]. Mutations identified on the surface of *CYP17A1* (R347C/H, R358Q) have been proposed to diminish the interaction with POR but could not explain the mechanism of their specific effect on 17,20 lyase activity [27,35].

Recently we have shown that in the earliest reported cases of apparent isolated 17,20 lyase deficiency, that were based solely on hormonal and morphological findings and without genetic analysis, the *CYP17A1* and *POR* genes were actually normal and mutations in *AKR1C2* and *AKR1C4* were found to cause a similar phenotype [36–38]. In the current report, we are describing a novel active site mutation in CYP17A1 that specifically abolishes the 17,20 lyase activity.

2. Results

2.1. Case Report and Genetic Analysis of the Patient

The patient was born at term, with normal female external genitalia, after a normal spontaneous pregnancy, whereas an older sister was the product of an insemination with donor semen to avoid retinitis pigmentosa carried by the father's family. At 2 months of age, the patient was operated for a right inguinal hernia. No female internal sex organs were found and karyotype was 46, XY. During the procedure, a gonad was detected and biopsied showing to be a testis (Figure 3). Electrolytes were normal and baseline hormone values at 3 months of age revealed moderately elevated ACTH, highly elevated PROG, normal/low 17OH-PREG, 17OH-PROG, 11-deoxycortisol and cortisol, undetectable androstenedione (Δ_4A) and normal DHEA-S and Testosterone for female sex (Table 2). At the age of 5 months a human chorionic gonadotropin (hCG) test (500 IU/d $\times$ 3) was performed which showed no increase of Δ_4A and T upon stimulation (Table 2). At 20 months of age an ACTH test (Synacthen®) revealed a moderately elevated baseline ACTH and a normal baseline plasma renin activity (PRA), Prog was highly elevated and further increased upon stimulation, whereas baseline 17OH-PREG, 17OH-PROG, cortisol, 11-deoxycortisol, and aldosterone were normal/low, and did not increase after stimulation (Table 2). Baseline DHEA-S and baseline and stimulated Δ_4A were undetectable. Because of female phenotype and obvious biochemical lack of androgens, female sex of rearing was confirmed and a gonadectomy was performed at the age of 20 months. Testes morphology showed abnormal findings similar to those found in androgen-insensitive patients (Figure 4a). Blood pressure (BP) control was recommended as a precautionary measure while hydrocortisone replacement therapy was postponed depending on follow-up. BP controls revealed normal values. Baseline BP controls revealed normal values up to 11 years of age as well a 24-h ambulatory BP monitoring performed at 8 years of age (baseline and at the end of 3 months of therapy with hydrocortisone: 6 mg/m^2 in 3 daily doses).

Initial genetic analysis of the genes for *AR* and *SRD5A2* were normal [39,40] and hormonal findings suggested partial 17α-hydroxylase and complete 17,20 lyase deficiencies (Table 2). The *CYP17A1* gene was analyzed and compound heterozygous point mutations c.1096G > A (V366M) and c.1321T > C (S441P) in exons 6 and 8 were identified (Figure 4b). The healthy fertile mother was found to carry the V366M mutation, a residue which is highly conserved across species (Figure 4c), while the father was normal. Therefore, *CYP17A1* S441P might be a de novo mutation in the patient although paternity testing was not performed. The mutations in the patient are likely to be on different alleles as even total disruption of one copy of *CYP17A1* does not result in disease. As both *CYP17A1* mutations have not been described previously, and as our patient presented with a very rare phenotype of apparent isolated 17,20 lyase deficiency, we performed further investigations to characterize these novel mutations.

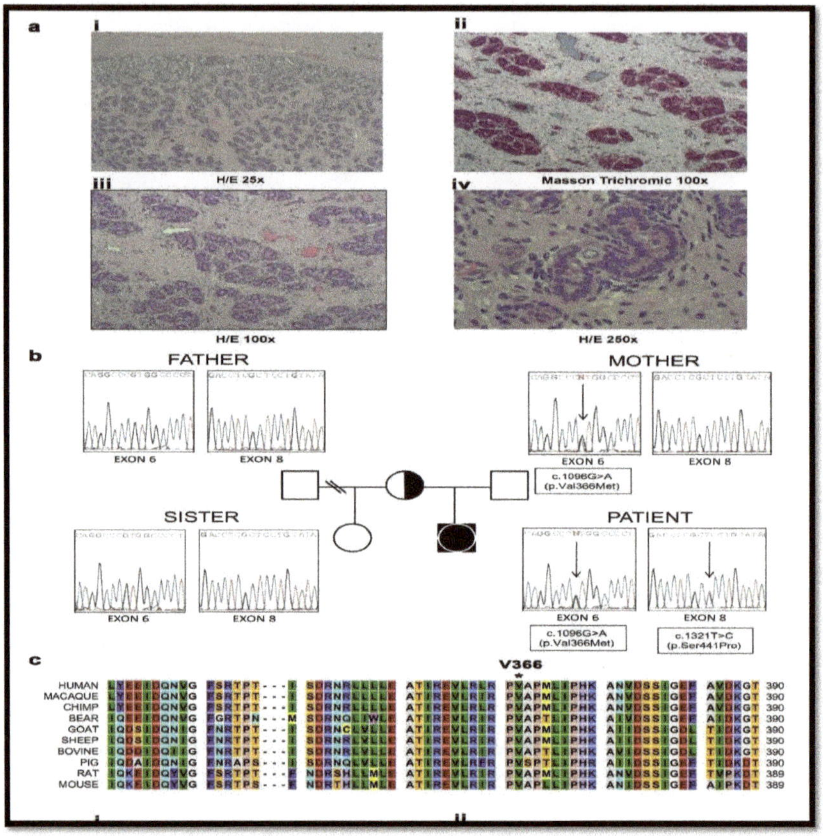

Figure 3. Genetic characterization and testis histology of the 46, XY disorder of sexual development (DSD) patient with a female phenotype. (**a**) Histopathologic studies revealed that both gonads consisted of atrophic and immature seminiferous tubules which were filled almost exclusively with pre-Sertoli cells. The fertility index was 5% with abortive and fetal type spermatogonia (i–iv); iii. in some areas, the tubules formed lobule-like structures similar to pseudo-hamartomas surrounded by collagen fibrous tissue; iv. nests of fibroblastic pre-Leydig cells were found in the interstitium. Albuginea and epidydimus were unremarkable. H/E-hematoxylin-eosin stain. (**b**) Family tree and electropherograms showing the index patient, the parents and the half-sister. Both, the patient and mother harbored the heterozygote c.1096G > A (p.Val366Met) mutation in exon 6, while the heterozygote c.1321T > C (p.Ser441Pro) mutation in exon 8 was only present in the patient. The father and the half-sister were both non-carriers of either mutation. (**c**) Alignment of human CYP17A1 amino acid sequence with a range of CYP17A1 proteins from other species found in the Universal Protein Knowledgebase (UniProt) database. The Valine 366 residue is highly conserved in all species studied.

Table 2. Laboratory findings in our patient harboring compound heterozygote *CYP17A1* mutations.

Age		3 Months		5 Months		20 Months			5 Years	6.5 Years	
Parameter	**Unit**	**Basal**	*Normal Range*	**hCG Test (500 IU/d × 3)**	*Normal Range*	**Basal**	*Normal Range*	**ACTH-Stimulated**	**Basal**	**Basal**	*Normal Range*
Sodium	mEq/L	140	136–145	-		141	136–145		-	144	136–145
Potassium	mEq/L	4.0	3.5–5.1	-		4.6	3.5–5.1		-	4.7	3.5–5.1
ACTH	pg/mL	81	9–50	82	9–50	66	9–50	-	62	46	9–50
Progesterone	ng/dL	222	5–80	-		251	10–50	425	522	339	10–50
17OH Preg	ng/dL	132	60–830	27	60–830	13	10–50	-	-	-	
17OHProg	ng/dL	300	40–460	40	40–460	29	19–159	35	110	80	10–470
DHEA-S	µg/dL	<5	5–62	<5	5–62	<5	5–190	-	<5	<5	5–95
11-Deoxycortisol	ng/dL	1100	1450 ± 790	200	1450 ± 790	140	186 ± 116	-	87	-	205 ± 108
Cortisol	µg/dL	3.7	4.3–22.2	8.6	4.3–22.2	8.9	4.3–22.2	7.8	7.1	4.1	4.3–22.4
Δ4A	ng/dL	<30	63 ± 39	<3	63 ± 39	<30	30–330	<30	-	<30	30–330
Testosterone	ng/dL	7	140 ± 132	<4	140 ± 132	28	15–30	16	-	-	
LH	IU/L	-		-		0.3	0.2–1.0	-	<0.07	-	0.2–1.0
FSH	IU/L	-		-		9	0.4–2.0	-	4.3	-	0.4–2.0
PRA	ng/mL/h	-		-		1.8	0.6–21.3	-	-	0.1	0.3–6.4
Aldosterone	ng/dL	-		-		12.1	14–114	11.5		6.2	9–66

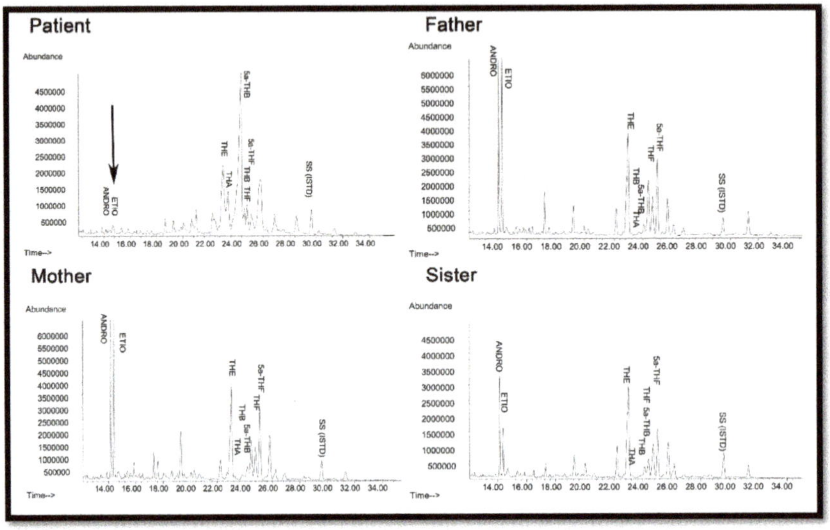

Figure 4. Urine steroid profile of the patient, heterozygote mother, father, and sister. The steroid analysis was performed on 24 h urine samples by GC/MS. Note the lack of androgens (ETIO, ANDRO) and the relative increase in corticosterone metabolites (THA, THB, 5α-THB) in the steroid profile of the patient compared to mother and father. THA—tetrahydro-11-dehydrocorticosterone; THB—tetrahydro corticosterone; 5a-THB-5α-tetrahydro corticosterone; THE—tetrahydrocortisone; THF—tetrahydrocortisol; 5a-THF-5α-tetrahydrocortisol; ETIO—etiocholanolone; ANDRO—androsterone; SS (ISTD)—internal standard.

2.2. *Steroid Analysis*

Urine steroid profiling of the patient revealed almost complete loss of androgen metabolites, low-normal cortisol and elevated corticosterone metabolites (Figure 5), suggesting partial 17α-hydroxylase and complete 17,20 lyase deficiency. All other family members had normal steroid profiles (Figure 4).

2.3. *Loss of 17,20 Lyase Activity of* CYP17A1 *by the V366M Mutation*

To investigate the molecular basis of these mutations we produced both mutant and the wild-type CYP17A1 proteins and performed enzyme kinetic assays (Table 3).

Comparison of mutant and wild-type proteins revealed that both mutations V366M and S441P affected CYP17A1 enzyme activities and therefore qualified as disease-causing mutations. The S441P mutation was found to cause a complete loss of both 17α-hydroxylase and 17,20 lyase activities of CYP17A1. Structural analysis of the S441P mutation indicated that heme binding may be affected (Figure 5), and quantification of heme in the S441P mutant revealed that it contained less than 5% of heme compared to the wild-type enzyme (Table 4).

The CYP17A1-V366M protein retained >40% of WT activity in the 17α-hydroxylase assay but had no activity in the 17,20 lyase assay using 17OH-PREG as substrate (Table 3). Therefore, S441P is a loss-of-function *CYP17A1* mutation whereas V366M qualifies as a rare mutation predominantly affecting CYP17A1-17,20 lyase activity *in vitro*. Therefore, the S441P mutation effectively created a non-functional allele and allowed us to explore the specific effects of the V366M mutation in greater detail.

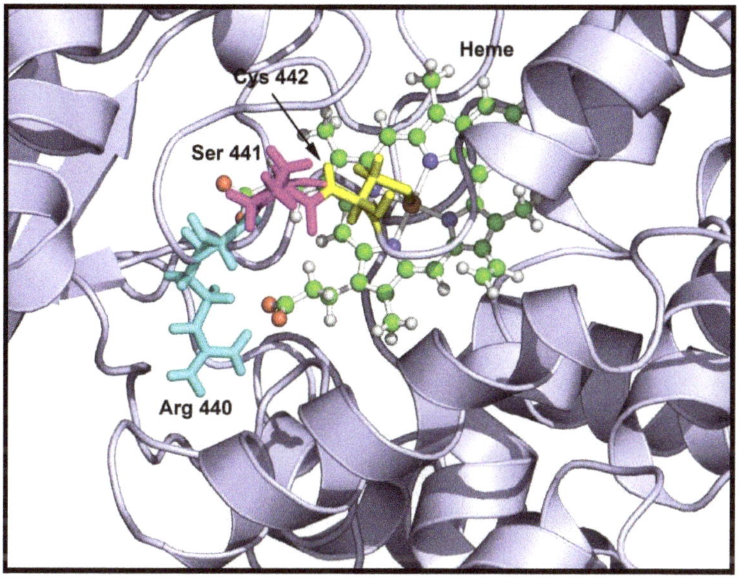

Figure 5. Location of S441P mutation in CYP17A1 structure showing the affected amino acids. The cysteine 442 is shown in yellow, serine 441 is in magenta and arginine 440 is in cyan. Both the cysteine 442 and arginine 440 are required for heme binding and the serine 441 to proline mutation creates a bend in the loop containing the cysteine 442 and arginine 440 residues, resulting in loss of heme binding that leads to an inactive enzyme.

Table 3. Kinetic parameters for the metabolism of PROG to 17OH-PROG (17hydroxylation) and 17OH-PREG to DHEA (17,20 lyase reaction) by WT and V366M mutant of CYP17A1.

CYP17A1 Variant	17α-Hydroxylase PROG to 17OH-PROG			17,20 Lyase17 OH-PREG to DHEA	
	Km (μM)	Vmax (min^{-1})	Cat Eff (%)	Km (μM)	Vmax (min^{-1})
WT	6.1 ± 0.7	0.71	100	0.92 ± 0.07	0.025 ± 0.004
V366M	8.4 ± 0.9	0.42	43	-	-
S441P	-	-	-	-	-

Table 4. Heme content of proteins used in assays.

Protein Preparation	Heme Content (nnol/nmol of Protein)
CYP17A1 WT	0.93
CYP17A1_V366M	0.95
CYP17A1-S441P	<0.05
CYB5A	1.0

2.4. The 17OH-PREG is Not an Effective Inhibitor of 17α-Hydroxylase Reaction by the V366M Mutant

For the human CYP17A1, PREG, 17OH-PREG, and PROG are all very good substrates and, therefore, are expected to compete for the binding to CYP17A1 when more than one substrate is present at the same time. To test if there is a difference between the WT versus the V366M mutant of CYP17A1, we used 17OH-PREG as an inhibitor for the 17α-hydroxylase reaction of CYP17A1 using radiolabeled

[^{3}H]PROG as substrate. For the WT CYP17A1, 17OH-PREG inhibited the 17α-hydroxylation of PROG with an observed IC_{50} value of 1.7 μM (Table 5).

Table 5. Binding and inhibition studies of WT and the V366M mutant of *CYP17A1*.

	CYP17A1_WT	CYP17A1_V366M
Binding studies	**Kd (nM)**	**Kd (nM)**
Binding of PROG	163 ± 29	287 ± 35
Binding of PREG	62 ± 17	92 ± 15
Binding of 17OH-PREG	142 ± 38	-
Binding of Abiraterone	85 ± 23	-
Inhibition studies	**IC_{50} (μM)**	**IC_{50} (μM)**
Inhibition of PROG 17α-hydroxylation by Abiraterone	0.04 ± 0.01	-
Inhibition of PROG 17α-hydroxylation by 17OH-PREG	1.7 ± 0.2	-
Inhibition of PROG 17α-hydroxylation by PREG	0.9 ± 0.15	1.4 ± 0.2

For the V366M mutant of *CYP17A1*, no inhibition of the 17α-hydroxylation of PROG was observed by 17OH-PREG within the range of concentration used in the assay (0–100 μM). These results indicated difficulty in the binding of 17OH-PREG to the V366M mutant of CYP17A1. By contrast, when PREG was used as an inhibitor in the 17α-hydroxylation reaction catalyzed by CYP17A1 using PROG as a substrate, both the WT as well as V366M mutant enzymes were inhibited with apparent IC_{50} values of 0.9 μM for the WT enzyme versus 1.4 μM for the V366M mutant (Table 5). This suggests that both PREG and PROG can bind and be metabolized by the V366M variant of CYP17A1 but 17OH-PREG could not be used as a substrate by the mutant enzyme.

2.5. Computational Structural Analysis by Molecular Dynamics

We used the recently solved crystal structures of the human CYP17A1 [22,23] to make in-silico mutations and analyzed the changes through molecular dynamics (MD) simulations. In the CYP17A1 crystal structure, the active site for the binding of steroids is characterized by the positioning of residues V366, N202 and E305 (Figure 6). This led us to hypothesize that the specific space requirements exist for correct positioning of 17α-hydroxysteroids. The larger side chain of methionine in the V366M mutant protruded into the active site of CYP17A1 (Figure 7). Interestingly the shape of the protruding side chain of methionine 366 indicated that it might restrict the movement of steroids only in one direction, allowing the 17-hydroxy-steroids to leave the active site by the flexibility of movement in one direction, but creating a strong steric hindrance in the path of incoming steroids.

One of the most intriguing questions about CYP17A1 activities has been whether the 17α-hydroxysteroid can stay in the catalytic site and be metabolized again to androgen precursors, or whether the product of 17α-hydroxylase reaction leaves the active site and re-enters for the second reaction (Figure 7a). The one-way valve created by V366M mutation provides some answers to this question for the human CYP17A1. The presence of 17α-hydroxylase activity in the V366M variant suggested that PREG can get into the active site and be converted to 17OH-PREG (Figure 7b). If the 17OH-PREG was not able to leave the active site, it would have created an irreversible inhibition and the enzyme would have been unable to carry out further reactions. However, the 17α-hydroxylase reaction progressed (Figure 4 and Table 3), indicating that 17OH-PREG can exit the active site. Furthermore, if the 17OH-PREG could be converted without exiting the active site, then DHEA formation should have been observed as in case of the wild-type enzyme.

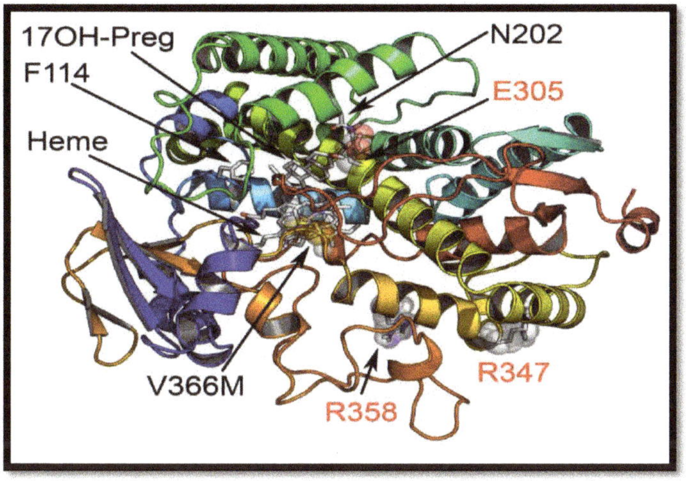

Figure 6. Comparison of novel V366M mutation with the previously reported isolated CYP17A1-17,20 lyase mutations. Only three other residues in CYP17A1 have been reported to be mutated in patients with isolated 17,20 lyase deficiency. The R347 and R358 are at the redox partner binding sites and their mutations may interfere with binding of POR and /or cytochrome b_5. The E305 residue at the active site is important for orientation of the substrate and its mutation has been shown to alter substrate specificity and lead to a preference for progesterone as the more efficient substrate. The V366 is located exactly at the active site of the CYP17A1.

However, DHEA was absent in both the *in vitro* enzyme reactions of the V366M mutant of CYP17A1 (Table 3) as well as in the urine of the patient (Figure 4), clearly indicating that 17OH-PREG must exit the active site after the 17α-hydroxylase reaction. If the problem was with the exit of DHEA, then that would also have created an irreversible inhibition by blocking the active site with one molecule of DHEA per unit of enzyme and further enzymatic activity would have come to a halt, but that was clearly not the case from the *in vitro* enzyme analysis as well as the patient's urine steroid profile (Figure 4 and Table 3). In the case of bovine CYP17A1, about 20% of pregnenolone consumed in the reaction could be converted to DHEA without exiting the active site [41]. When PROG was used as a substrate, compared to 17OH-PREG the dissociation of 17OH-PROG was 10 times faster. The release of the intermediate reaction was much faster than 17,20 lyase reaction and that prevented the direct formation of androstenedione from PROG. There are significant differences in activities of CYP17A1 between different species and the human enzyme has a very poor affinity for 17OH-PROG as substrate [25,42,43].

To further study this mechanism, we employed molecular dynamics simulations for the analysis of steroid binding in the active site of wild-type and the V366M mutant of CYP17A1. This was confirmed by the ensemble docking experiments which (for wild-type protein) yielded ligand poses in close proximity to the heme and highly resembling the co-crystallized abiraterone in the *CYP17A1* (PDB: 3RUK) structure [22]. The validity of our docking protocol was supported by a set of additional CYP17A1 crystal structures containing all the ligands of interest (PDB codes: 4NKW, 4NKX, 4NKY, and 4NKZ) in very similar poses enabling hydrogen-bonding to a distal N202 residue for PROG/PREG but not for 17OH-PREG [23]. Based on these observations, we hypothesized that the methionine side-chain could prevent a closer proximity to the heme iron necessary for the substrates undergoing lyase reaction [23,24]. To check this, we performed an additional pair of simulations with 17OH-PREG docked into the wild-type and mutant binding sites. Thus, we could indeed measure that the average distance between the ligand C17 atom and the heme iron differed in these systems (4.4 Å for wild-type and 6.3 Å for V366M mutant) (Figure 8c,d). While these results cannot be compared directly to the crystal structure of CYP17A1 with 17OH-PREG (PDB code 4NKZ; the O17-Fe distance between 3.4 and 3.9 Å depending on the chain), this hypothesis is well in line with all our experimental data and recently reported structures of human CYP17A1 in complexes with steroid substrates. In addition, the simulations, as well as the docking to the mutant protein, provided a possible explanation for the decreased reaction rates of the pregnenolone hydroxylation. Specifically, these structures (Figure 7b,d,f) hinted at an electrostatic interaction between the methionine methyl group (positively polarized by the preceding sulfur atom) and the negatively-charged carboxylate found in all ligands we studied. We propose that this added interaction slows down ligand dissociation/exit and thus slows down the reaction. Our MD simulation and docking results agree with greatly reduced Vmax but only marginally increased Km of both the wild-type and V366M mutant of CYP17A1 for the PROG (Table 3), indicating that binding of PREG and PROG is not affected but the exit of the 17α-hydroxy steroid from the active site may be slower in the V366M variant.

2.6. Substrate- and Inhibitor-Binding Analysis

Abiraterone bound to the WT CYP17A1 with a Kd value of 95 nM and showed the typical soret peak at 427 nm, indicative of nitrogen co-ordination with heme iron (Table 5). However, in case of the V366M mutant of CYP17A1, this binding pattern was not observed. To test the integrity of the protein, we used imidazole to check the binding and found that imidazole itself could bind to the V366M mutant. This confirmed our hypothesis that the introduction of the bulky methionine to replace the valine at position 366 creates steric hindrance and perturbs the binding pattern of drugs and steroids. These results also point to structural considerations for future inhibitor development which may utilize the spatial arrangement of binding-site residues to design tight-fitting inhibitors. Progesterone bound with slightly decreased affinity to the V366M mutant (Kd 287 nM compared to 162 nM for the WT enzyme). Binding of 17OH-PREG was not observed for the V366M mutation and explained the lack of 17,20 lyase activity, while for the WT CYP17A1 a Kd value 142 nM was observed. It is possible that some apparent binding of 17OH-PREG may occur at exceedingly high, non-physiological levels due to the nature of the structural hindrance from the V366M mutation which is at the very end of the binding site and close to the heme iron and water molecules that occupy the binding pocket.

Since the spectral binding of steroid substrates to CYP17A1 is observed by the replacement of water molecules at the active site, it is possible for some apparent binding to emerge from titration studies using very high enzyme and substrate concentrations, but due to unfavorable binding poses and distances, as revealed by further computational structure analysis, such apparent binding is not likely to result in an enzyme-substrate complex that can lead to product (DHEA) formation. This is further evidenced by lack of inhibition by 17OH-PREG in the 17hydroxylation reaction using PROG as substrate. In the case of inhibitor abiraterone, which needs to form an iron-nitrogen co-ordination and gets much closer to heme iron than steroid substrates (2.9 Å compared to 4.4–4.8 Å) (Figures 8 and S1), no binding was observed. Taken together these data indicate a steric hindrance for the binding of 17OH-PREG which may result in poor interaction with the enzyme and loss of 17,20 lyase activity.

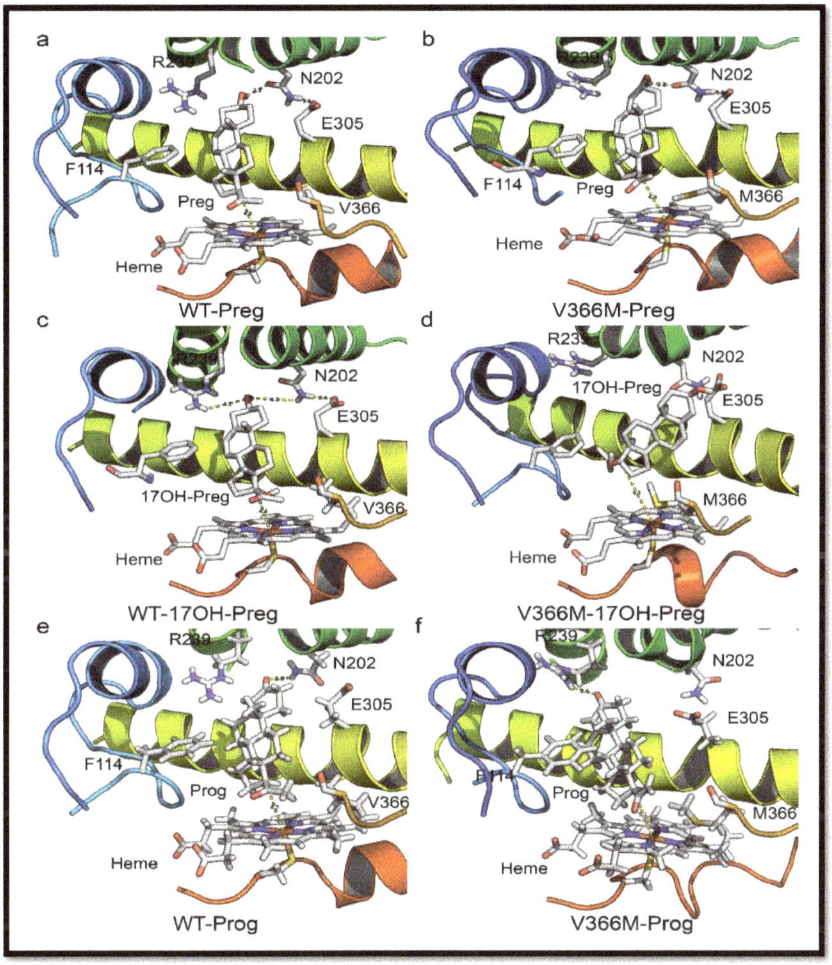

Figure 7. Structure analysis of the V366M mutation. (**a**) Binding of pregnenolone in CYP17A1 active site. Pregnenolone binds perpendicular to heme and is converted to 17OH-PREG. (**b**) Binding of pregnenolone to V366M variant of CYP17A1. Pregnenolone can still bind to V366M variant and is metabolized to 17OH-PREG. The side chain of methionine 366 in the mutant structure protrudes into the active site but still allows 17OH-PREG to exit. This is likely to slow down the reaction velocity of the 17α-hydroxylase reaction, which was confirmed by enzyme kinetic experiments (Table 1). (**c**) Binding of 17OH-PREG to WT CYP17A1. (**d**) Docking of 17OH-PREG to V366M variant of CYP17A1. The 17OH-PREG could not bind in the proximity to heme and distances between the heme iron and C17 atom increased for the mutant enzyme (6.3 Å in the mutant vs. 4.4 Å for the WT enzyme). Increased iron-C17 distances are observed together with N202-O3 interactions which are considered undesirable for optimal binding of 17hydroxy steroids for 17,20 lyase reaction. The methionine 366 side chain in the mutant protein blocks the entry of 17α-hydroxy steroid into the active site, resulting in loss of 17,20 lyase activity. (**e**,**f**) Comparison of WT and V366M variant of CYP17A1 binding to PROG.

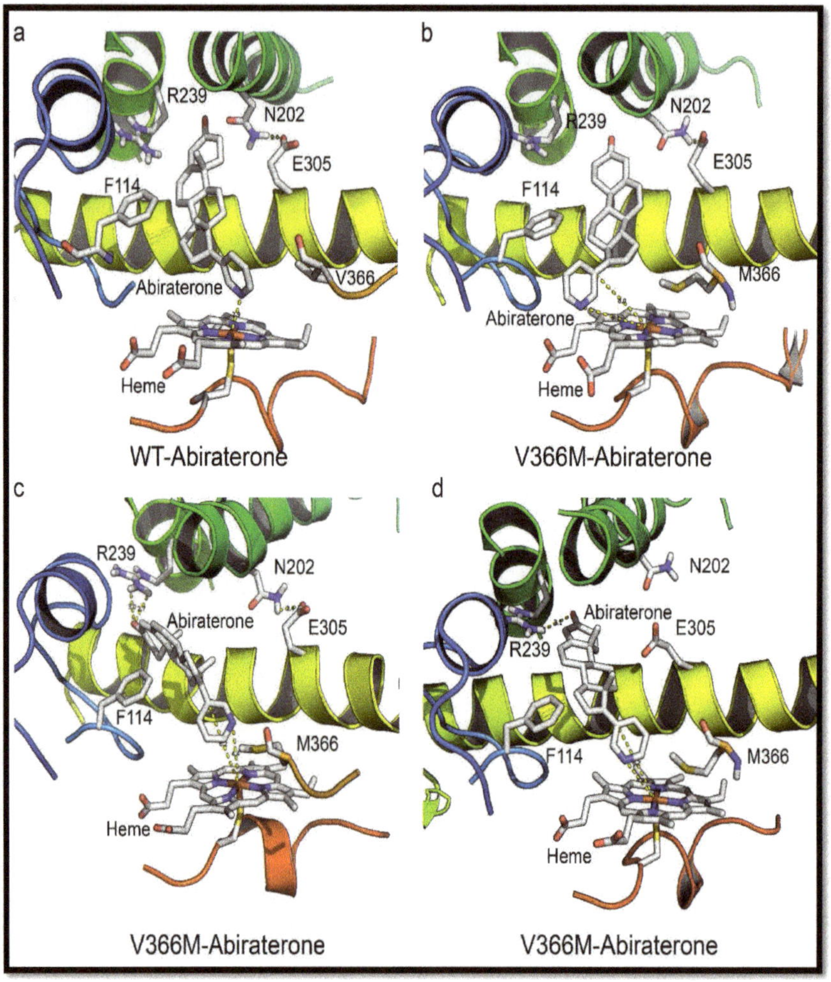

Figure 8. Comparison of abiraterone interaction with the WT and V366M variant of CYP17A1. (**a**) In the WT CYP17A1 abiraterone binds by forming a nitrogen-iron co-ordination (2.9 Å) with the central heme. (**b–d**) Different poses of abiraterone seen during docking into the V366M mutant of CYP17A1. In the V366M mutant, the methionine side chain prevents the binding of abiraterone and increased distances between the C17 atom and heme iron are observed together with binding poses that are different from the WT.

2.7. Mechanism of Steroid/Abiraterone Binding and Action in Relation to the V366M Mutation

Docking was performed with all ligands to WT as well as the V366M mutant of CYP17A1. Thr306 is reported to be a vital residue for the hydroxylation reaction (part of an alcohol pair donating protons). It is also very close to the heme and, like residue 366, is near the bound ligands. Asn202 is reported to interact with the distal side of the molecules. It is at the end of the cavity formed around the bound steroids/abiraterone (Figure 6) and most likely one of the residues inside the access channel. Ensemble docking of all relevant ligands implies that docking poses mimic the co-crystallized abiraterone (CH3 groups to the left when looking from the direction of residue 366) and allow interaction with the residue 202 highlighted in recent structures of human CYP17A1 (Figures 8 and 9) [23].

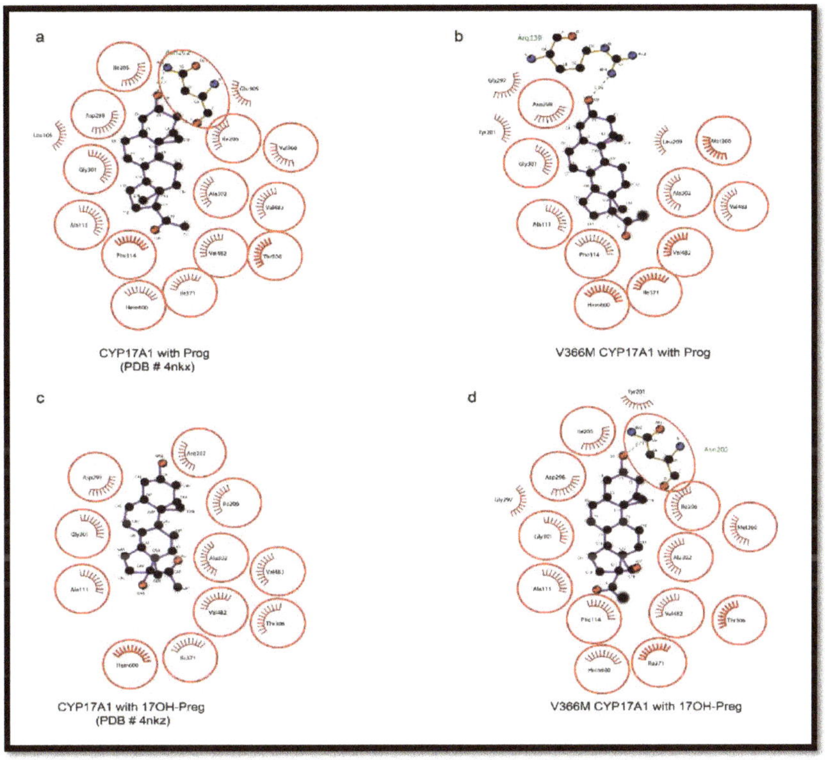

Figure 9. Comparison of PROG and 17OH-PREG bound in crystal structures of human CYP17A1 with the docked steroids into the V366M mutant. (**a**,**b**) PROG is found to bind similarly to WT as well as the mutant enzyme. (**c**,**d**) Mutation of V366 to M leads to non-optimal interactions with the N202 group in the V366M mutant compared to WT where this interaction is absent in poses which have 17OH-PREG close to the heme.

The pose from which 17α-hydroxy steroid leaves the site (after being formed) may differ from the one it assumes upon coming back. There are also possible differences between 17OH-PREG and PROG/PREG binding (Figures 7 and 9). Angular analysis of apo and relaxation V366M simulations imply that the methionine moves around a single conformation (chi2 and 3 angles roughly in 20-degree windows—a good match to the rotamers reported by http://www.dynameomics.org). It seems most likely that the CH3 group is involved in steric effects. The sulfur group in methionine may further polarize it, enhancing interaction with the carboxylate of 17α-hydroxy steroids. In some MD poses the methionine could be seen moving away from the heme, indicating it has conformational flexibility and in the presence of the metabolized PREG/PROG the 17α-hydroxylated ligand may exit without excessive hindrance. The reduced velocity of the PROG to 17OH-PROG reaction indicates that there could be an interaction between the carboxylate and the (likely-polarized) CH3 group of the methionine, which may slow down the exit of the product. Some other differences in the binding pattern were observed, like the involvement of Arg239 in the interaction of PROG with the V366M variant which may create bottlenecks during the exit of the product. Computationally calculated binding constants and binding energy calculations also supported the experimental results of reduced binding affinities for 17OH-PREG and abiraterone for the V366M mutant (Table 6). All this implies a general steric hindrance by the bigger residue (methionine vs. valine).

Table 6. Computational binding energy, computationally calculated dissociation constants, and interacting residues for steroid substrates and abiraterone with WT and the V366M mutant of *CYP17A1*. Key residues identified in different studies are shown in bold.

CYP17A1 Protein	Binding Energy (kcal/mol)	Dissociation Constant (nM)	Contacting Residues
WT with Prog	10.6	14.66	ALA113 PHE114 **ASN202** ILE205 ILE206 LEU209 **ARG239** GLY297 ASP298 GLY301 ALA302 THR306 ALA367 ILE371 VAL482 VAL483 **HEME**
M366 with Prog	9.75	43.71	ALA113 PHE114 **ASN202** ILE205 ILE206 LEU209 **ARG239** GLY297 ASP298 GLY301 ALA302 THR306 **MET366** ALA367 ILE371 VAL482 VAL483 **HEME**
WT with Preg	10.7	13.29	ALA105 ALA113 PHE114 ILE205 ILE206 LEU209 VAL236 **ARG239** GLY297 ASP298 GLY301 ALA302 **GLU305** THR306 **VAL366** ILE371 VAL482 VAL483 **HEME**
M366 with Preg	10.3	27.11	ALA105 SER106 ALA113 PHE114 ILE205 ILE206 LEU209 VAL236 **ARG239** GLY297 ASP298 GLY301 ALA302 THR306 **MET366** ILE371 VAL482 VAL483 **HEME**
WT with 17OH-Preg	11.3	5.22	ALA113 PHE114 TYR201 **ASN202** ILE205 ILE206 LEU209 LEU214 **ARG239** GLY297 ASP298 GLY301 ALA302 THR306 **VAL366** ALA367 ILE371 VAL482 VAL483 **HEME**
M366 with 17OH-Preg	7.0	60.4	ALA113 PHE114 TYR201 **ASN202** ILE205 ILE206 LEU209 **ARG239** GLY297 ASP298 GLY301 ALA302 **GLU305** THR306 **MET366** ALA367 ILE371 VAL482 VAL483
WT with Abiraterone	12.5	0.69	ALA113 PHE114 TYR201 **ASN202** ILE205 ILE206 LEU209 **ARG239** GLY297 ASP298 GLY301 ALA302 **GLU305** THR306 **VAL366** ALA367 LEU370 ILE371 VAL482 VAL483 **HEME**
V366 with Abiraterone	8.1	1112.9	ALA105 SER106 ASN107 ALA113 PHE114 TYR201 ILE205 ILE206 LEU209 **ARG239** THR294 GLY297 ASP298 GLY301 ALA302 THR306 **MET366** ILE371 VAL482 VAL483

Given the information from crystal structure of human CYP17A1 with abiraterone (nitrogen at 2.9 Å from the heme iron) (Figure 8), this implies that PREG either does not have to get this close to the heme or can accesses it from a different angle and is hence relatively unimpaired by the methionine. Recent structures of the human CYP17A1 bound with different steroid substrates confirm this hypothesis and show that 17OH-PREG binds much closer to the heme iron than PROG or PREG (Figures 7 and 9) [23,24]. For the 17OH-PREG we observed the existence of poses with the hydroxyl positioned very close to the CH3 of the methionine, indicating the bulky methionine residue could be preventing the ligand from getting close enough to the heme (Figures 7d and S2).

In addition, we also observed shorter distances suitable for hydrogen bonds with N202 and R239 groups and 17OH-PREG in the docking poses of V366M mutant (2.6 Å compared to 4.4 Å for the WT) (Figures 7d and S2, Table 6); it has been proposed that these interactions are required for PROG/PREG but are considered suboptimal for 17,20 lyase reaction and are found together with increased distances of C17 in 17α-hydroxy steroid substrate and the heme iron. Increased distances between the C17 of 17OH-PREG/Abiraterone and the heme iron, together with the extra/undesired interactions with N202/R239, were consistently observed in our simulations (Figures 7c, 8 S1 and S2).

It is more likely that the ligands cannot get into the binding site rather than have too much difficulty in leaving it since that would block the active site and prevent the 17α-hydroxylation reaction from occurring (which is not severely affected as observed by enzymatic analysis as well as the urine steroid profile of the patient). Also, DHEA is the smallest of all steroids involved, making it the most likely to leave, so it is the entry of 17OH-PREG into the active site that is likely to be impaired. Many different poses of abiraterone and 17OH-PREG were observed for the V366M mutant which illustrates the non-optimal binding pattern for the mutant enzyme (Figures 8 and S2). The inhibitor abiraterone (similar scaffold but bigger than the steroid substrates) also has trouble binding (Figures 8 and S1, Table 5) and does not act as an inhibitor for the 17α-hydroxylation reaction catalyzed by the V366M mutant of *CYP17A1* (Table 5).

3. Discussion

Among the previously reported mutations causing isolated 17,20 lyase deficiency, the R347C, R347H and R358Q are located on the redox partner binding site (Figure 6) and seem to act by altering the interaction with POR. Generally, a defect in redox partner or loss of interaction with redox partner affects all cytochrome P450 activities in the endoplasmic reticulum as well as in mitochondria [31,36,44–48]. In the case of R347H and R358Q mutations in CYP17A1, why this loss of interaction with POR affects the 17,20 lyase activity in a more severe fashion than the 17α-hydroxylase activity is not clear, since both activities of CYP17A1 require electrons supplied by NADPH through POR for their catalytic function [49]. The only other mutation in CYP17A1 that had been reported to selectively impair the 17,20 lyase activity is E305G which is part of the substrate access channel of CYP17A1 (Figures 6 and 8) [28,30]. The E305G mutation had been reported to affect the binding of 17α-hydroxy steroids while showing even higher than normal 17α-hydroxylase activities [28]; however a later analysis of the patient's steroid metabolic profile [30] showed that 17α-hydroxylase activity was also impaired, contradicting the earlier claims of isolated 17,20 lyase deficiency [30]. A more efficient coupling with POR and efficient use of NADPH have recently been proposed to favor the 17,20 lyase reaction [49]. Multiple potential mechanisms for the selectivity of the 17,20 lyase reaction have been proposed in recent works from different laboratories [23,26,49–53].

The V366M is an active site mutation in CYP17A1 that not only preferentially targets 17,20 lyase activity but also provides insights into the structural basis of the 17,20 lyase reaction, the key regulator of sex steroid biosynthesis in humans (Figures 2 and 7). The specificity of the human CYP17A1 active site allows the binding of PREG and its 17hydroxy metabolite (17OH-PREG) to bind in different conformations and exit the active site after the reactions (Figure 7a,c), and the mutation of valine 366 to methionine alters the active site and hinders the binding of 17α-hydroxy-steroids (Figure 8d). The V366M mutant also explains the effectiveness of the anti-prostate-cancer drug abiraterone as a potent inhibitor of CYP17A1. Abiraterone fills the active site of CYP17A1 (Figures 8 and S1) and becomes irreversibly bound to the enzyme (Supplementary Figure S1c), stopping any further substrate binding and activity [22]. This location of V366 at the catalytic center provides a structural basis for improving and designing novel and specific CYP17A1 inhibitors by targeting spatial selectivity of the active site with imidazole or other suitable chemical moieties added to core steroid structures.

Structural modifications based on the above information may help in designing more specific and potent inhibitors directed only towards the 17,20 lyase activity of CYP17A1 that could produce tighter binding at the active site. The 17,20 lyase-specific inhibitors will have advantages over current compounds that target both the 17α-hydroxylase and the 17,20 lyase activities of CYP17A1 and require steroid supplementation [12,54–58]. The mechanistic and structural insights revealed by these studies will help in the development of better drugs against polycystic ovary syndrome and prostate cancer. These findings will also improve our understanding of the structural basis of the dual function of CYP17A1 as both a 17α-hydroxylase and 17,20 lyase, and the role of these activities in the regulation of steroid hormone production in different tissues.

4. Materials and Methods

4.1. Human Subjects

All clinical investigations were carried out following the Declaration of Helsinki principles. Written informed consent was received from the parents for genetic work-up of 46, XY DSD in their child in the pediatric endocrinology research laboratory in Barcelona which holds ethical approval for these studies.

4.2. Genetic Analysis

DNA was extracted from the peripheral blood leucocytes of the patient. Genetic analysis of the androgen receptor gene (*AR*) and for the 5αreductase type 2 gene (*SRD5A2*) were performed as described [39,40], yielding normal results. The *CYP17A1* gene was analyzed as reported [59] and identified sequence variations were compared to National Center for Biotechnology Information (NCBI, Bethesda, USA) entry NG_007955.1 (GI:189339218). The *CYP17A1* gene was subsequently also analyzed in the parents and the older half-sister, and one mutation was found in the mother. Since the second mutation is a completely inactivating mutation, its presence on a different allele was inferred (as the presence of both mutations on one allele will give a good working copy of the *CYP17A1* gene, and that does not cause disease).

4.3. Steroid Profiling from 24-h Urine Samples

Steroid metabolites in urine were measured by the gas chromatography-mass spectrometry (GC/MS) method as described previously [60,61].

4.4. Recombinant Protein Expression

Human wild-type and mutant *CYP17A1* proteins were produced in an *E. coli* expression system and purified for enzyme kinetic assays [15,17,18,62]. The pCWH17-mod(His)4 expression plasmid (a gift from Prof. Michael Waterman, Nashville, TN) containing the cDNA for human WT or mutant CYP17A1 [15], was transformed into the *E. coli* JM109 cells and colonies were selected under ampicillin control. Bacteria were grown at 37 °C to OD_{600} 0.6 and the CYP17A1 protein expression was induced by the addition of 0.5 mM IPTG followed by further incubation at 28 °C for 48 h. Purification of CYP17A1 was performed as described [15,17,18]. In brief, the spheroplasts prepared by the lysozyme treatment of bacterial cells were ruptured by sonication and cleared by centrifugation at 4000× *g* for 10 min, then the supernatant containing the CYP17A1 protein was extracted with 1.5% Triton X-114 and centrifuged at 100,000× *g* for 30 min. A reddish-brown colored detergent-rich supernatant fraction containing the CYP17A1 was isolated, diluted to reduce the detergent concentration to 0.1%, and passed over a Ni-NTA-sepharose column. The column was washed with 5 mM histidine to remove the non-specific binding and eluted with 200 mM histidine. Further purification was carried out by gel filtration chromatography to remove histidine and other protein contaminants.

4.5. In Vitro Enzyme Kinetic Analysis of Identified CYP17A1 Mutations

To assess 17α-hydroxylase activity, 10 pmol of CYP17A1 along with 20 pmol purified human POR [17,31,32,34,62] (at a 1:2 ratio) was incubated with 0.1–15 μM [^{14}C]PROG (80,000 cpm/reaction) and 1 mM NADPH in 50 mM potassium-phosphate buffer (pH 7.4) containing 6 mM potassium acetate, 10 mM $MgCl_2$, 1 mM reduced glutathione, 20% glycerol and 20 μg phosphatidylcholine for 60 min at 37 °C. Human CYP17A1 does not use 17OH-PROG as a major substrate and, therefore, PROG is considered a better substrate to monitor only 17α-hydroxylase activity due to very little further conversion of 17OH-PROG. To assess 17,20 lyase activity, CYP17A1 and POR proteins were incubated with 0.05–5 μM [^{3}H]17OH-PREG (100,000 cpm/reaction), 1 mM NADPH and 20 pmol cytochrome b_5/reaction in 50 mM K-phosphate buffer (pH 7.4) containing 6 mM potassium acetate,

10 mM MgC_{12}, 1 mM reduced glutathione, 20% glycerol and 20 μg phosphatidylcholine for 90 min at 37 °C. Steroids were extracted and resolved by thin layer chromatography before quantitative analysis for conversion to 17OH-PREG and DHEA respectively as described [19]. For inhibition assays, abiraterone, PREG as well as 17OH-PREG were used to compete with radioactive PROG for 17α-hydroxylase reaction. Enzyme kinetic calculations were performed using non-linear regression curve fitting with Prism (GraphPad Software Inc., San Diego, CA, USA). Data represent the mean of three independent experiments.

4.6. Heme and P450 Measurements

Heme content was measured as described previously by dissolving the protein in NaOH and measuring the heme absorbance in a triton-methanol mixture [63]. Cytochrome P450 and Cytochrome b_5 were measured as described previously [1,17]. Cytochrome b_5 content was estimated by monitoring the absorbance difference at 423–490 nm using an extinction coefficient of 181 mmol cm^{-1}.

4.7. Substrate-Binding Assay

Binding of steroid substrates to CYP17A1 was measured by recording the substrate-binding spectra in the range of 340–500 nm on a Perkin Elmer Lambda 25 spectrophotometer. A change in heme absorbance is observed when water molecules at the active site are replaced by steroid substrates [22]. In case of abiraterone, an increase in the soret peak at 427 nm is observed by co-ordination of the heme iron with pyridine nitrogen. To accurately measure the tight binding substrates and inhibitors, a cuvette with 100 mm path length was employed and protein concentration was kept at 50 nM. Binding of steroids, as well as abiraterone to CYP17A1, occurs with very high affinity and, as observed previously, Kd values measured are often close to protein concentration used in binding assays. All substrates and abiraterone were dissolved in ethanol and an equal amount of ethanol was added to the reference cuvette and the final concentration of ethanol added to the cuvettes was kept below 2%. After each addition of the compounds, cuvettes were incubated for 5 min at 22 °C before recording the spectra. The slit width was fixed at 1.0 nm and spectra were recorded at 50 nm/min with a series of increasing concentrations of different compounds (abiraterone: 0–200 nM; PREG: 0–500 nM; 17OH-PREG: 0–1000 nM; PROG: 0–1000 nM). Data were fitted with GraphPad Prism based on the tight binding pattern of substrates to a single binding site.

4.8. Protein Structure Analysis of WT and Mutant CYP17A1

The published 3D structures of human CYP17A1 [22,23] were downloaded from the protein structure repository (www.rcsb.org). We performed several rounds of multiple-sequence alignments with different CYP17A1 protein sequences from several organisms and created in-silico mutants using the programs YASARA [64] and WHATIF [65]. For all further experiments described, a 2.6 Å resolution crystal structure [22] (PDB code 3RUK) of CYP17A1 was used; with the abiraterone ligand, the membrane anchor (all residues preceding R45), and water molecules (aside from one conserved between residue 366 and the heme) removed. Missing hydrogen atoms were added to the structure with YASARA [64] which was also used for all other computations. The V366M mutant model was then constructed by replacing the original valine with the most favorable methionine conformation found with the in-built SCWALL method (rotamer library search followed by energy minimization) [66]. Afterward, both systems were subjected to 10 ns explicit solvent MD simulations at 310 K, which was preceded by 500 steps of steepest descent and simulated annealing minimization using the AMBER03 force field and the TIP3P water model [67,68]. All following MDs were performed with similar settings. The resulting simulation snapshots (100 per run) were used for the docking of steroids with the AutoDock Vina [69] ensemble-docking experiments using PREG, 17OH-PREG, PROG and 17OH-PROG (orthorhombic docking was grid-established around the central heme and the residues 105, 202, and 366 of the CYP17A1). The final selection of poses was based on their docking scores and similarities to the abiraterone ligand which was co-crystallized in the template structure (PDB: 3RUK) [22]. The docked steroid poses agreed with the binding site details highlighted by a recent set of CYP17A1 crystal structures [23]. Clustering of simulation snapshots was done using USCF Chimera [70]. Figures of the structure models were created with the program Pymol (www.pymol.org) and the chosen poses were rendered as ray-traced images with POVRAY (www.povray.org). Ligand interactions were analyzed and depicted with the program LIGPLOT+ (http://www.ebi.ac.uk/thornton-srv/software/LigPlus/).

Supplementary Materials: The following are available online at http://www.mdpi.com/1424-8247/11/2/37/s1, Supplementary Figures S1 and S2.

Author Contributions: C.E.F., L.A., and A.V.P. designed the experiments. A.V.P. supervised the study. M.F.C., N.C., and R.M., N.T., and L.A. performed genetic, histochemical and biochemical analysis. A.Z. performed computational modeling and molecular dynamics simulations. A.Z. and A.V.P. performed bioinformatic analysis. C.E.F. and A.V.P. expressed and purified the proteins and performed functional assays. B.D. and B.F. performed the mass spectrometric analysis of urine samples and analysed mass spectrometry data. M.F.C., N.C., C.E.F., A.Z., B.D., B.F., R.M., N.T., L.A. and A.V.P. analysed data and critically read the manuscript. A.V.P. wrote the paper with discussion, input and editing contributions from all the authors.

Acknowledgments: We thank Walter L Miller, University of California San Francisco, CA, USA for his generous gift of anti-human CYP17A1 antibodies. We thank Michael R Waterman, Nashville, TN, USA for human CYP17A1 bacterial expression system. This study has been funded by grants from the Instituto de Salud Carlos III (FIS PI06/0903), the Centre for Biomedical Research Network on Rare Diseases (CIBERER, Madrid), and the AGAUR—University and Research Management and Evaluation Agency SGR05-00908 and 2009SGR-31, Barcelona, Spain, to M.F.-C. and L.A., and by grants from the Swiss National Science Foundation (31003A-134926) to AVP, Bern University Research Foundation (to A.V.P.), Burgergemeinde Bern (to A.V.P.) and Department of Biomedical Research intramural support (to A.V.P.). N.C. was supported by a fellowship grant of the European Society of Paediatric Endocrinology, sponsored by Novo Nordisk A/S.

Conflicts of Interest: The authors declare no conflict of interest. The funding sponsors had no role in the design of the study; in the collection, analyses, or interpretation of data; in the writing of the manuscript, and in the decision to publish the results.

References

1. Omura, T.; Sato, R. The carbon monoxide-binding pigment of liver microsomes. I. Evidence for its hemoprotein nature. *J. Biol. Chem.* **1964**, *239*, 2370–2378. [PubMed]
2. Pandey, A.V.; Flück, C.E. NADPH P450 oxidoreductase: Structure, function, and pathology of diseases. *Pharmacol. Ther.* **2013**, *138*, 229–254. [CrossRef] [PubMed]
3. Zanger, U.M.; Schwab, M. Cytochrome P450 enzymes in drug metabolism: Regulation of gene expression, enzyme activities, and impact of genetic variation. *Pharmacol. Ther.* **2013**, *138*, 103–141. [CrossRef] [PubMed]
4. Miller, W.L.; Auchus, R.J. The molecular biology, biochemistry, and physiology of human steroidogenesis and its disorders. *Endocr. Rev.* **2011**, *32*, 81–151. [CrossRef] [PubMed]
5. Zuber, M.X.; Simpson, E.R.; Waterman, M.R. Expression of bovine 17 alpha-hydroxylase cytochrome P-450 cDNA in nonsteroidogenic (COS 1) cells. *Science* **1986**, *234*, 1258–1261. [CrossRef] [PubMed]
6. Chung, B.C.; Picado-Leonard, J.; Haniu, M.; Bienkowski, M.; Hall, P.F.; Shively, J.E.; Miller, W.L. Cytochrome P450c17 (steroid 17 alpha-hydroxylase/17,20 lyase): Cloning of human adrenal and testis cDNAs indicates the same gene is expressed in both tissues. *Proc. Natl. Acad. Sci. USA* **1987**, *84*, 407–411. [CrossRef] [PubMed]
7. Nakajin, S.; Shinoda, M.; Haniu, M.; Shively, J.E.; Hall, P.F. C21 steroid side chain cleavage enzyme from porcine adrenal microsomes. Purification and characterization of the 17 alpha-hydroxylase/C17,20-lyase cytochrome P-450. *J. Biol. Chem.* **1984**, *259*, 3971–3976. [PubMed]
8. Vasaitis, T.S.; Bruno, R.D.; Njar, V.C. CYP17 inhibitors for prostate cancer therapy. *J. Steroid Biochem. Mol. Biol.* **2011**, *125*, 23–31. [CrossRef] [PubMed]
9. Attard, G.; Reid, A.H.M.; Auchus, R.; Hughes, B.A.; Cassidy, A.M.; Thompson, E.; Oommen, N.B.; Folkerd, E.; Dowsett, M.; Arlt, W.; et al. Clinical and biochemical consequences of CYP17A1 inhibition with abiraterone given with and without exogenous glucocorticoids in castrate men with advanced prostate cancer. *J. Clin. Endocrinol. Metab.* **2012**, *97*, 507–516. [CrossRef] [PubMed]
10. De Bono, J.S.; Logothetiset, C.J.; Molinaal, A.; Fizazi, K.; North, S.; Chu, L.; Chi, K.N.; Jones, R.J.; Goodman, O.B.; Saad, F.; et al. Abiraterone and Increased Survival in Metastatic Prostate Cancer. *N. Engl. J. Med.* **2011**, *364*, 1995–2005. [CrossRef] [PubMed]

11. Attard, G.; Reid, A.H.; Yap, T.A.; Raynaud, F.; Dowsett, M.; Settatree, S.; Barrett, M.; Parker, C.; Martins, V.; Folkerd, E.; et al. Phase I clinical trial of a selective inhibitor of CYP17, abiraterone acetate, confirms that castration-resistant prostate cancer commonly remains hormone driven. *J. Clin. Oncol.* **2008**, *26*, 4563–4571. [CrossRef] [PubMed]
12. Malikova, J.; Brixius-Anderko, S.; Udhane, S.S.; Parween, S.; Dick, B.; Bernhardt, R.; Pandey, A.V. CYP17A1 inhibitor abiraterone, an anti-prostate cancer drug, also inhibits the 21-hydroxylase activity of CYP21A2. *J. Steroid Biochem. Mol. Biol.* **2017**, *174*, 192–200. [CrossRef] [PubMed]
13. Lu, A.Y.; Junk, K.W.; Coon, M.J. Resolution of the cytochrome P-450-containing w-hydroxylation system of liver microsomes into three components. *J. Biol. Chem.* **1969**, *244*, 3714–3721. [PubMed]
14. Flück, C.E.; Tajima, T.; Pandey, A.V.; Arlt, W.; Okuhara, K.; Verge, C.F.; Jabs, E.W.; Mendonça, B.B.; Fujieda, K.; Miller, W.L. Mutant P450 oxidoreductase causes disordered steroidogenesis with and without Antley-Bixler syndrome. *Nat. Genet.* **2004**, *36*, 228–230. [CrossRef] [PubMed]
15. Imai, T.; Globerman, H.; Gertner, J.M.; Kagawa, N.; Waterman, M.R. Expression and purification of functional human 17 alpha-hydroxylase/17,20-lyase (P450c17) in Escherichia coli. Use of this system for study of a novel form of combined 17 alpha-hydroxylase/17,20-lyase deficiency. *J. Biol. Chem.* **1993**, *268*, 19681–19689. [PubMed]
16. Burkhard, F.Z.; Parween, S.; Udhane, S.S.; Flück, C.E.; Pandey, A.V. P450 Oxidoreductase deficiency: Analysis of mutations and polymorphisms. *J. Steroid Biochem. Mol. Biol.* **2017**, *165 Pt A*, 38–50. [CrossRef] [PubMed]
17. Pandey, A.V.; Miller, W.L. Regulation of 17,20 lyase activity by cytochrome b5 and by serine phosphorylation of P450c17. *J. Biol. Chem.* **2005**, *280*, 13265–13271. [CrossRef] [PubMed]
18. Pandey, A.V.; Mellon, S.H.; Miller, W.L. Protein phosphatase 2A and phosphoprotein SET regulate androgen production by P450c17. *J. Biol. Chem.* **2003**, *278*, 2837–2844. [CrossRef] [PubMed]
19. Auchus, R.J.; Lee, T.C.; Miller, W.L. Cytochrome b5 augments the 17,20-lyase activity of human P450c17 without direct electron transfer. *J. Biol. Chem.* **1998**, *273*, 3158–3165. [CrossRef] [PubMed]
20. Zhang, L.H.; Rodriguez, H.; Ohno, S.; Miller, W.L. Serine phosphorylation of human P450c17 increases 17,20-lyase activity: Implications for adrenarche and the polycystic ovary syndrome. *Proc. Natl. Acad. Sci. USA* **1995**, *92*, 10619–10623. [CrossRef] [PubMed]
21. Idkowiak, J.; Randell, T.; Dhir, V.; Patel, P.; Shackleton, C.H.; Taylor, N.F.; Krone, N.; Arlt, W. A missense mutation in the human cytochrome b5 gene causes 46,XY disorder of sex development due to true isolated 17,20 lyase deficiency. *J. Clin. Endocrinol. Metab.* **2012**, *97*, E465–E475. [CrossRef] [PubMed]
22. DeVore, N.M.; Scott, E.E. Structures of cytochrome P450 17A1 with prostate cancer drugs abiraterone and TOK-001. *Nature* **2012**, *482*, 116–119. [CrossRef] [PubMed]
23. Petrunak, E.M.; DeVore, N.M.; Porubsky, P.R.; Scott, E.E. Structures of human steroidogenic cytochrome P450 17A1 with substrates. *J. Biol. Chem.* **2014**, *289*, 32952–32964. [CrossRef] [PubMed]
24. Yadav, R.; Petrunak, E.M.; Estrada, D.F.; Scott, E.E. Structural insights into the function of steroidogenic cytochrome P450 17A1. *Mol. Cell Endocrinol.* **2017**, *441*, 68–75. [CrossRef] [PubMed]
25. Auchus, R.J. Steroid 17-hydroxylase and 17,20-lyase deficiencies, genetic and pharmacologic. *J. Steroid Biochem. Mol. Biol.* **2017**, *165*, 71–78. [CrossRef] [PubMed]
26. Mak, P.J.; Gregory, M.C.; Denisov, I.G.; Sligar, S.G.; Kincaid, J.R. Unveiling the crucial intermediates in androgen production. *Proc. Natl. Acad. Sci. USA* **2015**, *112*, 15856–15861. [CrossRef] [PubMed]
27. Geller, D.H.; Auchus, R.J.; Mendonça, B.B.; Miller, W.L. The genetic and functional basis of isolated 17,20-lyase deficiency. *Nat. Genet.* **1997**, *17*, 201–205. [CrossRef] [PubMed]
28. Sherbet, D.P.; Tiosano, D.; Kwist, K.M.; Hochberg, Z.; Auchus, R.J. CYP17 mutation E305G causes isolated 17,20-lyase deficiency by selectively altering substrate binding. *J. Biol. Chem.* **2003**, *278*, 48563–48569. [CrossRef] [PubMed]
29. Van Den Akker, E.L.; Koper, J.W.; Boehmer, A.L.; Themmen, A.P.; Verhoef-Post, M.; Timmerman, M.A.; Otten, B.J.; Drop, S.L.; De Jong, F.H. Differential inhibition of 17alpha-hydroxylase and 17,20-lyase activities by three novel missense CYP17 mutations identified in patients with P450c17 deficiency. *J. Clin. Endocrinol. Metab.* **2002**, *87*, 5714–5721. [CrossRef] [PubMed]
30. Tiosano, D.; Knopf, C.; Koren, I.; Wudy, S.A. Metabolic evidence for impaired 17alpha-hydroxylase activity in a kindred bearing the E305G mutation for isolate 17,20-lyase activity. *Eur. J. Endocrinol.* **2008**, *158*, 385–392. [CrossRef] [PubMed]

31. Parween, S.; Roucher-Boulez, F.; Flück, C.E.; Lienhardt-Roussie, A.; Mallet, D.; Morel, Y.; Pandey, A.V. P450 Oxidoreductase Deficiency: Loss of Activity Caused by Protein Instability From a Novel L374H Mutation. *J. Clin. Endocrinol. Metab.* **2016**, *101*, 4789–4798. [CrossRef] [PubMed]
32. Flück, C.E.; Pandey, A.V. Impact on CYP19A1 activity by mutations in NADPH cytochrome P450 oxidoreductase. *J. Steroid Biochem. Mol. Biol.* **2017**, *165 Pt A*, 64–70. [CrossRef] [PubMed]
33. Pandey, A.V.; Sproll, P. Pharmacogenomics of human P450 oxidoreductase. *Front. Pharmacol.* **2014**, *5*, 103. [CrossRef] [PubMed]
34. Udhane, S.S.; Parween, S.; Kagawa, N.; Pandey, A.V. Altered CYP19A1 and CYP3A4 Activities Due to Mutations A115V, T142A, Q153R and P284L in the Human P450 Oxidoreductase. *Front. Pharmacol.* **2017**, *8*, 580. [CrossRef] [PubMed]
35. Geller, D.H.; Auchus, R.J.; Miller, W.L. P450c17 mutations R347H and R358Q selectively disrupt 17,20-lyase activity by disrupting interactions with P450 oxidoreductase and cytochrome b5. *Mol. Endocrinol.* **1999**, *13*, 167–175. [CrossRef] [PubMed]
36. Flück, C.E.; Meyer-Böni, M.; Pandey, A.V.; Kempná, P.; Miller, W.L.; Schoenle, E.J.; Biason-Lauber, A. Why boys will be boys: Two pathways of fetal testicular androgen biosynthesis are needed for male sexual differentiation. *Am. J. Hum. Genet.* **2011**, *89*, 201–218. [CrossRef] [PubMed]
37. Flück, C.E.; Pandey, A.V. Steroidogenesis of the testis—New genes and pathways. *Ann. Endocrinol.* **2014**, *75*, 40–47. [CrossRef] [PubMed]
38. Biason-Lauber, A.; Miller, W.L.; Pandey, A.V.; Fluck, C.E. Of marsupials and men: "Backdoor" dihydrotestosterone synthesis in male sexual differentiation. *Mol. Cell Endocrinol.* **2013**, *371*, 124–132. [CrossRef] [PubMed]
39. Audi, L.; Fernández-Cancio, M.; Carrascosa, A.; Andaluz, P.; Torán, N.; Piró, C.; Vilaró, E.; Vicens-Calvet, E.; Gussinyé, M.; Albisu, M.A.; et al. Novel (60%) and recurrent (40%) androgen receptor gene mutations in a series of 59 patients with a 46,XY disorder of sex development. *J. Clin. Endocrinol. Metab.* **2010**, *95*, 1876–1888. [CrossRef] [PubMed]
40. Fernandez-Cancio, M.; Audí, L.; Andaluz, P.; Torán, N.; Piró, C.; Albisu, M.; Gussinyé, M.; Yeste, D.; Clemente, M.; Martínez-Mora, J.; et al. SRD5A2 gene mutations and polymorphisms in Spanish 46,XY patients with a disorder of sex differentiation. *Int. J. Androl.* **2011**, *34 Pt 2*, e526–e535. [CrossRef] [PubMed]
41. Yamazaki, T.; Ohno, T.; Sakaki, T.; Akiyoshi-Shibata, M.; Yabusaki, Y.; Imai, T.; Kominami, S. Kinetic analysis of successive reactions catalyzed by bovine cytochrome p450(17alpha,lyase). *Biochemistry* **1998**, *37*, 2800–2806. [CrossRef] [PubMed]
42. Soucy, P.; Van, L.-T. Conversion of pregnenolone to DHEA by human 17α-hydroxylase/17,20-lyase (P450c17). *Eur. J. Biochem.* **2000**, *267*, 3243–3247. [CrossRef] [PubMed]
43. Brock, B.J.; Waterman, M.R. Biochemical Differences between Rat and Human Cytochrome P450c17 Support the Different Steroidogenic Needs of These Two Species. *Biochemistry* **1999**, *38*, 1598–1606. [CrossRef] [PubMed]
44. Pandey, A.V.; Kempná, P.; Hofer, G.; Mullis, P.E.; Flück, C.E. Modulation of human CYP19A1 activity by mutant NADPH P450 oxidoreductase. *Mol. Endocrinol.* **2007**, *21*, 2579–2595. [CrossRef] [PubMed]
45. Flück, C.E.; Mullis, P.E.; Pandey, A.V. Reduction in hepatic drug metabolizing CYP3A4 activities caused by P450 oxidoreductase mutations identified in patients with disordered steroid metabolism. *Biochem. Biophys. Res. Commun.* **2010**, *401*, 149–153. [CrossRef] [PubMed]
46. Nicolo, C.; Flück, C.E.; Mullis, P.E.; Pandey, A.V. Restoration of mutant cytochrome P450 reductase activity by external flavin. *Mol. Cell Endocrinol.* **2010**, *321*, 245–252. [CrossRef] [PubMed]
47. Riddick, D.S.; Ding, X.; Wolf, C.R.; Porter, T.D.; Pandey, A.V.; Zhang, Q.; Gu, J.; Finn, R.D.; Ronseaux, S.; McLaughlin, L.A.; et al. NADPH-cytochrome P450 oxidoreductase: Roles in physiology, pharmacology, and toxicology. *Drug Metab. Dispos.* **2013**, *41*, 12–23. [CrossRef] [PubMed]
48. Zalewski, A.; Ma, N.S.; Legeza, B.; Renthal, N.; Flück, C.E.; Pandey, A.V. Vitamin D-Dependent Rickets Type 1 Caused by Mutations in CYP27B1 Affecting Protein Interactions With Adrenodoxin. *J. Clin. Endocrinol. Metab.* **2016**, *101*, 3409–3418. [CrossRef] [PubMed]
49. Peng, H.M.; Im, Sa.; Pearl, N.M.; Turcu, A.F.; Waskell, J.R.L.; Auchus, R.J. Cytochrome b5 Activates the 17,20-Lyase Activity of Human Cytochrome P450 17A1 by Increasing the Coupling of NADPH Consumption to Androgen Production. *Biochemistry* **2016**, *55*, 4356–4365. [CrossRef] [PubMed]

50. Yoshimoto, F.K.; Gonzalez, E.; Auchus, R.J.; Guengerich, F.P. Mechanism of 17alpha,20-Lyase and New Hydroxylation Reactions of Human Cytochrome P450 17A1: 18O Labeling And Oxygen Surrogate Evidence For A Role Of A Perferryl Oxygen. *J. Biol. Chem.* **2016**, *291*, 17143–17164. [CrossRef] [PubMed]
51. Duggal, R.; Liu, Y.; Gregory, M.C.; Denisov, I.G.; Kincaid, J.R.; Sligar, S.G. Evidence that cytochrome b5 acts as a redox donor in CYP17A1 mediated androgen synthesis. *Biochem. Biophys. Res. Commun.* **2016**, *477*, 202–208. [CrossRef] [PubMed]
52. Estrada, D.F.; Skinner, A.L.; Laurence, J.S.; Scott, E.E. Human cytochrome P450 17A1 conformational selection: Modulation by ligand and cytochrome b5. *J. Biol. Chem.* **2014**, *289*, 14310–14320. [CrossRef] [PubMed]
53. Pallan, P.S.; Nagy, L.D.; Lei, L.; Gonzalez, E.; Kramlinger, V.M.; Azumaya, C.M.; Wawrzak, Z.; Waterman, M.R.; Guengerich, F.P.; Egli, M. Structural and kinetic basis of steroid 17alpha,20-lyase activity in teleost fish cytochrome P450 17A1 and its absence in cytochrome P450 17A2. *J. Biol. Chem.* **2015**, *290*, 3248–3268. [CrossRef] [PubMed]
54. Ramudo Cela, L.; Balea-Filgueiras, J.; Vizoso-Hermida, J.R.; Martín-Herranz, I. Study of cases of abiraterone discontinuation due to toxicity in pre-chemotherapy after 1 year's experience. *J. Oncol. Pharm. Pract.* **2017**, *23*, 615–619. [CrossRef] [PubMed]
55. Li, Z.; Alyamani, M.; Li, J.; Rogacki, K.; Abazeed, M.; Upadhyay, S.K.; Balk, S.P.; Taplin, M.E.; Auchus, R.J.; Sharifi, N. Redirecting abiraterone metabolism to fine-tune prostate cancer anti-androgen therapy. *Nature* **2016**, *533*, 547–551. [CrossRef] [PubMed]
56. Bonomo, S.; Hansen, C.H.; Petrunak, E.M.; Scott, E.E.; Styrishave, B.; Jørgensen, F.S.; Olsen, L. Promising Tools in Prostate Cancer Research: Selective Non-Steroidal Cytochrome P450 17A1 Inhibitors. *Sci. Rep.* **2016**, *6*, 29468. [CrossRef] [PubMed]
57. Sharifi, N. Prostate cancer: CYP17A1 inhibitor failure-lessons for future drug development. *Nat. Rev. Urol.* **2015**, *12*, 245–246. [CrossRef] [PubMed]
58. Udhane, S.S.; Dick, B.; Hu, Q.; Hartmann, R.W.; Pandey, A.V. Specificity of anti-prostate cancer CYP17A1 inhibitors on androgen biosynthesis. *Biochem. Biophys. Res. Commun.* **2016**, *477*, 1005–1010. [CrossRef] [PubMed]
59. Monno, S.; Ogawa, H.; Date, T.; Fujioka, M.; Miller, W.L.; Kobayashi, M. Mutation of histidine 373 to leucine in cytochrome P450c17 causes 17 alpha-hydroxylase deficiency. *J. Biol. Chem.* **1993**, *268*, 25811–25817. [PubMed]
60. Quattropani, C.; Vogt, B.; Odermatt, A.; Dick, B.; Frey, B.M.; Frey, F.J. Reduced activity of 11 beta-hydroxysteroid dehydrogenase in patients with cholestasis. *J. Clin. Investig.* **2001**, *108*, 1299–1305. [CrossRef] [PubMed]
61. Shackleton, C.H. Mass spectrometry in the diagnosis of steroid-related disorders and in hypertension research. *J. Steroid Biochem. Mol. Biol.* **1993**, *45*, 127–140. [CrossRef]
62. Huang, N.; Pandey, A.V.; Agrawal, V.; Reardon, W.; Lapunzina, P.D.; Mowat, D.; Jabs, E.W.; Van Vliet, G.; Sack, J.; Flück, C.E.; et al. Diversity and function of mutations in p450 oxidoreductase in patients with Antley-Bixler syndrome and disordered steroidogenesis. *Am. J. Hum. Genet.* **2005**, *76*, 729–749. [CrossRef] [PubMed]
63. Pandey, A.V.; Joshi, S.K.; Tekwani, B.L.; Chauhan, V.S. A colorimetric assay for heme in biological samples using 96-well plates. *Anal. Biochem.* **1999**, *268*, 159–161. [CrossRef] [PubMed]
64. Krieger, E.; Darden, T.; Nabuurs, S.B.; Finkelstein, A.; Vriend, G. Making optimal use of empirical energy functions: Force-field parameterization in crystal space. *Proteins* **2004**, *57*, 678–683. [CrossRef] [PubMed]
65. Vriend, G. WHAT IF: A molecular modeling and drug design program. *J. Mol. Graph.* **1990**, *8*, 52–56. [CrossRef]
66. Canutescu, A.A.; Shelenkov, A.A.; Dunbrack, R.L. A graph-theory algorithm for rapid protein side-chain prediction. *Protein Science* **2003**, *12*, 2001–2014. [CrossRef] [PubMed]
67. Duan, Y.; Wu, C.; Chowdhury, S.; Lee, M.C.; Xiong, G.; Zhang, W.; Yang, R.; Cieplak, P.; Luo, R.; Lee, T.; et al. A point-charge force field for molecular mechanics simulations of proteins based on condensed-phase quantum mechanical calculations. *J. Comput. Chem.* **2003**, *24*, 1999–2012. [CrossRef] [PubMed]
68. Jorgensen, W.L.; Tirado-Rives, J. Potential energy functions for atomic-level simulations of water and organic and biomolecular systems. *Proc. Natl. Acad. Sci. USA* **2005**, *102*, 6665–6670. [CrossRef] [PubMed]

69. Trott, O.; Olson, A.J. AutoDock Vina: Improving the speed and accuracy of docking with a new scoring function, efficient optimization, and multithreading. *J. Comput. Chem.* **2010**, *31*, 455–461. [CrossRef] [PubMed]
70. Pettersen, E.F.; Goddard, T.D.; Huang, C.C.; Couch, G.S.; Greenblatt, D.M.; Meng, E.C.; Ferrin, T.E. UCSF Chimera—A visualization system for exploratory research and analysis. *J. Comput. Chem.* **2004**, *25*, 1605–1612. [CrossRef] [PubMed]

pharmaceuticals

Review

Can the Efficacy of [^{18}F]FDG-PET/CT in Clinical Oncology Be Enhanced by Screening Biomolecular Profiles?

Hazel O'Neill [1,*], Vinod Malik [2], Ciaran Johnston [2], John V Reynolds [1] and Jacintha O'Sullivan [1]

[1] Trinity Translational Medicine Institute, Department of Surgery, Trinity College Dublin, D08W9RT Dublin, Ireland; reynoldsjv@stjames.ie (J.V.R.); osullij4@tcd.ie (J.O.S.)
[2] Department of Radiology, St. James's Hospital, D08 X4RX Dublin, Ireland; malikvi@tcd.ie (V.M.); cjohnston@stjames.ie (C.J.)
* Correspondence: oneillhm@tcd.ie

Received: 18 December 2018; Accepted: 14 January 2019; Published: 23 January 2019

Abstract: Positron Emission Tomography (PET) is a functional imaging modality widely used in clinical oncology. Over the years the sensitivity and specificity of PET has improved with the advent of specific radiotracers, increased technical accuracy of PET scanners and incremental experience of Radiologists. However, significant limitations exist—most notably false positives and false negatives. Additionally, the accuracy of PET varies between cancer types and in some cancers, is no longer considered a standard imaging modality. This review considers the relative influence of macroscopic tumour features such as size and morphology on 2-Deoxy-2-[^{18}F]fluoroglucose ([^{18}F]FDG) uptake by tumours which, though well described in the literature, lacks a comprehensive assessment of biomolecular features which may influence [^{18}F]FDG uptake. The review aims to discuss the potential influence of individual molecular markers of glucose transport, glycolysis, hypoxia and angiogenesis in addition to the relationships between these key cellular processes and their influence on [^{18}F]FDG uptake. Finally, the potential role for biomolecular profiling of individual tumours to predict positivity on PET imaging is discussed to enhance accuracy and clinical utility.

Keywords: [^{18}F]FDG PET/CT; biomarker profiling; cancer

1. Introduction

1.1. Positron Emission Tomography

Positron emission tomography (PET) is an imaging modality used in the diagnosis, staging, restaging and monitoring of cancer. It involves the administration of selected labelled molecules that localise in malignant tissues. These molecules integrate into metabolic pathways or act as receptor ligands in cancer cells, concentrating in tumours. Examples include non-specific tracers of metabolism and cell membrane synthesis such as [^{11}C]Choline, [^{11}C]Acetate and 2-Deoxy-2-[^{18}F]fluoroglucose ([^{18}F]FDG) and specific tracers such as tyrosine kinase inhibitors that localise exclusively to overexpressed epithelial growth factor receptors on cancer cells [1]. Clinically the most widely used tracer is glucose analogue [^{18}F]FDG, a marker of cellular metabolism. Detection of [^{18}F]FDG is the basis of functional cancer imaging and is the focus of this review.

1.2. 2-Deoxy-2-[^{18}F]fluoroglucose ([^{18}F]FDG)

[^{18}F]FDG undergoes cellular uptake via the same mechanisms as glucose and other hexoses: passive diffusion, sodium dependent transport mechanisms and via specific glucose uptake transporters (GLUTs). GLUTs are expressed on the membranes of most cells and facilitate transmembrane glucose transport [2]. Thirteen GLUT subtypes are described with GLUT-1 and GLUT-3 most commonly expressed on cancer cells [2]. Upon entering the cell, [^{18}F]FDG undergoes an initial phosphorylation reaction via hexokinase. Structural modifications produced by the hexose-[^{18}F]FDG bond prevent its catabolism or extracellular transport at a high rate via glucose-6-phosphatase, hence metabolically "trapping" [^{18}F]FDG [3].

The detection of [^{18}F]FDG uptake relies on the ability of the PET detector to detect the natural radioactive decay of fluorine-18 attached to this glucose analogue. This occurs by beta+ decay which involves the conversion of fluorine to oxygen, releasing a positron which travels approximately 1mm before colliding with an electron, becoming neutralised and undergoing an annihilation reaction, producing a pair of gamma rays emitted at 180° from each other. These are detected by the scanner which draws a line of response between the rays. The crossing point of several lines of response indicates the area of greatest [^{18}F]FDG uptake. Abnormal regions of [^{18}F]FDG uptake are detected by comparison with the low overall background activity [3]. Standard uptake value (SUV) is a measure of [^{18}F]FDG uptake by tissues and this is calculated by the division of the activity detected in the region of interest by the injected dose per unit body weight [3].

[^{18}F]FDG competes with glucose for uptake by metabolically active tissue. It localises in tissues with a greater metabolic rate such as tumours, brain, salivary glands, myocardium, gastrointestinal tract, bladder, thyroid and gonads. [^{18}F]FDG uptake has also been noted in brown adipose tissue in 2.3–4% of patients [3]. Thus, PET is not specific to cancerous tissues but those tissues with a greater than average metabolic rate offering functional information about the metabolic state of tissues. The advent of PET-CT has made it feasible to visualize the anatomical and metabolic properties of the tumour simultaneously.

1.3. Limitations: False Positives and Negatives

[^{18}F]FDG-PET scanning is not without limitations, in particular false positives and false negatives impacting on sensitivity and specificity. False positives occur in tissues more metabolically active than background tissue such as inflammatory foci, limiting the specificity of [^{18}F]FDG-PET. False positives can result in additional investigation, inappropriate treatment and altered clinical management with increased costs. Pancreatic cancer, commonly detected at a late stage, lacks an accurate method of detection often hindered by the difficulty in differentiating pancreatitis from pancreatic cancer and compounded by pancreatitis often accompanying cancer. Kubota et al. revealed that 24% of [^{18}F]FDG uptake in pancreatic cancer is consumed by local inflammatory cells, demonstrating the poor specificity of [^{18}F]FDG-PET in differentiating pancreatitis from cancer [4].

Thoracic diseases including tuberculomas, sarcoidosis, cryptococcosis and radiation fibrosis are a common source of false positive results, necessitating further invasive testing [3]. Immunosuppressed cancer patients or recipients of prior radiation are at increased risk of suffering from one of these conditions, effecting the efficacy of [^{18}F]FDG-PET in cancer follow up or diagnosis of lung metastases.

False negatives are another major limitation to [^{18}F]FDG-PET scanning where appropriate scanning fails to detect malignancy. Some of the underlying biology underpinning these false negative results will be outlined later in this review.

1.4. Clinical Importance

[^{18}F]FDG-PET has a significant role in the diagnosis, staging, restaging, prognosis and monitoring of response to therapy in cancer. The functional information on tissue metabolism allows for identification of tumours otherwise undetectable on standard imaging modalities. PET has also had an impact on the treatment planning of cancer patients. Identification of occult metastases by PET alters the clinical management of patients, by avoiding futile surgery in favour of palliative interventions. Despite its usefulness, there is scope to improve the accuracy of PET by addressing the limitations outlined above.

2. Factors Affecting the Clinical Efficacy of PET

2.1. Gross Features

2.1.1. Tumour Size

Small tumour size has been associated with decreased [^{18}F]FDG uptake, accounting for false negative results in many studies [5–9]. This is most notable in the breast cancer setting where the persistent correlation between small tumour size and false negativity has meant that the National Comprehensive Cancer Network (NCCN) no longer endorses PET for evaluating stage I, II or operable stage III invasive disease [10]. A recent systematic review confirmed that [^{18}F]FDG-PET does not have sufficient sensitivity to detect breast tumours <10 mm and is therefore not a recommended first line imaging modality for the initial assessment of primary breast tumours [5]. In bronchoalveolar lung cancer, a study with lung nodules <10 mm identified a negative PET scan in 20% of patients [8]. [^{18}F]FDG uptake in cervical cancer is also influenced by size with a significant association between SUV and tumour size (r = 0.456, p = 0.025) [9]. In oral squamous cell carcinoma (SCC) higher T stage (3 and 4) have increased [^{18}F]FDG uptake compared to lower T stages (1 and 2) [2]. Despite the evidence, small tumour size cannot exclusively cause false negatives. Higashi et al. identified a large 33 mm false negative tumour in their pancreatic study and highlighted that size alone does not influence decreased tumour [^{18}F]FDG uptake [11].

2.1.2. Tumour Grade

Aggressive lesions are associated with higher metabolism and increased [^{18}F]FDG uptake compared to slow growing, less invasive types [5]. Tumour grade has been strongly associated with increased [^{18}F]FDG uptake in breast, musculoskeletal and brain tumours however no correlation exists with mucinous tumours of the GI tract and lung [12,13]. In cervical cancer, Yen et al. reported higher [^{18}F]FDG uptake in poorly differentiated, aggressive tumours compared to lower grade tumours in their 2004 study [9].

2.1.3. Cellularity

The content of the tumour mass, in particular the cellular concentration has an association with [^{18}F]FDG uptake. Poor [^{18}F]FDG uptake by cystic mucinous, or signet ring tumours is attributed to fewer tumour cells forming the tumour mass [13]. Kim et al. and Higashi et al. have both reported a large difference in peak SUVs in mucinous bronchoalveolar carcinoma compared to cell-dense SCC or adenocarcinoma (AC) cancer types [14,15]. One large study by Higashi et al. revealed 57% of bronchoalveolar carcinoma patients as negative on PET while Berger et al. noted false negatives in 40% of patients with mucinous tumours [13,15]. Cellularity is also postulated to be linked to more rapid proliferation, increased likelihood of hypoxia and glycolysis, translating into increased [^{18}F]FDG uptake [16].

2.2. Molecular Features

2.2.1. Heterogeneity

The heterogeneity of the tumour microenvironment dictates the varied intratumoral uptake of [^{18}F]FDG resulting in both false negatives and underestimations of tumour size [17]. Establishing these microenvironmental characteristics that influence [^{18}F]FDG uptake is therefore important in order to optimise the clinical reliability of PET.

Currently, intratumoral variations in [^{18}F]FDG uptake are not clearly defined in clinical practice when staging or planning radiation treatment in cancer, potentially misdiagnosing more extensive disease. Knowledge of tumour micro-environmental factors could augment PET efficacy with accurate prediction of tumour volume and disease extent with biomolecular profiles having a potential role [17].

2.2.2. Metabolism

The preferential role for glycolysis over oxidative phosphorylation in cancer cells forms the basis of effective PET imaging. Glycolysis associated protein expression has been extensively studied with GLUT-1 and GLUT-3 overexpressed in a range of cancer types [18,19]. The evidence for correlating GLUT expression and [^{18}F]FDG uptake is strong. Kurokawa et al. showed a positive correlation between [^{18}F]FDG uptake and GLUT-1 expression [20]. Similarly Kunkel et al. associated high GLUT-1 to increased SUV in oral SCC [21] while Tian et al. confirmed this, no linear relationship between expression and [^{18}F]FDG uptake was noted rather only overexpression facilitates increased SUVs [2].

The increased expression of GLUT-1 and GLUT-3 compared with other GLUT subtypes in cancer cells is in theory due to their significance in facilitating basal glucose transport in cells. They are vital in maintaining glycolysis despite a relative deficiency of glucose in the poorly perfused tumour microenvironment. GLUT-1 and GLUT-3 are therefore largely responsible for facilitating the Warburg effect, that is the preferential use of aerobic glycolysis by tumours compared with oxidative phosphorylation- and satisfying the abnormal glucose requirements of cancer cells. This provides some explanation for increased [^{18}F]FDG uptake associated with these biomarkers of metabolism [2].

The metabolic profile of distant tumour metastasis differs from the primary tumour in some cases. Kurata et al. revealed elevated GLUT-3 and GLUT-5 in liver metastases compared to the primary lung cancer [22]. This differential expression of metabolic markers may present a limitation in biomolecular profiling for enhancing PET as some primary and secondary tumours appear to differ in their protein expression.

Despite several studies correlating high GLUT-1 and [^{18}F]FDG uptake, some studies have revealed discrepant results postulating involvement of other metabolic factors. In oesophageal squamous cell cancer (SCC) hexokinase (HK) II had a higher correlation with [^{18}F]FDG uptake than GLUT-1 expression [23]. Although not as prominent in influencing [^{18}F]FDG uptake as GLUT, HK have been noted to strengthen the statistical significance of GLUT correlation with increased [^{18}F]FDG uptake. Studies in oesophageal SCC and breast cancer could not demonstrate a significant correlation between tumour SUV and HK expression; on logistic regression however HK was identified as adding significance to the correlation between SUV and GLUT-1 expression [19]. This demonstrates the combined role of intracellular FDG transport via GLUTs with the commencement of glycolysis facilitated by HK.

The discordance in metabolic markers of [^{18}F]FDG uptake between studies may not be an artefact but a source of biological significance. Correlations have been documented between GLUT expression and tumour aggressiveness as well as inflammation of normal tissue. Experimental models have shown GLUT-1 and 3 to be overexpressed in both tumour and inflammation though GLUT-1 was higher in tumour tissue while GLUT-3 was higher in inflammatory lesions [24]. This differential expression of biomarkers between cancer and inflammation, both of which exhibit increased [^{18}F]FDG uptake on PET could potentially form some basis for differentiating benign from malignant lesions.

GLUT-1 appears to be the most prominently investigated GLUT in relation to [^{18}F]FDG uptake. Though the studies described above have identified that GLUT-1 overexpression relates to increased [^{18}F]FDG uptake, the correlation seems to vary between cancer types, something that may in part be attributable to the degree of tumour hypoxia (vide infra). Understanding and identifying cancers which exhibit the greatest correlation between GLUT-1 and [^{18}F]FDG uptake could help highlight these cancers by means of a viable biomarker.

2.2.3. Hypoxia

Hypoxia inducible factor 1-alpha (HIF-1α) is known to regulate glucose metabolism and consequently influence the regulation of [^{18}F]FDG uptake. In the absence of oxygen, HIF-1α binds hypoxia response elements (HREs) causing expression of hypoxia responding genes related to angiogenesis, glycolysis and oxygen delivery. The underlying reasoning behind this mechanism is the cell's attempt to prevent death; a mechanism manipulated by cancer in its expression of HIF-1α.

HIF-1α acts as an essential transcription factor involved in regulating metabolic functions by targeting a number of metabolism related proteins (Table 1) [25]. In addition, HIF-1α influences the relative contribution from metabolic function to overall energy production depending on the hypoxic state of the cell. Thus, the tumour hypoxic state affects the relative uptake of [^{18}F]FDG. Pugachev et al. showed a positive correlation between [^{18}F]FDG uptake and pimonidazole staining which identified hypoxic areas of tumour [17]. This supports the Dearling et al. study which revealed [^{18}F]FDG uptake 1.26 times higher in hypoxic tumour regions versus normoxic areas [26].

Tumour necrosis has also been positively associated with [^{18}F]FDG uptake in breast cancer [19]. This is probable due to the pre-necrotic hypoxic environment activating glycolysis and increasing [^{18}F]FDG uptake. This theory is supported by pre-necrotic changes in cancer demonstrating increased [^{18}F]FDG uptake.

Table 1. Targets of HIF-1α. Adapted from Denko et al. [25].

Target Genes	Metabolic Function
GLUT-1/GLUT-3	Cellular Glucose Entry
HKII	Phosphorylation
PGI, PFK1, Aldolase, TPI, GAPDH, PGK, PGM, enolase, PK, PFKFB1-4	Glycolysis
LDHA	Pyruvate>Lactate Conversion
MCT4	Cellular Lactate Removal
PDK1, MXI1	Decreased Mitochondrial Activity
COX4I2, Lon Protease	O_2 Consumption in Hypoxia

GLUT: Glucose uptake transporter; HK: Hexokinase; PGI: Glucose-6-phosphate isomerase; PFK: Phosphofructokinase; TPI: Triose phosphate isomerase; GAPDH: Glyceraldehyde 3-phosphate dehydrogenase; PGK: phosphoglycerate kinase; PGM: phosphoglucomutase; PK: pyruvate kinase; PFKFB: 6-phosphofructo-2-kinase/fructose-2,6-biphosphatase; LDHA: Lactate Dehydrogenase A; MCT: Monocarboxylate transporter; PDK: Pyruvate dehydrogenase kinase; MXI: MAX-interacting protein; COX: Cytochrome c oxidase.

2.2.4. Angiogenesis

Tumour blood vessel status including microvascular blood volume (measured on functional MRI) and microvessel density has also been associated with variations in [^{18}F]FDG uptake [19,27]. Though few studies exist regarding blood flow distribution in cancer, the evidence reveals that blood flow varies with the site, size, type of tumour and micro-vessel density [17]. Histologically identical tumours can also vary in their rates and distribution of blood flow [28]. The impact of angiogenesis on [^{18}F]FDG uptake has been established in few cancer types such as breast cancer and malignant glioma where micro-vessel density and microvascular blood volume have been associated with increased [^{18}F]FDG uptake [19,27].

The influence of angiogenesis on [^{18}F]FDG uptake has led to investigation of the potential role of [^{18}F]FDG PET in monitoring response to anti-angiogenic therapies such as bevacizumab. De Bruyne et al. demonstrated that low [^{18}F]FDG uptake following bevacizumab therapy was associated with improved progression free survival in metastatic colorectal cancer [29]. Additionally, Colavolpe et al. showed that low [^{18}F]FDG uptake on PET following bevacizumab treatment for glioma predicted longer progression-free survival, postulating reduced tumour angiogenesis, resulting in lower SUVs [30]. Similarly Goshen et al. concluded that pre and post bevacizumab [^{18}F]FDG PET was superior in predicting pathological response to bevacizumab compared to standard restaging CT for metastatic colorectal cancer [31].

2.3. Interplay of Biological Features

Identifying individual biological features that influence [^{18}F]FDG uptake is complicated by many of the biological processes being intricately linked. HIF-1α, expressed in hypoxia, regulates several key genes involved in angiogenesis and metabolism. Additionally, angiogenesis and metabolism influence each other and in turn have an impact of hypoxia.

For cellular [^{18}F]FDG uptake to occur, it must reach the tumour site, making perfusion of the tumour facilitated by angiogenesis a key feature in controlling [^{18}F]FDG metabolism [23]. Furthermore, metabolic demands in cancer influence hypoxia which induces vascular endothelial growth factor (VEGF) expression, facilitating blood vessel formation and tumour perfusion. Rapidly proliferating cells also require increased levels of glucose and differentiation has been correlated to [^{18}F]FDG uptake [12,32,33]. When metabolic needs go unaddressed necrosis occurs causing inflammation with additional glucose demands and hypoxia. This intricate interplay between biological features highlights factors influencing [^{18}F]FDG uptake are multifactorial and complex with interpretation of their combined effect on [^{18}F]FDG uptake more important than any individual feature. Figure 1 illustrates this complex interplay of cellular processes.

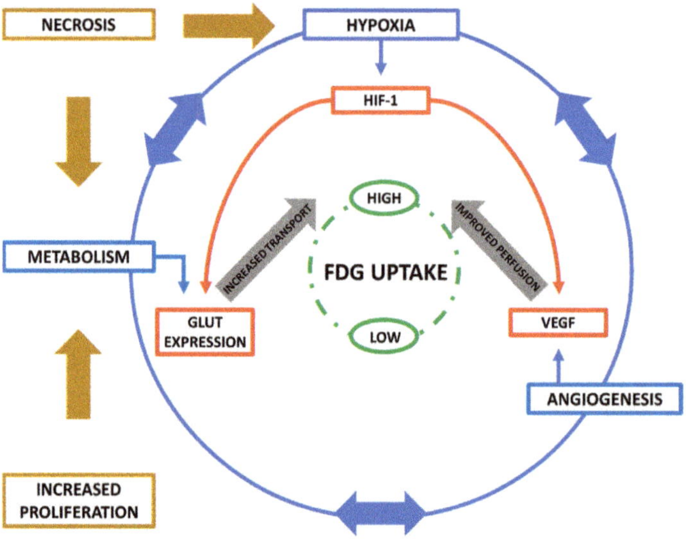

Figure 1. Biomolecular influences on [^{18}F]FDG uptake. Metabolism, hypoxia and angiogenesis all play a role in glucose and therefore [^{18}F]FDG uptake via their associated biomolecular proteins (GLUT, HIF-1α and VEGF respectively). Interrelationships exist between metabolism, hypoxia and angiogenesis such that they play a role in regulating each other. Proliferation and necrosis-induced inflammation increase overall tumoral energy requirements, also driving metabolism and contributing to this complex network.

2.4. Other Factors

2.4.1. P-glycoprotein

Elevated expression of P-glycoprotein has been associated with decreased [^{18}F]FDG uptake [34]. In hepatocellular carcinoma (HCC), both in vivo and in vitro models showed decreased [^{18}F]FDG uptake with increased P-glycoprotein expression [35]. This suggests that [^{18}F]FDG was a substrate of this drug efflux pump, with high levels of expression leading to reduced [^{18}F]FDG uptake. Decreased [^{18}F]FDG uptake and associate high P-glycoprotein expression have been observed in lung cancer and cholangiocarcinoma patients [34].

2.4.2. Tumour Suppressor Genes

Tumour suppressor gene expression has been shown to influence SUVs. Vousden et al. demonstrated that p53 plays a significant role in cell metabolism and other essential cellular functions [36]. As p53 is mutated in up to 50% of tumours, and wild type p53 is anti-Warburg, promoting mitochondrial oxidative phosphorylation, the impact of p53 in promoting glycolysis is consequently potentially of great importance. Several studies have observed that variations in [^{18}F]FDG uptake have been associated with mutated p53 [37,38]. In breast cancer, tumours with p53 mutations exhibit higher SUVs than those expressing the wild type protein [37]. In lung cancer, a statistically significant difference in [^{18}F]FDG uptake was noted between cancers with no mutated tumour suppressors (Rb, P16, P27 and P53) and cancers with alterations which exhibited higher uptake values [38].

2.4.3. Patient Factors

Multiple patient related factors are known to cause variable [^{18}F]FDG uptake [39]. Patient size and body composition affects distribution of [^{18}F]FDG and this is important considering the increasing prevalence of obesity and obesity-associated cancers [39]. Furthermore, high plasma glucose levels reduce [^{18}F]FDG uptake [23]—an issue to account for in the diabetic and pre-diabetic setting. It is proposed that decreased [^{18}F]FDG uptake is a result of the high glucose levels competing with [^{18}F]FDG for cellular uptake [40]. The significance of glucose levels on FDG uptake remains controversial—while some studies report a significant effect of glucose levels on SUV, others dispute this [40–43]. The introduction of a 'glycaemia modified SUV' has been proposed, though there is no evidence of a linear relationship between glycaemia and SUV [11].

As blood glucose levels influence [^{18}F]FDG uptake, drugs that can alter these levels need to be considered. In diabetics, drugs such as insulin or metformin, their dosage and administration time from commencement of PET scan could affect the reliability of PET. Consequently, cancer patients with comorbidities and drugs used to treat them can play a role in influencing [^{18}F]FDG uptake. Corticosteroids may also affect [^{18}F]FDG uptake. Zhao et al. compared the effect of prednisolone therapy on [^{18}F]FDG uptake in granuloma and cancer xenograft rat models identifying that corticosteroids decreased [^{18}F]FDG uptake in the granuloma models but not the cancerous lesions [44]. The potential that corticosteroids could help differentiate between inflammatory and cancerous lesions needs to be further validated as it could enhance the accuracy of PET scanning.

3. Optimising PET with Biomolecular Profiling

3.1. Stratification

It is evident from the literature that PET is a clinically useful diagnostic and prognostic imaging modality in oncology. However, variations in [^{18}F]FDG uptake between patients highlight the apparent influence of tumour biology on PET accuracy and thus its efficacy. As stated herein, gross and molecular tumour features in addition to inherent patient characteristics play a role in influencing [^{18}F]FDG uptake. If the relative influence of each of these factors could be ascertained both clinically and molecularly, it could be employed to enhance the accuracy of PET. The addition of biomolecular testing to PET imaging could also improve the sensitivity in identifying certain tumours. In an era where multimodal therapy is becoming increasingly utilized, the improved information obtained on the tumour could facilitate development of diagnostic algorithms for stratification of patients into appropriate treatment regimens.

This theory has been trailed by Hoeben et al. who investigated the significance of biomolecular profiling in mouse xenograft models, aiming to determine if combining immunohistochemistry (IHC) and [^{18}F]FDG-PET parameters could reliably stratify Head and Neck cancers (HNC) into clusters [45]. By using [^{18}F]FDG-PET as a biomarker and adding an IHC criterion, this group aimed to enhance prognostic prediction and facilitate appropriate treatment selection. Using 14 HNC lines grafted into mice, they revealed a distinct selection of biomarkers related to metabolism, proliferation, hypoxia and perfusion that could match tumours consistently to the correct cell line with high reliability [45]. The potential of combining [^{18}F]FDG-PET with biomolecular profiling added value in terms of providing diagnostic and prognostic information.

3.2. Diagnosis and Predicting Prognosis

[^{18}F]FDG avidity on PET is in itself a 'biomarker,' with studies citing it as a predictor of prognosis at diagnosis and post treatment in head and neck cancer (HNC) and oesophageal cancer [46–48]. In HNC pre-treatment high [^{18}F]FDG uptake is associated with poor survival [49]. Conversely, HNC with an increased [^{18}F]FDG pre-treatment had a better response to radiotherapy [46].

In oesophageal cancer, increased [^{18}F]FDG uptake is also associated with poor prognosis compared to low [^{18}F]FDG uptake [47,48]. Studies have also revealed however that SUVmax is nota prognostic parameter [50,51].

[^{18}F]FDG uptake in oesophageal cancer is also identified as a predictor of lymph node disease, disease free survival (DFS) and recurrence [50,51]. A significant correlation between [^{18}F]FDG uptake and tumour recurrence has also been noted in other cancer types [23,52–54]. The prognostic potential of [^{18}F]FDG uptake in combination with biomarkers of tumour metabolism has also been evaluated. In oral SCC associations were found between increased [^{18}F]FDG uptake in combination with increased GLUT-1 expression and poorer survival while another study showed similar results with GLUT-3 [21,55].

As described above, FDG uptake has been proposed as a prognostic biomarker in some small HNC and oesophageal cancer studies. Whether increased SUVs in smaller tumours predict a worse prognosis compared to decreased SUVs in larger tumours is not clearly defined from this research. It appears that several factors are responsible for predicting outcomes in combination with [^{18}F]FDG uptake. By identifying molecular features that affect [^{18}F]FDG uptake for individual cancers, biomolecular profiling could advance the role of PET in stratifying tumours and increase its efficacy. Table 2 outlines biomarkers and their associated influence on [^{18}F]FDG uptake published to date.

4. Profiling Specific Cancer Types

The relationship between [^{18}F]FDG uptake and tumour biology is not clearly defined with conflicting results between cancer types and subtypes with no definite consensus on which biomarkers are relevant for specific cancer types.

Discordance between studies regarding PET biomarkers can be attributed to variations in study design. Higashi et al. demonstrated in their pancreatic study that the numerical value of SUVs varied between different studies and between PET machines [11]. They suggest that SUV should not be used as an absolute value in the evaluation of [^{18}F]FDG uptake rather broader categories of positive or negative uptake results are more important than absolute values [11].

Biological features and technical differences have both caused discordance in establishing the most appropriate and reliable biomarkers in relation to PET. However, there is evidence for specific biomarkers to predict levels of FDG uptake in some cancer types which are outlined below.

4.1. Oesophageal Cancer

PET's ability to identify metastases not detected by conventional workup have been highlighted in oesophageal cancer [52]. Prediction of prognosis based on tumour SUVs has been shown with pathologic response and DFS correlated with SUV changes following induction therapy [53,54]. Importantly, 10–20% of oesophageal cancers are [^{18}F]FDG negative on PET, demonstrating the need for biomolecular profiling to help identify this sub-group of tumours [56].

Potential biomarkers include size and GLUT-1 expression which positively correlate with SUV [23]. Taylor et al. could not identify a correlation between several prominent tumour markers and SUVmax, namely EGRF, P53, cyclin D1 and VEGF [57]. Although Schreurs et al. observed a significant relationship between HKII and SUVmax there were no significant relationships between GLUT-1, HK-1, HIF-Iα 1, VEGF-C, p53 and Ki-67 with SUV [58].

4.2. Breast Cancer

PET is not recommended for staging or follow-up in operable breast cancer as per the NCCN guidelines on account of the high rate of false negatives, largely attributed to small tumour size [10,59]. As a result, PET is not available to all breast cancer patients. Development of biomolecular profiles could help increase its accuracy by identifying tumours with likely poor [^{18}F]FDG uptake. Recommended markers which indicate increased [^{18}F]FDG uptake are GLUT-1 and HK-1 [19].

4.3. Non-Small Cell Lung Cancer (NSCLC)

The histological differences between NSCLC subtypes have revealed varied results in relation to PET accuracy. Several studies have suggested a high frequency of false negatives in bronchoalveolar carcinoma is due to decreased cellularity an assertion disproved by Yap et al. They showed sensitivity of [^{18}F]FDG PET in bronchoalveolar carcinoma to be high overall with the introduction of more precise classification guidelines by the World Health Organisation [60]. GLUT-1, GLUT-3 and Ki-67 are potential biomarkers which have been positively correlated with increased [^{18}F]FDG uptake in NSCLC [61].

4.4. Glioma

A SR on glioma revealed that [^{18}F]FDG-PET has a sensitivity of 0.77 (95% CI, 0.66–0.85) and specificity of 0.78 (95% CI, 0.54–0.91) [62]. The only biomarker identified influencing [^{18}F]FDG uptake is VEGF [63]. The practicality of using biomolecular profiling to increase sensitivity is made difficult by the inability to obtaining tumour samples as these tumours are often unresectable.

4.5. Head and Neck Cancer

Gronroos et al. revealed that an increased [^{18}F]FDG uptake is associated with a more aggressive phenotype and therefore high P53 and VEGF expression [64]. Detecting the presence or absence of these markers in HNC could enhance accuracy of PET. A recent study by Rasmussen et al. reported a positive correlation between SUVmax and β-tubulin-1 index and significant negative correlations between SUV max and Bcl-2 and P16 [65].

Table 2. Metabolic, hypoxic and angiogenic biomarkers affecting [^{18}F]FDG uptake in different cancer types. A positive association (+) indicates [^{18}F]FDG uptake increased with biomarker. A negative association (−) indicates [^{18}F]FDG uptake decreased with biomarker. A null association (0) indicates biomarker expression was unrelated to [^{18}F]FDG uptake.

Cancer Type	[^{18}F]FDG Uptake Association	Biomarker	Function	Reference
Oesophageal SCC	+	HK-I	Metabolism	[19]
	+	HK-II *	Metabolism	[19]
	−	HK-II	Metabolism	[58]
	+	VEGF	Angiogenesis	[66]
	0	VEGF	Angiogenesis	[57,66]
	0	KI67	Proliferation	[23]
Oesophageal AC	+	GLUT-1	Metabolism	[23,57]
	−	HK-II	Metabolism	[58]
	0	HIF-1α	Hypoxia	[58]
	0	VEGF	Angiogenesis	[23]
	0	P53	TSG	[58]
	0	Ki67	Proliferation	[58]

Table 2. *Cont.*

Cancer Type	[18F]FDG Uptake Association	Biomarker	Function	Reference
Breast	+	GLUT-1	Metabolism	[19]
	+	HK-1	Metabolism	[19]
	0	HK-II **	Metabolism	[19]
	0	HK-III	Metabolism	[19]
	0	HIF-1α	Hypoxia	[19]
	0	VEGF	Angiogenesis	[19]
Head and Neck	−	GLUT-1	Metabolism	[2,21,64]
	+	GLUT-3	Metabolism	[2]
	+	VEGF	Angiogenesis	[64]
Oral SCC	+	GLUT-1 **	Metabolism	[2,21,67]
	+	GLUT-3 **	Metabolism	[2,21]
	+	HK-II	Metabolism	[67]
	+	HIF-1α	Hypoxia	[67]
Cervical	+	GLUT-1	Metabolism	[9,68]
	+	HK-II	Metabolism	[68]
Pancreatic	+	GLUT-1	Metabolism	[18]
Ovarian	+	GLUT-1	Metabolism	[20]
NSCLC	+	GLUT-1	Metabolism	[61,69]
	+	GLUT-3	Metabolism	[61]
	0	GLUT-3	Metabolism	[69]
	+	HIF-1α	Hypoxia	[69]
	0	Ki-67	Proliferation	[69]
Glioma	+	VEGF	Angiogenesis	[63]
Gastric	0	GLUT-1	Metabolism	[70]
	0	HKII	Metabolism	[70]
	+	HIF-1α	Hypoxia	[70]
	0	PCNA	Proliferation	[70]
Colorectal	+	HIF-1α	Hypoxia	[71]
	0	PCNA	Proliferation	[71]
Musculoskeletal	+	GLUT-1	Metabolism	[72]
	+	HK-II	Metabolism	[72]
Hodgkin's Lymphoma	+	GLUT-1	Metabolism	[73]
	0	GLUT-3	Metabolism	[73]
	0	HK-II	Metabolism	[73]
Thyroid	0	GLUT-1	Metabolism	[74]
	0	GLUT-3	Metabolism	[74]
	0	HK-II	Metabolism	[74]
	+	VEGF	Angiogenesis	[74]

* No significant correlation between these biomarkers and SUV though in logistic regression they added value to GLUT-1 correlation. ** These biomarkers were only found to correlate with increased SUV when overexpressed.

5. Conclusions and Future Directions

The influence of biomolecular markers on [18F]FDG uptake has been established and is clearly linked with hypoxia, metabolism and angiogenesis. Despite this, a definite consensus is lacking on associations between biomarkers, [18F]FDG uptake and cancer. Considerable variation and heterogeneity in study design including small sample size, variation in PET algorithms employed between centres; the diverse molecular markers examined and the lack of validation are clearly an issue limiting firm conclusions, and further research is clearly warranted. Biomolecular profiling can articulate the true significance of [18F]FDG uptake while also addressing the limitations of PET in clinical oncology such as false negative results. There is a compelling case that the integration of biomolecular profiling and [^{18}F]FDG PET could enhance diagnosis, improve prognosis prediction and facilitate appropriate stratification of patients to treatment regimens based on a clear characterisation of the tumour, but this needs to be validated in rigorous scientific study.

Author Contributions: Conceptualization: J.V.R., J.O.S., C.J.; Methodology: V.M., H.O.N., J.O.S.; Software: N/A; Validation: N/A; Formal Analysis: N/A; Investigation: H.O.N., V.M., J.O.S.; Resources: J.O.S.; Data Curation: N/A; Writing—original draft preparation: H.O.N.; Writing—review and editing: C.J., J.V.R.; Visualization: H.O.N., J.O.S., V.M.; Supervision: J.V.R., J.O.S., C.J.; Project; Administration: J.O.S.; Funding Acquisition: N/A.

Funding: Hazel O'Neill was supported on the MSc. in Translational Oncology, Trinity College Dublin, Ireland. This research received no additional external funding.

Conflicts of Interest: The authors declare no conflict of interest.

References

1. Slobbe, P.; Windhorst, A.D.; Stigter-van Walsum, M.; Schuit, R.C.; Smit, E.F.; Niessen, H.G.; Solca, F.; Stehle, G.; van Dongen, G.A.; Poot, A.J. Development of [^{18}f]afatinib as new tki-pet tracer for egfr positive tumours. *Nucl. Med. Boil.* **2014**, *41*, 749–757. [CrossRef]
2. Tian, M.; Zhang, H.; Nakasone, Y.; Mogi, K.; Endo, K. Expression of glut-1 and glut-3 in untreated oral squamous cell carcinoma compared with fdg accumulation in a pet study. *Eur. J. Nucl. Med. Mol. Imaging* **2004**, *31*, 5–12. [CrossRef] [PubMed]
3. Chang, J.M.; Lee, H.J.; Goo, J.M.; Lee, H.Y.; Lee, J.J.; Chung, J.K.; Im, J.G. False positive and false negative fdg-pet scans in various thoracic diseases. *Korean J. Radiol.* **2006**, *7*, 57–69. [CrossRef] [PubMed]
4. Kubota, R.; Kubota, K.; Yamada, S.; Tada, M.; Ido, T.; Tamahashi, N. Active and passive mechanisms of [fluorine-18] fluorodeoxyglucose uptake by proliferating and prenecrotic cancer cells in vivo: A microautoradiographic study. *J. Nucl. Med.* **1994**, *35*, 1067–1075. [PubMed]
5. Warning, K.; Hildebrandt, M.G.; Kristensen, B.; Ewertz, M. Utility of 18fdg-pet/ct in breast cancer diagnostics—A systematic review. *Dan. Med. Bull.* **2011**, *58*, A4289.
6. Purohit, B.S.; Ailianou, A.; Dulguerov, N.; Becker, C.D.; Ratib, O.; Becker, M. Fdg-pet/ct pitfalls in oncological head and neck imaging. *Insights Imaging* **2014**, *5*, 585–602. [CrossRef] [PubMed]
7. Jo, I.; Zeon, S.K.; Kim, S.H.; Kim, H.W.; Kang, S.H.; Kwon, S.Y.; Kim, S.J. Correlation of primary tumour fdg uptake with clinicopathologic prognostic factors in invasive ductal carcinoma of the breast. *Nucl. Med. Mol. Imaging* **2015**, *49*, 19–25. [CrossRef] [PubMed]
8. Balogova, S.; Huchet, V.; Kerrou, K.; Nataf, V.; Gutman, F.; Antoine, M.; Ruppert, A.M.; Prignon, A.; Lavolee, A.; Montravers, F.; et al. Detection of bronchioloalveolar cancer by means of pet/ct and 18f-fluorocholine and comparison with 18f-fluorodeoxyglucose. *Nucl. Med. Commun.* **2010**, *31*, 389–397. [CrossRef] [PubMed]
9. Yen, T.C.; See, L.C.; Lai, C.H.; Yah-Huei, C.W.; Ng, K.K.; Ma, S.Y.; Lin, W.J.; Chen, J.T.; Chen, W.J.; Lai, C.R.; et al. ^{18}f-fdg uptake in squamous cell carcinoma of the cervix is correlated with glucose transporter 1 expression. *J. Nucl. Med.* **2004**, *45*, 22–29.
10. Society of Nuclear Medicine and Molecular Imaging. NCCN Practice Guidelines: Narrative Summary of Indications for FDG Pet and PET/CT; 2016. Available online: http://snmmi.files.cms-plus.com/images/NCCN%20Narrative%20Summary%20Feb%202016.pdf (accessed on 22 January 2019).
11. Higashi, T.; Saga, T.; Nakamoto, Y.; Ishimori, T.; Fujimoto, K.; Doi, R.; Imamura, M.; Konishi, J. Diagnosis of pancreatic cancer using fluorine-18 fluorodeoxyglucose positron emission tomography (fdg pet)—Usefulness and limitations in "clinical reality". *Ann. Nucl. Med.* **2003**, *17*, 261–279. [CrossRef] [PubMed]
12. Adler, L.P.; Blair, H.F.; Makley, J.T.; Williams, R.P.; Joyce, M.J.; Leisure, G.; al-Kaisi, N.; Miraldi, F. Noninvasive grading of musculoskeletal tumours using pet. *J. Nucl. Med.* **1991**, *32*, 1508–1512.
13. Berger, K.L.; Nicholson, S.A.; Dehdashti, F.; Siegel, B.A. Fdg pet evaluation of mucinous neoplasms: Correlation of fdg uptake with histopathologic features. *Am. J. Roentgenol.* **2000**, *174*, 1005–1008. [CrossRef] [PubMed]
14. Kim, B.T.; Kim, Y.; Lee, K.S.; Yoon, S.B.; Cheon, E.M.; Kwon, O.J.; Rhee, C.H.; Han, J.; Shin, M.H. Localized form of bronchioloalveolar carcinoma: Fdg pet findings. *Am. J. Roentgenol.* **1998**, *170*, 935–939. [CrossRef] [PubMed]

15. Higashi, K.; Ueda, Y.; Seki, H.; Yuasa, K.; Oguchi, M.; Noguchi, T.; Taniguchi, M.; Tonami, H.; Okimura, T.; Yamamoto, I. Fluorine-18-fdg pet imaging is negative in bronchioloalveolar lung carcinoma. *J. Nucl. Med.* **1998**, *39*, 1016–1020. [PubMed]
16. Norikane, T.; Yamamoto, Y.; Maeda, Y.; Kudomi, N.; Matsunaga, T.; Haba, R.; Iwasaki, A.; Hoshikawa, H.; Nishiyama, Y. Correlation of (18)f-fluoromisonidazole pet findings with hif-1alpha and p53 expressions in head and neck cancer: Comparison with (18)f-fdg pet. *Nucl. Med. Commun.* **2014**, *35*, 30–35. [CrossRef] [PubMed]
17. Pugachev, A.; Ruan, S.; Carlin, S.; Larson, S.M.; Campa, J.; Ling, C.C.; Humm, J.L. Dependence of fdg uptake on tumor microenvironment. *Int. J. Radiat. Oncol. Biol. Phys.* **2005**, *62*, 545–553. [CrossRef] [PubMed]
18. Higashi, T.; Tamaki, N.; Honda, T.; Torizuka, T.; Kimura, T.; Inokuma, T.; Ohshio, G.; Hosotani, R.; Imamura, M.; Konishi, J. Expression of glucose transporters in human pancreatic tumors compared with increased fdg accumulation in pet study. *J. Nucl. Med.* **1997**, *38*, 1337–1344.
19. Bos, R.; van Der Hoeven, J.J.; van Der Wall, E.; van Der Groep, P.; van Diest, P.J.; Comans, E.F.; Joshi, U.; Semenza, G.L.; Hoekstra, O.S.; Lammertsma, A.A.; et al. Biologic correlates of (18)fluorodeoxyglucose uptake in human breast cancer measured by positron emission tomography. *J. Clin. Oncol.* **2002**, *20*, 379–387. [CrossRef]
20. Kurokawa, T.; Yoshida, Y.; Kawahara, K.; Tsuchida, T.; Okazawa, H.; Fujibayashi, Y.; Yonekura, Y.; Kotsuji, F. Expression of glut-1 glucose transfer, cellular proliferation activity and grade of tumor correlate with [f-18]-fluorodeoxyglucose uptake by positron emission tomography in epithelial tumors of the ovary. *Int. J. Cancer* **2004**, *109*, 926–932. [CrossRef]
21. Kunkel, M.; Reichert, T.E.; Benz, P.; Lehr, H.A.; Jeong, J.H.; Wieand, S.; Bartenstein, P.; Wagner, W.; Whiteside, T.L. Overexpression of glut-1 and increased glucose metabolism in tumors are associated with a poor prognosis in patients with oral squamous cell carcinoma. *Cancer* **2003**, *97*, 1015–1024. [CrossRef]
22. Kurata, T.; Oguri, T.; Isobe, T.; Ishioka, S.; Yamakido, M. Differential expression of facilitative glucose transporter (glut) genes in primary lung cancers and their liver metastases. *Jpn. J. Cancer Res. GANN* **1999**, *90*, 1238–1243. [CrossRef] [PubMed]
23. Westerterp, M.; Sloof, G.W.; Hoekstra, O.S.; Ten Kate, F.J.; Meijer, G.A.; Reitsma, J.B.; Boellaard, R.; van Lanschot, J.J.; Molthoff, C.F. 18fdg uptake in oesophageal adenocarcinoma: Linking biology and outcome. *J. Cancer Res. Clin. Oncol.* **2008**, *134*, 227–236. [CrossRef] [PubMed]
24. Mochizuki, T.; Tsukamoto, E.; Kuge, Y.; Kanegae, K.; Zhao, S.; Hikosaka, K.; Hosokawa, M.; Kohanawa, M.; Tamaki, N. Fdg uptake and glucose transporter subtype expressions in experimental tumor and inflammation models. *J. Nucl. Med.* **2001**, *42*, 1551–1555. [PubMed]
25. Denko, N.C. Hypoxia, hif1 and glucose metabolism in the solid tumour. *Nat. Rev. Cancer* **2008**, *8*, 705–713. [CrossRef]
26. Dearling, J.L.; Flynn, A.A.; Sutcliffe-Goulden, J.; Petrie, I.A.; Boden, R.; Green, A.J.; Boxer, G.M.; Begent, R.H.; Pedley, R.B. Analysis of the regional uptake of radiolabeled deoxyglucose analogs in human tumor xenografts. *J. Nucl. Med.* **2004**, *45*, 101–107. [PubMed]
27. Aronen, H.J.; Pardo, F.S.; Kennedy, D.N.; Belliveau, J.W.; Packard, S.D.; Hsu, D.W.; Hochberg, F.H.; Fischman, A.J.; Rosen, B.R. High microvascular blood volume is associated with high glucose uptake and tumor angiogenesis in human gliomas. *Clin. Cancer Res.* **2000**, *6*, 2189–2200. [PubMed]
28. Laking, G.; Price, P. Radionuclide imaging of perfusion and hypoxia. *Eur. J. Nucl. Med. Mol. Imaging* **2010**, *37* (Suppl. 1), S20–S29. [CrossRef] [PubMed]
29. De Bruyne, S.; Van Damme, N.; Smeets, P.; Ferdinande, L.; Ceelen, W.; Mertens, J.; Van de Wiele, C.; Troisi, R.; Libbrecht, L.; Laurent, S.; et al. Value of dce-mri and fdg-pet/ct in the prediction of response to preoperative chemotherapy with bevacizumab for colorectal liver metastases. *Br. J. Cancer* **2012**, *106*, 1926–1933. [CrossRef]
30. Colavolpe, C.; Chinot, O.; Metellus, P.; Mancini, J.; Barrie, M.; Bequet-Boucard, C.; Tabouret, E.; Mundler, O.; Figarella-Branger, D.; Guedj, E. Fdg-pet predicts survival in recurrent high-grade gliomas treated with bevacizumab and irinotecan. *Neuro Oncol.* **2012**, *14*, 649–657. [CrossRef]
31. Goshen, E.; Davidson, T.; Zwas, S.T.; Aderka, D. Pet/ct in the evaluation of response to treatment of liver metastases from colorectal cancer with bevacizumab and irinotecan. *Technol. Cancer Res. Treat.* **2006**, *5*, 37–43. [CrossRef]

32. Crippa, F.; Seregni, E.; Agresti, R.; Chiesa, C.; Pascali, C.; Bogni, A.; Decise, D.; De Sanctis, V.; Greco, M.; Daidone, M.G.; et al. Association between [^{18}f]fluorodeoxyglucose uptake and postoperative histopathology, hormone receptor status, thymidine labelling index and p53 in primary breast cancer: A preliminary observation. *Eur. J. Nucl. Med.* **1998**, *25*, 1429–1434. [CrossRef] [PubMed]
33. Schulte, M.; Brecht-Krauss, D.; Heymer, B.; Guhlmann, A.; Hartwig, E.; Sarkar, M.R.; Diederichs, C.G.; Schultheiss, M.; Kotzerke, J.; Reske, S.N. Fluorodeoxyglucose positron emission tomography of soft tissue tumours: Is a non-invasive determination of biological activity possible? *Eur. J. Nucl. Med.* **1999**, *26*, 599–605. [CrossRef]
34. Smith, T.A. Influence of chemoresistance and p53 status on fluoro-2-deoxy-d-glucose incorporation in cancer. *Nucl. Med. Biol.* **2010**, *37*, 51–55. [CrossRef]
35. Seo, S.; Hatano, E.; Higashi, T.; Nakajima, A.; Nakamoto, Y.; Tada, M.; Tamaki, N.; Iwaisako, K.; Kitamura, K.; Ikai, I.; et al. P-glycoprotein expression affects 18f-fluorodeoxyglucose accumulation in hepatocellular carcinoma in vivo and in vitro. *Int. J. Oncol.* **2009**, *34*, 1303–1312.
36. Berkers, C.R.; Maddocks, O.D.; Cheung, E.C.; Mor, I.; Vousden, K.H. Metabolic regulation by p53 family members. *Cell Metab.* **2013**, *18*, 617–633. [CrossRef]
37. Groheux, D.; Giacchetti, S.; Moretti, J.L.; Porcher, R.; Espie, M.; Lehmann-Che, J.; de Roquancourt, A.; Hamy, A.S.; Cuvier, C.; Vercellino, L.; et al. Correlation of high 18f-fdg uptake to clinical, pathological and biological prognostic factors in breast cancer. *Eur. J. Nucl. Med. Mol. Imaging* **2011**, *38*, 426–435. [CrossRef]
38. Sasaki, M.; Sugio, K.; Kuwabara, Y.; Koga, H.; Nakagawa, M.; Chen, T.; Kaneko, K.; Hayashi, K.; Shioyama, Y.; Sakai, S.; et al. Alterations of tumor suppressor genes (rb, p16, p27 and p53) and an increased fdg uptake in lung cancer. *Ann. Nucl. Med.* **2003**, *17*, 189–196. [CrossRef] [PubMed]
39. Adams, M.C.; Turkington, T.G.; Wilson, J.M.; Wong, T.Z. A systematic review of the factors affecting accuracy of suv measurements. *Am. J. Roentgenol.* **2010**, *195*, 310–320. [CrossRef] [PubMed]
40. Bares, R.; Klever, P.; Hauptmann, S.; Hellwig, D.; Fass, J.; Cremerius, U.; Schumpelick, V.; Mittermayer, C.; Bull, U. F-18 fluorodeoxyglucose pet in vivo evaluation of pancreatic glucose metabolism for detection of pancreatic cancer. *Radiology* **1994**, *192*, 79–86. [CrossRef]
41. Friess, H.; Langhans, J.; Ebert, M.; Beger, H.G.; Stollfuss, J.; Reske, S.N.; Buchler, M.W. Diagnosis of pancreatic cancer by 2[^{18}f]-fluoro-2-deoxy-d-glucose positron emission tomography. *Gut* **1995**, *36*, 771–777. [CrossRef]
42. Zimny, M.; Bares, R.; Fass, J.; Adam, G.; Cremerius, U.; Dohmen, B.; Klever, P.; Sabri, O.; Schumpelick, V.; Buell, U. Fluorine-18 fluorodeoxyglucose positron emission tomography in the differential diagnosis of pancreatic carcinoma: A report of 106 cases. *Eur. J. Nucl. Med.* **1997**, *24*, 678–682. [CrossRef] [PubMed]
43. Diederichs, C.G.; Staib, L.; Glatting, G.; Beger, H.G.; Reske, S.N. Fdg pet: Elevated plasma glucose reduces both uptake and detection rate of pancreatic malignancies. *J. Nucl. Med.* **1998**, *39*, 1030–1033.
44. Zhao, S.; Kuge, Y.; Nakada, K.; Mochizuki, T.; Takei, T.; Okada, F.; Tamaki, N. Effect of steroids on [^{18}f]fluorodeoxyglucose uptake in an experimental tumour model. *Nucl. Med. Commun.* **2004**, *25*, 727–730. [CrossRef] [PubMed]
45. Hoeben, B.A.; Starmans, M.H.; Leijenaar, R.T.; Dubois, L.J.; van der Kogel, A.J.; Kaanders, J.H.; Boutros, P.C.; Lambin, P.; Bussink, J. Systematic analysis of 18f-fdg pet and metabolism, proliferation and hypoxia markers for classification of head and neck tumors. *BMC Cancer* **2014**, *14*, 130. [CrossRef] [PubMed]
46. Rege, S.; Safa, A.A.; Chaiken, L.; Hoh, C.; Juillard, G.; Withers, H.R. Positron emission tomography: An independent indicator of radiocurability in head and neck carcinomas. *Am. J. Clin. Oncol.* **2000**, *23*, 164–169. [CrossRef]
47. Sepesi, B.; Raymond, D.P.; Polomsky, M.; Watson, T.J.; Litle, V.R.; Jones, C.E.; Hu, R.; Qiu, X.; Peters, J.H. Does the value of pet-ct extend beyond pretreatment staging? An analysis of survival in surgical patients with esophageal cancer. *J. Gastrointest. Surg.* **2009**, *13*, 2121–2127. [CrossRef]
48. Suzuki, A.; Xiao, L.; Hayashi, Y.; Macapinlac, H.A.; Welsh, J.; Lin, S.H.; Lee, J.H.; Bhutani, M.S.; Maru, D.M.; Hofstetter, W.L.; et al. Prognostic significance of baseline positron emission tomography and importance of clinical complete response in patients with esophageal or gastroesophageal junction cancer treated with definitive chemoradiotherapy. *Cancer* **2011**, *117*, 4823–4833. [CrossRef]
49. Minn, H.; Lapela, M.; Klemi, P.J.; Grenman, R.; Leskinen, S.; Lindholm, P.; Bergman, J.; Eronen, E.; Haaparanta, M.; Joensuu, H. Prediction of survival with fluorine-18-fluoro-deoxyglucose and pet in head and neck cancer. *J. Nucl. Med.* **1997**, *38*, 1907–1911.

50. Chatterton, B.E.; Ho Shon, I.; Baldey, A.; Lenzo, N.; Patrikeos, A.; Kelley, B.; Wong, D.; Ramshaw, J.E.; Scott, A.M. Positron emission tomography changes management and prognostic stratification in patients with oesophageal cancer: Results of a multicentre prospective study. *Eur. J. Nucl. Med. Mol. Imaging* **2009**, *36*, 354–361. [CrossRef]
51. Gillies, R.S.; Middleton, M.R.; Han, C.; Marshall, R.E.; Maynard, N.D.; Bradley, K.M.; Gleeson, F.V. Role of positron emission tomography-computed tomography in predicting survival after neoadjuvant chemotherapy and surgery for oesophageal adenocarcinoma. *Br. J. Surg.* **2012**, *99*, 239–245. [CrossRef]
52. Meyers, B.F.; Downey, R.J.; Decker, P.A.; Keenan, R.J.; Siegel, B.A.; Cerfolio, R.J.; Landreneau, R.J.; Reed, C.E.; Balfe, D.M.; Dehdashti, F.; et al. The utility of positron emission tomography in staging of potentially operable carcinoma of the thoracic esophagus: Results of the american college of surgeons oncology group z0060 trial. *J. Thorac. Cardiovasc. Surg.* **2007**, *133*, 738–745. [CrossRef] [PubMed]
53. Cerfolio, R.J.; Bryant, A.S. Maximum standardized uptake values on positron emission tomography of esophageal cancer predicts stage, tumor biology and survival. *Ann. Thorac. Surg.* **2006**, *82*, 391–394; discussion 394–395. [CrossRef] [PubMed]
54. Rizk, N.; Downey, R.J.; Akhurst, T.; Gonen, M.; Bains, M.S.; Larson, S.; Rusch, V. Preoperative ^{18}[f]-fluorodeoxyglucose positron emission tomography standardized uptake values predict survival after esophageal adenocarcinoma resection. *Ann. Thorac. Surg.* **2006**, *81*, 1076–1081. [CrossRef] [PubMed]
55. Baer, S.; Casaubon, L.; Schwartz, M.R.; Marcogliese, A.; Younes, M. Glut3 expression in biopsy specimens of laryngeal carcinoma is associated with poor survival. *Laryngoscope* **2002**, *112*, 393–396. [CrossRef]
56. Van Westreenen, H.L.; Heeren, P.A.; van Dullemen, H.M.; van der Jagt, E.J.; Jager, P.L.; Groen, H.; Plukker, J.T. Positron emission tomography with f-18-fluorodeoxyglucose in a combined staging strategy of esophageal cancer prevents unnecessary surgical explorations. *J. Gastrointest. Surg.* **2005**, *9*, 54–61. [CrossRef] [PubMed]
57. Taylor, M.D.; Smith, P.W.; Brix, W.K.; Wick, M.R.; Theodosakis, N.; Swenson, B.R.; Kozower, B.D.; Jones, D.R. Correlations between selected tumor markers and fluorodeoxyglucose maximal standardized uptake values in esophageal cancer. *Eur. J. Cardio-Thorac. Surg.* **2009**, *35*, 699–705. [CrossRef] [PubMed]
58. Schreurs, L.M.; Smit, J.K.; Pavlov, K.; Pultrum, B.B.; Pruim, J.; Groen, H.; Hollema, H.; Plukker, J.T. Prognostic impact of clinicopathological features and expression of biomarkers related to (18)f-fdg uptake in esophageal cancer. *Ann. Surg. Oncol.* **2014**, *21*, 3751–3757. [CrossRef] [PubMed]
59. Kumar, R.; Chauhan, A.; Zhuang, H.; Chandra, P.; Schnall, M.; Alavi, A. Clinicopathologic factors associated with false negative fdg-pet in primary breast cancer. *Breast Cancer Res. Treat.* **2006**, *98*, 267–274. [CrossRef]
60. Yap, C.S.; Schiepers, C.; Fishbein, M.C.; Phelps, M.E.; Czernin, J. Fdg-pet imaging in lung cancer: How sensitive is it for bronchioloalveolar carcinoma? *Eur. J. Nucl. Med. Mol. Imaging* **2002**, *29*, 1166–1173. [CrossRef] [PubMed]
61. Marom, E.M.; Aloia, T.A.; Moore, M.B.; Hara, M.; Herndon, J.E., 2nd; Harpole, D.H., Jr.; Goodman, P.C.; Patz, E.F., Jr. Correlation of fdg-pet imaging with glut-1 and glut-3 expression in early-stage non-small cell lung cancer. *Lung Cancer* **2001**, *33*, 99–107. [CrossRef]
62. Nihashi, T.; Dahabreh, I.J.; Terasawa, T. Diagnostic accuracy of pet for recurrent glioma diagnosis: A meta-analysis. *Am. J. Neuroradiol.* **2013**, *34*, 944–950, s941-911. [CrossRef] [PubMed]
63. Cher, L.M.; Murone, C.; Lawrentschuk, N.; Ramdave, S.; Papenfuss, A.; Hannah, A.; O'Keefe, G.J.; Sachinidis, J.I.; Berlangieri, S.U.; Fabinyi, G.; et al. Correlation of hypoxic cell fraction and angiogenesis with glucose metabolic rate in gliomas using 18f-fluoromisonidazole, 18f-fdg pet and immunohistochemical studies. *J. Nucl. Med.* **2006**, *47*, 410–418. [PubMed]
64. Grönroos, T.J.; Lehtiö, K.; Söderström, K.-O.; Kronqvist, P.; Laine, J.; Eskola, O.; Viljanen, T.; Grénman, R.; Solin, O.; Minn, H. Hypoxia, blood flow and metabolism in squamous-cell carcinoma of the head and neck: Correlations between multiple immunohistochemical parameters and pet. *BMC Cancer* **2014**, *14*, 876. [CrossRef] [PubMed]
65. Rasmussen, G.B.; Vogelius, I.R.; Rasmussen, J.H.; Schumaker, L.; Ioffe, O.; Cullen, K.; Fischer, B.M.; Therkildsen, M.H.; Specht, L.; Bentzen, S.M. Immunohistochemical biomarkers and fdg uptake on pet/ct in head and neck squamous cell carcinoma. *Acta Oncol.* **2015**, *54*, 1408–1415. [CrossRef] [PubMed]
66. Kobayashi, M.; Kaida, H.; Kawahara, A.; Hattori, S.; Kurata, S.; Hayakawa, M.; Hirose, Y.; Uchida, M.; Kage, M.; Fujita, H.; et al. The relationship between glut-1 and vascular endothelial growth factor expression and 18f-fdg uptake in esophageal squamous cell cancer patients. *Clin. Nucl. Med.* **2012**, *37*, 447–452. [CrossRef] [PubMed]

67. Yamada, T.; Uchida, M.; Kwang-Lee, K.; Kitamura, N.; Yoshimura, T.; Sasabe, E.; Yamamoto, T. Correlation of metabolism/hypoxia markers and fluorodeoxyglucose uptake in oral squamous cell carcinomas. *Oral Surg. Oral Med. Oral Pathol. Oral Radiol.* **2012**, *113*, 464–471. [CrossRef] [PubMed]
68. Tong, S.Y.; Lee, J.M.; Ki, K.D.; Choi, Y.J.; Seol, H.J.; Lee, S.K.; Huh, C.Y.; Kim, G.Y.; Lim, S.J. Correlation between fdg uptake by pet/ct and the expressions of glucose transporter type 1 and hexokinase ii in cervical cancer. *Int. J. Gynecol. Cancer* **2012**, *22*, 654–658. [CrossRef]
69. Van Baardwijk, A.; Dooms, C.; van Suylen, R.J.; Verbeken, E.; Hochstenbag, M.; Dehing-Oberije, C.; Rupa, D.; Pastorekova, S.; Stroobants, S.; Buell, U.; et al. The maximum uptake of (18)f-deoxyglucose on positron emission tomography scan correlates with survival, hypoxia inducible factor-1alpha and glut-1 in non-small cell lung cancer. *Eur. J. Cancer* **2007**, *43*, 1392–1398. [CrossRef]
70. Takebayashi, R.; Izuishi, K.; Yamamoto, Y.; Kameyama, R.; Mori, H.; Masaki, T.; Suzuki, Y. [^{18}f]fluorodeoxyglucose accumulation as a biological marker of hypoxic status but not glucose transport ability in gastric cancer. *J. Exp. Clin. Cancer Res.* **2013**, *32*, 34. [CrossRef]
71. Izuishi, K.; Yamamoto, Y.; Sano, T.; Takebayashi, R.; Nishiyama, Y.; Mori, H.; Masaki, T.; Morishita, A.; Suzuki, Y. Molecular mechanism underlying the detection of colorectal cancer by 18f-2-fluoro-2-deoxy-d-glucose positron emission tomography. *J. Gastrointest. Surg.* **2012**, *16*, 394–400. [CrossRef]
72. Hamada, K.; Tomita, Y.; Qiu, Y.; Zhang, B.; Ueda, T.; Myoui, A.; Higuchi, I.; Yoshikawa, H.; Aozasa, K.; Hatazawa, J. 18f-fdg-pet of musculoskeletal tumors: A correlation with the expression of glucose transporter 1 and hexokinase II. *Ann. Nucl. Med.* **2008**, *22*, 699–705. [CrossRef] [PubMed]
73. Shim, H.K.; Lee, W.W.; Park, S.Y.; Kim, H.; Kim, S.E. Relationship between fdg uptake and expressions of glucose transporter type 1, type 3 and hexokinase-ii in reed-sternberg cells of hodgkin lymphoma. *Oncol. Res.* **2009**, *17*, 331–337. [CrossRef] [PubMed]
74. Kim, B.H.; Kim, I.J.; Kim, S.S.; Kim, S.J.; Lee, C.H.; Kim, Y.K. Relationship between biological marker expression and fluorine-18 fluorodeoxyglucose uptake in incidentally detected thyroid cancer. *Cancer Biother. Radiopharm.* **2010**, *25*, 309–315. [CrossRef] [PubMed]

pharmaceuticals

MDPI

Review

Cyclooxygenase-1 (COX-1) and COX-1 Inhibitors in Cancer: A Review of Oncology and Medicinal Chemistry Literature

Alessandra Pannunzio and Mauro Coluccia *

Department of Pharmacy-Drug Sciences, University of Bari "Aldo Moro", Via E. Orabona 4, I-70125 Bari, Italy; alessandra.pannunzio@uniba.it

* Correspondence: mauro.coluccia@uniba.it; Tel.: +39-080-544-2788

Received: 4 September 2018; Accepted: 9 October 2018; Published: 11 October 2018

Abstract: Prostaglandins and thromboxane are lipid signaling molecules deriving from arachidonic acid by the action of the cyclooxygenase isoenzymes COX-1 and COX-2. The role of cyclooxygenases (particularly COX-2) and prostaglandins (particularly PGE_2) in cancer-related inflammation has been extensively investigated. In contrast, COX-1 has received less attention, although its expression increases in several human cancers and a pathogenetic role emerges from experimental models. COX-1 and COX-2 isoforms seem to operate in a coordinate manner in cancer pathophysiology, especially in the tumorigenesis process. However, in some cases, exemplified by the serous ovarian carcinoma, COX-1 plays a pivotal role, suggesting that other histopathological and molecular subtypes of cancer disease could share this feature. Importantly, the analysis of functional implications of COX-1-signaling, as well as of pharmacological action of COX-1-selective inhibitors, should not be restricted to the COX pathway and to the effects of prostaglandins already known for their ability of affecting the tumor phenotype. A knowledge-based choice of the most appropriate tumor cell models, and a major effort in investigating the COX-1 issue in the more general context of arachidonic acid metabolic network by using the systems biology approaches, should be strongly encouraged.

Keywords: cyclooxygenase-1; cyclooxygenase-2; cancer; inflammation; tumorigenesis; COX-1 inhibitor

1. Introduction

Already in 1863, the German pathologist Rudolf C. Virchow had observed that some cancers were inherently associated with white blood cell infiltration [1]. However, it was only at the end of 20th century that an increasing body of research led to propose chronic inflammation as one of the enabling characteristics of cancer development [2,3], and the complex inflammatory network in premalignant and frankly malignant disease is now actively explored with the aim of translating epidemiological and experimental evidence into clinical practice [4].

Cancer may originate in the chronic inflammation setting associated with persistent infections, immune-mediated damage, or prolonged exposure to irritants. On the other hand, the genetic and epigenetic alterations underlying the cancerogenesis process inevitably modify the tissue homeostasis and may induce a chronic inflammatory response. Irrespective of the presumed primary or secondary nature of the process, inflammatory cells and mediators can be detected in most tumor tissues, where they act on both tumor and stromal cells and contribute to determine a tumor-promoting microenvironment [5].

In the general complexity of the inflammatory response (hundreds of chemical mediators have been identified, but how they function in a coordinated manner is still not fully understood), the arachidonic acid (AA) metabolites play a relevant role which appears intertwined with their functions in cell and tissue homeostasis [6]. Prostaglandins (PGs), including PGD_2, PGE_2, PGF_{2a},

PGI_2 and thromboxane $(TX)A_2$ (collectively known also as prostanoids) are produced from arachidonic acid by sequential actions of cyclooxygenases (COX-1 or COX-2) and specific synthases, and they exert their effects in autocrine and/or paracrine manner mainly through G protein-coupled receptors (GPCRs) at the cell surface [7].

The involvement of prostaglandins in cancer was first evidenced in human esophageal carcinoma cells, when their invasive and metastatic potential in nude mice was found to be related to PGE_2 and PGF_{2a} production [8]. Elevated levels of PGE_2 have been found in numerous cancers, and its effects on multiple cell signaling pathways involved in tumor malignant phenotype induction and maintenance have been thereafter demonstrated [9–13]. However, PGE_2 is not the only PG involved in carcinogenesis. PGD_2 potentially contributes to the colon cancer risk in ulcerative colitis [14]; more recently, $(TX)A_2$ was found to be involved in colorectal cancer pathophysiology [15,16], as well as in multiple myeloma [17] and lung [18] cancer cell proliferation.

The committed step of PG biosynthesis is catalyzed by COX-1 and COX-2 isoforms. These enzymes display many similarities in structure and catalytic properties and yield the same product, PGH_2. However, COX-1 and COX-2 are different in their regulation of expression, tissue distribution, and associated synthases, thus subserving distinct biological tasks. COX-1 is constitutively expressed in most tissues (e.g., platelets, lung, prostate, brain, gastrointestinal tract, kidney, liver and spleen), where the COX-1-derived prostanoids are involved in homeostatic functions. It is generally accepted that COX-1 activity maintains the prostanoid production at a basal rate, and allows a rapid increase when cell membrane remodeling produces a rise of free AA. In contrast, COX-2 is generally considered as the inducible isoform, responsible for enhanced prostanoid production in response to inflammatory stimuli and growth factors during inflammation and various pathological conditions, including cancer [19,20]. It should be noted, however, that the concept of "constitutive" and "inducible" isoforms has been challenged by growing evidence indicating that both isoforms are present in normal tissues and can be up-regulated in various pathological conditions [21]. Both the expression and regulation of COX isoforms have been intensively investigated, and reviews about transcriptional regulatory mechanisms [22], and the regulation of gene expression at the co- or post-transcriptional level [23] have been recently published.

The role of cyclooxygenases (in particular COX-2) and prostaglandin products (in particular PGE_2) in cancer-related inflammation has been extensively investigated in many neoplastic diseases, including esophageal [24], gastrointestinal [25,26] and pancreatic [27] cancers, breast [28] and cervical [29] cancers, renal [30], prostate [31], and bladder [32] cancers, skin [33,34] and head and neck [35] cancers, hematological tumors [36], and mesothelioma [37]. Tumor cells are often characterized by COX-2 aberrant expression [38,39], resulting from transcriptional and/or post-transcriptional alterations and contributing to tumor diseases, such as in colorectal cancer [40]. Importantly, the tumor-associated aberrant expression of COX-2 is often related to epigenetic alterations affecting COX-2 gene (PTGS2) as well as other genes involved into biosynthesis and signaling of its main prostaglandin products [41].

Epidemiological data are convincingly supported by various in vivo experimental systems, including chemically induced or transgenic models of colorectal, breast, and other types of cancer [42]. Finally, the therapeutic potential of aspirin, traditional nonsteroidal anti-inflammatory drugs (NSAIDs) and COX-2-selective inhibitors (coxibs) in human cancer has also been widely explored. A very large body of research, including about 2000 relevant publications only for aspirin, proposes that the anticancer activity of these drugs depends upon their ability to interfere with multiple pro-tumorigenic signaling pathways, some of them COX-dependent [38] and others COX-independent [43].

Unlike COX-2, the role of COX-1 in cancer has generally received less attention. Being usually considered as the constitutively expressed isoform that is involved in homeostatic cell and tissue functions, COX-1 was thought not be involved in carcinogenesis. However, increased levels of COX-1 expression have been occasionally reported in several cancers [44], and it has been shown that the genetic disruption of COX-1 is as effective as COX-2 disruption in reducing intestinal [45] and skin tumorigenesis [46] in mouse models, thus suggesting that both COX isoforms could cooperate in the cancerogenesis process. In the following, an overview of the available evidence about COX-1 expression and involvement in different neoplastic diseases will be presented. The objective of this review is to go through the COX-1-relevant literature in oncology and medicinal chemistry, thus attempting to fill the existing gap and highlighting the potential future studies.

2. COX-1 Involvement in Neoplastic Diseases

Renal cell carcinoma. The pathophysiological relevance of COX-2 in renal cell carcinoma (RCC) is generally acknowledged, and recently, it has been shown that COX-2 inhibition enhances the efficacy of immunotherapy and tyrosine kinase inhibitor-based treatment [30]. COX-1 expression, however, has been practically unexplored, except for a report on COX-1 mRNA overexpression in an RCC rat model [47]. Interestingly, two recent immunohistochemical investigations have shown a correlation between COX-1 overexpression and poor prognosis in RCC [48], and the validity of the combined use of COX-1 and VEGF in RCC histopathologic prognosis [49].

Skin cancer. The role of cyclooxygenase-dependent signaling in skin pathophysiology and non-melanoma carcinogenesis has been recently reviewed [33]. There is accumulating evidence that cyclooxygenase-2 may be involved in the pathogenesis of non-melanoma skin cancer, whereas COX-1 expression appears unaltered with respect to healthy tissue. At preclinical level, however, genetic studies show that the activity of both COX isoforms is mechanistically involved in the basal cell carcinoma pathogenesis [50,51].

Head and neck cancer. There are few data regarding COX-1 in head and neck cancer. A comparison of cyclooxygenase-1 expression levels between cancerous tissue from head and neck cancer patients and normal mucosa was performed by immunohistochemistry, Western blotting, and real-time RT-PCR (reverse transcription polymerase chain reaction), showing COX-1 overexpression in cancer cells and no expression in normal mucosa [52]. A progression-associated up-regulation of COX-1 expression was detected by immunohistochemistry in patients with hyperplasia, dysplasia, and carcinoma of oral mucosa [53] and a major expression of either COX-1 or COX-2 was reported in patients with oral squamous cell carcinoma with respect to normal mucosa [54]. More recently, tumor samples from patients with sebaceous gland carcinoma, an aggressive tumor commonly localized at Meibomian or Zeis glands, were examined by high-throughput tissue microarray for the expression of proteins involved in angiogenesis, inflammation, apoptosis, cell proliferation, cell-to-cell contact, and carcinogenesis. High expression of COX-1 and COX-2 was reported in 97% and 82% of patients, respectively [55]. Interesting implications on the COX-1 role derive also from in vitro investigations in head and neck squamous cell carcinoma (HNSCC) cell lines, in which the effects of pharmacologic inhibitors of cyclooxygenases were compared to those of small-interfering RNA as far as cell-growth, vascular endothelial growth factor (VEGF) production, and intracellular signaling are concerned [56,57]. The results showed that COX-2 inhibition blocked VEGF productions in some HNSCC cells; in contrast, other COX-2 (and PGE_2) expressing HNSCC cells showed little response to COX-2 inhibition, this effect depending upon a differential expression of COX-1.

Esophageal cancer. Barrett's esophagus, a complication of the chronic gastro-esophageal reflux disease, represents the best-known risk factor for esophageal adenocarcinoma development. Esophageal cancer prevention strategies [58], the role of inflammatory mediators in the disease pathophysiology [24], as well as encouraging experimental and epidemiological data on chemoprophylaxis with NSAIDs in patients with Barrett's esophagus have been recently reviewed [59], along with a body of evidence supporting a role for COX-2 in the pathogenetic sequence leading to esophageal adenocarcinoma [60,61]. Interestingly, a possible involvement of COX-1 in the disease pathophysiology had already been suggested by the co-expression of both COX isoforms and angiogenic (VEGF-A) and lymphangiogenic (VEGF-C) growth factors in primary human tumor samples [62]. More recently, a possible cooperation of COX-1 and COX-2 isoforms has been suggested in an investigation of the PGE_2 pathway in a rat model of esophageal adenocarcinoma induced by gastroduodenal reflux resulting from esophagojejunostomy [63], as well as by the finding that in the same experimental model indomethacin (a dual COX-1/COX-2 inhibitor) reduced the inflammatory lesions and tumor development, whereas a selective COX-2 inhibitor (MF-tricyclic) was ineffective [64]. Interestingly, a recent meta-analysis of nine observational studies has shown that both low-dose aspirin and non-aspirin COX inhibitor use is associated with a reduced risk of developing esophageal adenocarcinoma in patients with Barrett's esophagus [65].

Colorectal cancer. In the colorectal carcinogenesis, the long-term transition process from normal mucosa to benign adenoma and final carcinoma provides the possibility to adopt preventive measures. Many evidences exist underlying the pathophysiological link between chronic inflammation and colorectal cancer [66], and the role of COX-2 in the carcinogenesis process has been extensively investigated [67,68]. COX-1 and COX-2 mRNA expression profiles were examined in tumor tissue in comparison to normal mucosa in stage III (Dukes' C) colorectal cancer patients by Church et al. [69]. In contrast to the general opinion that constitutive COX-1 was not subject to variable expression, an altered regulation of COX-1 expression between normal and malignant tissues was reported, consistent with a COX-1 role in tumorigenesis. A significant correlation between levels of mRNA for COX-1, COX-2, TGF-beta1 and PGES, and those for proangiogenic factors VEGF-A and VEGF-C were also found in primary adenocarcinomas of the small intestine, thus suggesting a role for these factors in the propagation this rare neoplasia [70]. Interestingly, experimental mouse studies using genetic disruption of COX-1 or COX-2 plus *Apc* genes already 15 years ago suggested that both isoforms were involved in intestinal polyp formation [45]. Moreover, up-regulation of COX-1 protects intestinal stem cells from the DNA-damaging effect of azoxymethane and may play a key role in the early phase of intestinal tumorigenesis [71]. Furthermore, analysis of the expression levels of COX-1, COX-2, and mPGES (the downstream prostaglandin E synthase) in COX-$1^{-/-}$ and COX-$2^{-/-}$ ApcΔ716 double-knockout mice revealed that COX-1 was required from the early stage of intestinal polyp development, and that additional expression of COX-2 together with mPGES was necessary for subsequent accelerated growth of polyps [72]. On this basis, a mechanistic cooperation between COX-1 in the early stage of tumorigenesis and COX-2 in the subsequent polyp growth was proposed. In early stage of intestinal carcinogenesis, COX-1-PGE_2 signaling associated with a suppression of the PG-catabolizing enzyme, 15-prostaglandin-dehydrogenase (15-PGDH), has been proposed to occur before COX-2 induction [73]. Recent studies have also shown that COX-1 is required for the maintenance of anchorage-independent growth ability of colon cancer cells (a key feature of malignant phenotype), as well as for tumor promoter-induced transformation of preneoplastic cells [74]. Interestingly, Li et al. in the same work identified a novel selective COX-1 inhibitor, 6-C-(E-phenylethenyl)-naringenin, a derivative of the flavonoid naringenin, also showing its chemopreventive efficacy in a colon cancer xenograft model.

Breast cancer. In the breast cancer microenvironment, there is a complex interplay between tumor and stromal cells, and a relevant contribute of COX-2-derived prostanoids is generally acknowledged [24,75,76]. However, both isoforms are expressed in breast cancer clinical samples, COX-1 being primarily localized in stromal cells [77,78]. Up-regulation of COX-1 gene expression in tumor tissues compared to normal tissue has been demonstrated also by whole genome expression analysis of breast carcinomas [79]. Moreover, induction of cell growth arrest and apoptosis are induced in MCF-7 human breast cell line in vitro by the COX-1 inhibitor FR122047 [80], and additive effects on tumor cell growth by COX-1 and COX-2 inhibitors are induced in vitro [81] and in vivo [82].

Cervical cancer. Human papilloma virus (HPV) infection of the cervical epithelium is well regarded as the main cause of cervical cancer [83], and a link between HPV E6 and E7 oncoproteins and COX-2 transcription has been established [84,85]. However, current data supporting a benefit for NSAIDs in the treatment of cervical intraepithelial neoplasia—the premalignant cervical lesion—are uncertain [86]. COX-1 up-regulation in cervical carcinoma was reported more than 10 years ago, and COX-1-dependent autocrine/paracrine regulation of COX-2, PGE_2 receptors, and angiogenic factors was demonstrated in vitro [87]. Interestingly, it has been recently demonstrated that seminal plasma can promote cervical tumor cell growth in vitro and in vivo through the activation of inflammatory pathways involving both COX isoforms [88] and the expression of angiogenic chemokines [89]. Moreover, in an in vitro investigation of the co-regulation of COX-1 and downstream prostaglandin E synthases (mPGES-1, mPGES-2 and cPGES) in several tumor cell lines including cervical cancer, it was found that COX-1 and mPGES-1 messenger RNA (mRNA) are co-regulated and functionally coupled in basal PGE_2 synthesis [90]. Although few clinical investigations of COX isoforms expression in cervical cancer are available [91,92], these experimental results, along with previous findings on the relationships between COX isoforms expression and radiosensitivity of cervical cancer cell lines [93] suggest that also the COX-1 role in cervical cancer prevention and treatment could be reevaluated [94].

Endometrial cancer. It is generally accepted that production of prostaglandins by endometrial epithelial cells under resting conditions is regulated through the constitutive expression of COX-1, whereas under stimulated conditions prostaglandin production is a result of the up-regulation of COX-2. A critical role for COX-2 isoform in the maintenance of endometrial tissue during the menstrual cycle as well as in the progression of endometrial cancer has been already observed [95,96], along with the potential clinical benefit of a selective COX-2 inhibitor in COX-2 positive endometrial cancers [97]. However, a possible involvement of COX-1 in the early stage of endometrial cancer development has been suggested, based on a higher COX-1 mRNA expression in patients with WHO (World Health Organization)-grade G1 and G2 endometrial cancer [98]. Moreover, a possible role for COX-1 in endometrial cancerogenesis has been suggested [99]. In a mechanistic investigation of the oxytocin ability of modulating the invasive properties of human endometrial carcinoma cells, the results showed that the hormone increased the invasive properties of tumor cells through the activation of PIK3/AKT pathway; this in turn led to up-regulation of both COX isoforms and subsequent PGE_2 production. Interestingly, both COX isoforms were necessary and acted cooperatively for the oxytocin-induced invasion, COX-1 triggering the pro-invasive matrix metalloproteinase (MMP)-14 (a major MMP-2 activator), and COX-2 up-regulating MMP-2 expression. Importantly, an over-expression of oxytocin receptor was detected in endometrial cancer patients, thus indicating the clinical relevance of the oxytocin pathway in endometrial cancer progression.

Ovarian cancer. Epithelial ovarian cancer (EOC), the most lethal gynecological malignancy mainly occurring in older (postmenopausal) woman, is a highly heterogeneous disease [100], and includes distinct histological subtypes. A number of inflammatory cells and mediators are involved in EOC development and progression, and accumulating clinical and experimental evidence strongly suggests that inflammation might represent a unifying pathophysiological mechanism of ovarian carcinogenesis [101,102]. Interestingly, COX-1 was first identified as ovarian cancer marker two decades ago [103]. Since then, COX-1 over-expression has been reported by several groups in multiple human, mouse, as well as hen models of ovarian cancer [104–109]. COX-1 has been suggested as the major enzyme regulating PGE_2 production in ovarian cancer cells [110], and along with COX-2 it plays an essential role in gonadotropin-induced tumor cell migration and invasion [111]. Thus, it is not surprising that both COX-1 and COX-2 have been included in a panel of inflammatory markers that characterize the rapidly growing and highly aggressive (type II) ovarian carcinomas [112]. Accordingly, the expression of COX-1 is higher in ovarian cancer patients with low CD8+ (cytotoxic T cells) and high CD1a+ (dendritic cells) cell density than in those with high CD8+ cell density [113], and COX-1 overexpression is the characterizing element in a cluster of ovarian cancer patients in which the poor prognosis is associated with an immunosuppressive status [114]. However, a role for COX-2 isoform in ovarian cancer has been also reported in clinical [115], as well as experimental investigations [116,117]. A major contribution for clarifying this apparent controversy comes from a very recent large-scale quantitative analysis of the expression of COX isoforms through The Cancer Genome Atlas (TCGA) dataset [118]. This study revealed markedly higher COX-1 expression than COX-2 in high-grade serous ovarian cancer (HGSOC)—the most aggressive EOC histotype—along with higher COX-1 expression in HGSOC tumors than 10 other tumor types in TCGA. Interestingly, a similar or higher expression of COX-2 isoform was instead observed for endometrioid, mucinous and clear cell tumors in an independent tissue microarray, thus suggesting a more relevant role for COX-2 in other EOC histotypes. Importantly, genetic knockdown of COX-1 in ovarian cancer cell lines resulted in down-regulation of both PG signaling and multiple pro-tumorigenic pathways, thus strongly encouraging further development of methods to selectively target COX-1 in the management of HGSOC tumors. The COX-1 relevance in ovarian cancer is also indirectly witnessed by the major efficacy of aspirin, a stronger COX-1 than COX-2 inhibitor, in COX-1-overexpressing in vitro and in vivo models of ovarian cancer [119–122].

Hematological tumors. COX-2 expression in hematological malignancies, including chronic lymphocytic leukemia, chronic myeloid leukemia, lymphoma, and multiple myeloma, favors tumor cell growth and survival, and represents a poor prognostic indicator [36]. As for myeloid and lymphoid acute leukemia, the transcription of both COX-1 and COX-2 isoforms in human leukemic blast cells from acute myeloid (AML) and acute lymphoid (ALL) patients has been well documented, but only COX-1 protein is expressed and active. COX-1-derived PGE_2 stimulates the spontaneous growth of AML leukemic blasts in vitro [123]. Among the various COX-derived metabolites, only PGE_2 appears to be endowed with a stimulating effect on the growth of leukemic blast cells in vitro [124], this suggesting a potential benefit stemming from COX-1 selective inhibition. COX-1, but not COX-2, is expressed and enzymatically active also in primary blasts from patients affected by acute promyelocytic leukemia (APL), a distinct AML subtype characterized by the t(15;17) translocation involving the PML gene on chromosome 15 and the retinoic acid receptor-alpha (RAR-alpha) gene on chromosome 17. A major component of APL therapy is all-*trans* retinoic acid (ATRA), based on its ability of activating gene transcription and tumor cell differentiation [125]. The ATRA-induced cell differentiation program is very complex, as shown by systems analysis of transcriptome and proteome [126], and includes also COX-1, but not COX-2, upregulation [127]. In this respect, it should be noted that the COX-1 selective inhibitor SC-560, as well as the non-selective indomethacin, impair both PGE_2 production and ATRA-dependent differentiation of NB4 leukemic cells, a model of acute promyelocytic leukemia, thus suggesting that COX-1-inhibiting NSAIDs should be avoided in APL patients under ATRA treatment [128].

COX-1 and cancer stem cells. According to the cancer stem cell (CSC) model, tumor tissues are hierarchically organized as normal tissues, the cancer stem cells being able to fuel or reinitiate tumor growth, giving rise to the progeny which constitutes the bulk of tumor mass. The CSC niche homeostasis is regulated by a complex system of molecular signals, which include also the COX-derived AA metabolites [129,130]. In more detail, COX-2 is up-regulated in CSCs isolated from distinct tumor histotypes (e.g., in breast, colon and bone tumors), is co-expressed with stemness molecular markers, and promotes CSC growth in vitro systems, as recently reviewed by Pang L.Y. et al. [131]. This is not surprising, considering the relevance of COX-2-PGE_2 system in stem cell biology of normal tissues [132], as well as the well-known relevance of COX-2 in cancer. However, some experimental evidence of COX-1 involvement in CSC biology also exists. In the azoxymethane (AOM) murine colon cancer model, the early molecular response of intestinal stem cells to genotoxic insult is driven by COX-1-PGE_2 signaling, and results in increased stem cell survival [71]. In breast CSCs, isolated from primary cultures of spontaneous tumors from HER2/Neu transgenic mice, and characterized by proteomic analysis, both COX-1 and COX-2 genes are overexpressed with respect to non-CSCs. Moreover, both COX isoforms belong to an eight-gene signature that correlates with breast cancer patient survival, thus suggesting a role of both isoforms in breast cancers with HER2 overexpression [133]. More recently, the development of anticancer drug resistance has been demonstrated to depend also upon the activation of mesenchymal stem cells (MSCs), which are able of modulating in many ways the response to chemotherapy [134]. A peculiar occurrence after cisplatin treatment is the secretion of specific polyunsaturated fatty acids (12-oxo-5,8,10-heptadecatrienoic acid and hexadeca-4,7,10,13-tetraenoic acid) that are able to confer resistance to various anticancer drugs. Interestingly, the central enzymes involved in the synthesis of MSC-derived chemoprotective factors are COX-1 and thromboxane synthase [135], thus suggesting that enzyme inhibition could restore cancer cell sensitivity.

To summarize, there is a rich body of evidence suggesting that also COX-1 is involved in multiple aspects of cancer pathophysiology. In most cases, it seems that COX-1 and COX-2 isoforms operate in a coordinated manner, while in specific conditions a prominent role for COX-1 has been demonstrated. Functional consequences of COX-1 activation have been poorly investigated as compared to COX-2 activation, even though the effects of COX-1-PGE_2 signaling on tumor cell phenotype have been described. However, a proper consideration should be given to the distinct functional modifications associated to COX-1 (or COX-2) expression [136], as shown also by a very recent genomic, lipidomic and metabolomic analysis of cyclooxygenase-null murine fibroblasts [137]. This study, which describes the common and dissimilar functional interactions of the COX isoforms at the cellular level by using a systems biology approach, demonstrates that COX-1 up-regulation results in a distinct "eicosanoid storm" along with an "anti-inflammatory, proinflammatory, and redox-activated" signatures. Even though fibroblasts are not cancer cells, these results suggest that COX-1 activity, when placed in pivotal position, can affect cell behavior even beyond eicosanoid metabolism.

3. Antitumor Activity of COX-1 Selective Inhibitors

Specific inhibition of COX-2 has been extensively investigated, and many highly selective COX-2 inhibitors are available [138]. In contrast, relatively few COX-1-selective inhibitors have been described [139], and only some of them have been investigated for anticancer activity (Figure 1).

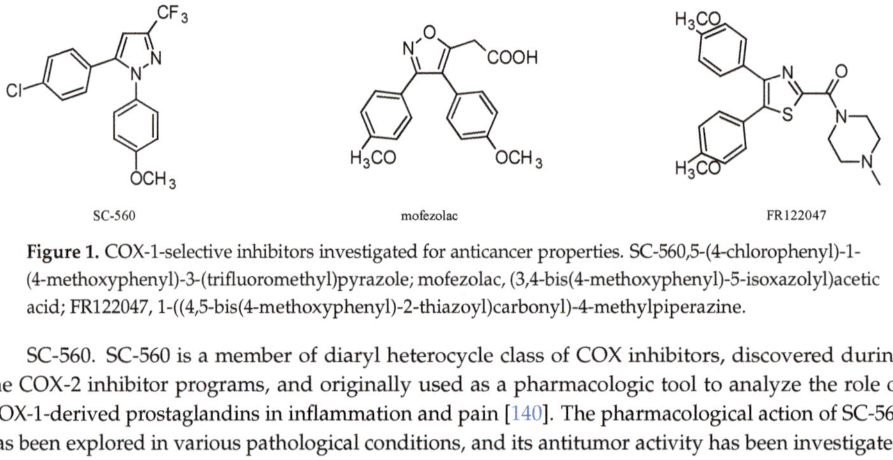

Figure 1. COX-1-selective inhibitors investigated for anticancer properties. SC-560,5-(4-chlorophenyl)-1-(4-methoxyphenyl)-3-(trifluoromethyl)pyrazole; mofezolac, (3,4-bis(4-methoxyphenyl)-5-isoxazolyl)acetic acid; FR122047, 1-((4,5-bis(4-methoxyphenyl)-2-thiazoyl)carbonyl)-4-methylpiperazine.

SC-560. SC-560 is a member of diaryl heterocycle class of COX inhibitors, discovered during the COX-2 inhibitor programs, and originally used as a pharmacologic tool to analyze the role of COX-1-derived prostaglandins in inflammation and pain [140]. The pharmacological action of SC-560 has been explored in various pathological conditions, and its antitumor activity has been investigated in multiple in vitro and in vivo experimental models of ovarian cancer and colorectal cancer, as well as other tumor histotypes, as described in the following.

Based upon a peculiar histopathological pattern showing elevated levels of COX-1 (not COX-2) in the epithelial compartment of ovarian tumor tissue undergoing extensive angiogenesis, the pharmacological action of SC-560 in ovarian cancer models was first investigated by Gupta R.A. et al. [104]. On ovarian cancer cell lines characterized for COX isoforms expression and activity, SC-560 showed in vitro antiproliferative effects similar to those of indomethacin and celecoxib (non-COX isoform selective and COX-2-selective, respectively), and only at doses 50–100 times greater than those achieved in in vivo systems [140]. In contrast, only SC-560 was found to inhibit arachidonic acid-induced VEGF secretion at low doses, an effect that was dose-dependently reverted by PGE_2. The in vivo tumor growth inhibitory efficacy of SC-560 was then demonstrated by Daikoku T. et al. in genetically engineered ovarian cancer murine models, in which COX-1 overexpression was common to various disease-associated genetic alterations [105,106]. As far as COX-1 downstream targets are concerned, experimental evidence for PPARδ–ERK signaling involvement was provided in murine, as well as in human ovarian cancer [119]. The in vivo activity of SC-560 alone or in various combination protocols has been extensively investigated by Li W. et al. in the SKOV-3 xenograft model [141–147]. In this model, SKOV-3 cells predominantly express the COX-1 isoform, as determined by immunohistochemical analysis of tumor samples [142], and SC-560 treatment at COX-1-specific inhibitory dosages produced a slight to moderate reduction of tumor growth. Interestingly, combination treatment of SC-560 with cisplatin [147] or taxol [144–147] generally provided greater efficacy than individual agents on various pharmacological end-points, including angiogenesis, proliferation and apoptosis. Not surprisingly, a combination of SC-560 with the non-selective inhibitor ibuprofen [141] or the COX-2-selective celecoxib [143] also showed major efficacy in the SKOV-3 system, suggesting that the inhibition of both COX-1 and COX-2 could overcome a potential compensation between the two isoforms in the SKOV-3 xenograft biology. From a mechanistic point of view, the in vivo effects of SC-560 in the SKOV-3 system may be related to the treatment-dependent reduction of PGE_2 production and to the associated inhibition of angiogenesis. However, a clear evidence for an exclusive or prevailing COX-1 dependence of prostaglandin production in SKOV-3 cells is lacking. Moreover, it cannot be excluded that in in vivo systems SC-560 could inhibit also COX-2 [148], and that COX-independent effects could contribute to antitumor activity. Some concern is partly due to the SKOV-3 cell line itself, which in some cases is reported as negative for COX-1 expression [104]. This is not actually unusual in the cyclooxygenase literature; the contrasting results variably depend upon a different source of the cell line, antibody cross-reactivity or other technical issues [149], and distinct experimental conditions (i.e., in vitro versus in vivo). Interestingly, SC-560 increases also paclitaxel sensitivity of taxane-resistant ovarian cancer cell lines characterized by MDR1/P-glycoprotein upregulation. A similar effect was produced by the COX-2 selective inhibitor NS398, not modified by PGE_2 addition, thus suggesting a prostaglandin- and COX-independent mechanism [150]. The concrete possibility that SC-560 could represent a promising lead for ovarian cancer treatment is also suggested by the SC-560 belonging to a group of small molecule compounds that are potentially able to target ovarian cancer stem cell (OVCSC)-specific genes [151]. This interesting feature has been recently discovered through the characterization of OVCSC-specific gene expression profiling and a co-expression extrapolation with CMAP, a massive repository of gene expression data that provides information on gene expression modification of several cell lines treated with >1000 bioactive compounds [152].

In vitro and in vivo activity of SC-560 in comparison to celecoxib against colorectal cancer cells was investigated by Grosch S. et al. [153], by evaluating their effects on survival, cell cycle progression, and apoptosis of colon cancer cell characterized for COX-1 and COX-2 expression. Independently from COX status, both SC-560 and celecoxib affected in vitro cell survival and induced a G0/G1 block, whereas only celecoxib induced apoptosis. In vivo, both compounds were active towards a HCT-15 (COX-2 deficient) xenograft, but devoid of significant effect on HT-29 (COX-2 expressing) tumors, overall indicating a COX-independent mechanism of action. The effects of SC-560 on HT-29 colon cancer cells have been investigated also by Wu W. K. et al. [154], showing that the growth inhibitory effect was accompanied by G1-S transition arrest and phosphoinositide 3-kinase (PI3K)-induced autophagy. Proliferation inhibition and cell-cycle progression arrest induced in vitro by SC-560 has been investigated also on HCT-116 colon cancer cells, which had been previously characterized by a total absence of COX expression and activity [155]. Lee et al. showed that the growth inhibitory effect towards HCT-116 cells was affected by the cell cycle regulator protein p21CIP1 [156]. Moreover, Sakoguchi-Okada N. et al. showed that the growth inhibitory and apoptotic effect of SC-560 (and other non-selective and COX-2-selective inhibitors) on HCT-116 cells was associated with inhibition of survivin expression and Wnt/beta-catenin signaling pathway [157]. With the aim of identifying possible COX-independent mechanisms of action of NSAIDs, treatment-induced gene expression modifications of HCT-116 cells were investigated by using suppression subtractive hybridization [158]. Interestingly, two cancer-related genes, NAG-1 (officially known as GDF15), and thymosin β-4 (TMSB4X), were induced by SC-560, thus suggesting potentially contrasting effects on its antitumor activity. NAG-1 codes indeed for a pleiotropic cytokine of the TGF-β superfamily expressed in a broad range of cell types and involved in the cellular stress response program. NAG-1 induction effect may either be tumor-growth suppressive or enhancing, depending upon its induction pattern (acute or sustained) and pathophysiological context [159]. The induction of thymosin β-4 too could potentially compromise the anticancer activity of SC-560, being thymosin β-4 mechanistically involved in the metastatic process [160,161] and associated with poor prognosis in CRC [162]. Cyclooxygenase- and prostaglandin-independent growth inhibitory effects of SC-560 have been reported in vitro in cells representing various other tumor histotypes. The growth and cell-cycle progression of human A549, H460, and H358 lung cancer cells is affected by SC-560 at doses that are definitely higher than those required for COX-inhibiting activity. Interestingly, the growth suppression induced by SC-560, but not celecoxib treatment, was associated with reactive oxygen species production [163]. Multiple myeloma cell proliferation is also inhibited by SC-560 at doses that are 10 times higher than those necessary for enzymatic inhibition [164]. SC-560 treatment of HuH-6 and HA22T/VGH human hepatocellular carcinoma cell lines, expressing both COX isoforms at mRNA and protein level, led to growth inhibition and apoptosis, and inhibited anchorage-independent growth of HuH-6 cells in soft agar, an in vitro marker for malignancy of cancer cells [165]. From a mechanistic point of view, treatment of tumor cells with SC-560, as well as with the coxib CAY10404, was associated with activation of ERK1/2 signaling pathway.

Mofezolac. Among the few selective COX-1 inhibitors investigated as potential analgesics and anti-platelet agents, mofezolac has been developed and marketed in Japan as a powerful pain killer [166], and its anticancer activity has been investigated almost exclusively in colorectal cancer experimental models. In vitro treatment of a COX-1-expressing RGMI cell line (non-transformed cells derived from rat gastric mucosa) by mofezolac induces a weak apoptotic effect, substantially prostaglandin-synthesis independent, with respect to indomethacin or sodium diclofenac [167], and a similar behavior was also observed in AGS gastric adenocarcinoma cells, treated at concentrations that were similar to those found at gastric mucosa after oral administration [168]. With regard to in vivo models of colorectal cancer, mofezolac treatment suppresses the development of aberrant crypt foci (putative preneoplastic lesions) induced by azoxymethane (AOM) and reduces the number of intestinal polyps in Apc knockout mice. In both murine models, the efficacy of mofezolac was similar to that of nimesulide, this indicating a tumorigenic role for both cyclooxygenase isoforms in this experimental model [169]. Accordingly, a combination treatment with COX-1- and COX-2-selective inhibitors more effectively suppressed polyp growth than either of the single treatments alone in Apc knockout mice [170]. Besides inhibiting preneoplastic lesions, mofezolac significantly reduces the incidence, multiplicity and volume of azoxymethane-induced rat colon carcinomas [171], thus confirming the COX-1 pathophysiological role in the AOM-induced intestinal carcinogenesis. Interestingly, Mofezolac is also effective in suppressing beef tallow-promoted colon carcinogenesis in rats, thus suggesting a potential benefit for populations with high fat intake [172].

FR122047. The COX-1-selective inhibitor, 4,5-bis(4-methoxyphenyl)-2-[(1-methylpiperazin-4-yl) carbonyl]thiazole (FR122047) was originally developed as antiplatelet agent devoid of ulcerogenic effects [173], and investigated as analgesic agent [174], or used as tool for studying the involvement of COX-1 as well as the role of prostanoids generated along the COX-1 and COX-2 pathways in various models of inflammation [175,176]. The antitumor activity of FR122047 has been investigated in vitro on MCF-7 breast cancer cells [80]. FR122047 treatment inhibits in vitro cell growth of MCF-7 cells, and induces apoptotic cell death that is mechanistically independent from treatment-associated ROS production, as well as from PGE_2 production inhibition. Mechanisms of MCF-7 cell death induced by FR12207 were further investigated by the same group [177], showing that FR122047 treatment induces caspase-mediated apoptosis and at the same time stimulates a defensive autophagic response of MCF-7 cells. Interestingly, the inhibition of caspase-9 blocks the cytoprotective autophagic process, thus increasing the susceptibility of MCF-7 cells to FR-122047-induced cell death.

In general, in vitro and in vivo antitumor properties of COX-1-selective inhibitors resemble those of other NSAIDs and coxibs; in some cases, COX-dependent, and in others, COX-independent mechanisms having been reported. Preliminary screening of the anticancer properties of COX inhibitors is usually performed by investigating the in vitro effect upon cell proliferation and cell cycle progression of tumor cells characterized for COX expression and activity. COX-1-selective inhibitors, not different from other NSAIDs or coxibs, impair cell growth and proliferation, this biological end-point being most often associated with cell cycle G1-phase arrest and cell death. These effects are usually observed at compound concentrations that are much higher than those of common cytotoxic drugs [178], and very often higher than clinically relevant COX-inhibitor concentrations. The true effective concentration of COX inhibitors in in vitro systems could actually be lower than that indicated, owing to a subtractive interaction with the serum proteins of culture medium [179]. However, whilst considering the protein interaction caveat, it is not surprising that COX-1 inhibitors (as well as traditional NSAIDs and coxibs) have weak antiproliferative effects related to enzymatic inhibition. This probably reflects the weak impact of COX-derived PGs in the maintenance of in vitro growth and proliferation condition. In the various inflammatory pathological conditions in which the PG activity has been investigated, these molecules do not operate as primary signals of homeostasis modification, but rather as amplification signals at the tissue level [19]. There is no reason to believe that in vitro tumor cell proliferation could be a different situation, as shown also by the lack of efficacy of COX inhibitors against resting tumor cells [180]. Therefore, to obtain more useful information from a basic antitumor assay such as cell growth and proliferation inhibition, it would be preferable to use tumor cells that increase their proliferation rate as a result of PG addition, and to demonstrate that this effect is impaired by the COX inhibitor under investigation. In this context, it would be preferable to integrate the COX expression and activity data into a more general knowledge of genes and gene products that are associated with AA metabolism in the tumor cells under investigation. This information is available to the scientific community in public databases, e.g., the Cancer Cell Line Encyclopedia [181], and it is essential for a reasoned choice of tumor cells to be used, also in relation to their suitability as models of human clinical disease [182]. The elegant paper of Wilson A.J. et al. [118] on the relevance of COX-1 in HGSOC witnesses the effectiveness of this strategy. Moreover, treatment effects upon cell cycle progression and the cell survival–death homeostasis could be more conveniently investigated in the same experimental setting by using modern multiparametric imaging technologies [183], thereby obtaining a comprehensive picture of treatment-associated phenotypic modifications. In in vitro systems again, specific investigations could be planned by using 3D tumor cell models enriched with stromal cells, to more closely mimic the tissue-like condition in which PGs usually operate. As far as other tumor phenotype hallmarks potentially affected by COX-derived PGs, such as angiogenesis, invasion and metastasis, and immune effects, they all would only be observed in in vivo systems, although some useful indication can be provided by in vitro assays measuring cell adhesion properties, migration, invasion, and colony formation [178]. As far as the COX-independent mechanism, which are often described for COX-1-selective inhibitors, they could also be of interest. Unlike what occurred with the COX-independent pharmacological actions of coxibs [184], which gave rise to substantial research and development activity [43], the results so far reported for COX-1-selective inhibitors have not triggered systematic research on this topic. This is not surprising, considering the small number COX-1-selective compounds available. On the other hand, a COX-independent mechanism occurs in an unpredictable manner, and sometimes in a different context, as in the case of the ability of mofezolac to interact with c-myc oncoprotein [185].

4. Conclusions

The involvement of COX-1 activity in cancer seems to have, in most cases, a pathophysiological role that is consistent and coordinated with COX-2, as in other inflammation-associated pathological conditions. However, in some cases, as exemplified by serous ovarian carcinoma, COX-1 overexpression plays a pivotal role, stimulating more in-depth studies on its function in this specific condition, and suggesting that other histopathological and molecular subtypes of cancer disease could share this feature. However, it seems clear that the analysis of functional implications of COX-1-signaling, as well as of the pharmacological action of COX-1-selective inhibitors, should not be restricted to the COX pathway, and to the effects of prostaglandins that are already known for their ability to affect the tumor phenotype. A knowledge-based choice of the most appropriate tumor cell models, and a major effort in investigating the COX-1 issue in the more general context of the arachidonic acid metabolic network by using systems biology approaches, should be strongly encouraged.

Author Contributions: Conceptualization, M.C.; Writing–Original draft, M.C. and A.P.; Writing–Review and Editing, M.C. and A.P.; Funding Acquisition, M.C.

Funding: This research was funded by PRIN, 2009WCNS5C.

Acknowledgments: The authors thank Federica Campanella for her help in the literature research.

Conflicts of Interest: The authors declare no conflict of interest.

References

1. Balkwill, F.; Mantovani, A. Inflammation and cancer: Back to Virchow? *Lancet* **2001**, *357*, 539–545. [CrossRef]
2. Hanahan, D.; Weinberg, R.A. Hallmarks of cancer: The next generation. *Cell* **2011**, *144*, 646–674. [CrossRef] [PubMed]
3. Ben-Neriah, Y.; Karin, M. Inflammation meets cancer, with NF-κB as the matchmaker. *Nat. Immunol.* **2011**, *12*, 715–723. [CrossRef] [PubMed]
4. Crusz, S.M.; Balkwill, F.R. Inflammation and cancer: Advances and new agents. *Nat. Rev. Clin. Oncol.* **2015**, *12*, 584–596. [CrossRef] [PubMed]
5. Coussens, L.M.; Zitvogel, L.; Palucka, A.K. Neutralizing tumor-promoting chronic inflammation: A magic bullet? *Science* **2013**, *339*, 286–291. [CrossRef] [PubMed]
6. Dennis, E.A.; Norris, P.C. Eicosanoid storm in infection and inflammation. *Nat. Rev. Immunol.* **2015**, *15*, 511–523. [CrossRef] [PubMed]
7. Hirata, T.; Narumiya, S. Prostanoid receptors. *Chem. Rev.* **2011**, *111*, 6209–6230. [CrossRef] [PubMed]
8. Botha, J.H.; Bobinson, K.M.; Ramchurren, N.; Reddi, K.; Norman, R.J. Human esophageal carcinoma cell lines: Prostaglandin production, biological properties, and behavior in nude mice. *J. Natl. Cancer Inst.* **1986**, *76*, 1053–1056. [PubMed]
9. Wang, D.; Dubois, R.N. Eicosanoids and cancer. *Nat. Rev. Cancer* **2010**, *10*, 181–193. [CrossRef] [PubMed]
10. Nakanishi, M.; Rosenberg, D.W. Multifaceted roles of PGE2 in inflammation and cancer. *Semin. Immunopathol.* **2013**, *35*, 123–137. [CrossRef] [PubMed]
11. Sha, W.; Brüne, B.; Weigert, A. The multi-faceted roles of prostaglandin E2 in cancer-infiltrating mononuclear phagocyte biology. *Immunobiology* **2012**, *217*, 1225–1232. [CrossRef] [PubMed]
12. Oshima, H.; Oshima, M. The inflammatory network in the gastrointestinal tumor microenvironment: Lessons from mouse models. *J. Gastroenterol.* **2012**, *47*, 97–106. [CrossRef] [PubMed]
13. Kalinski, P. Regulation of immune responses by prostaglandin E2. *J. Immunol.* **2012**, *188*, 21–28. [CrossRef] [PubMed]
14. Vong, L.; Ferraz, J.G.; Panaccione, R.; Beck, P.L.; Wallace, J.L. A pro-resolution mediator, prostaglandin D(2), is specifically up-regulated in individuals in long-term remission from ulcerative colitis. *Proc. Natl. Acad. Sci. USA* **2010**, *107*, 12023–12027. [CrossRef] [PubMed]
15. Li, H.; Liu, K.; Boardman, L.A.; Zhao, Y.; Wang, L.; Sheng, Y.; Oi, N.; Limburg, P.J.; Bode, A.M.; Dong, Z. Circulating prostaglandin biosynthesis in colorectal cancer and potential clinical significance. *EBioMedicine* **2015**, *2*, 165–171. [CrossRef] [PubMed]
16. Dovizio, M.; Tacconelli, S.; Ricciotti, E.; Bruno, A.; Maier, T.J.; Anzellotti, P.; Di Francesco, L.; Sala, P.; Signoroni, S.; Bertario, L.; et al. Effects of celecoxib on prostanoid biosyntesis and circulating angiogenesis proteins in familial adenomatous polyposis. *J. Pharmacol. Exp. Ther.* **2012**, *341*, 242–250. [CrossRef] [PubMed]

17. Liu, Q.; Tao, B.; Liu, G.; Chen, G.; Zhu, Q.; Yu, Y.; Yu, Y.; Xiong, H. Thromboxane A2 receptor inhibition suppresses multiple myeloma cell proliferation by inducing p38/c-Jun N-terminal Kinase (JNK) Mitogen-activated Protein Kinase (MAPK)-mediated G2/M progression delay and cell apoptosis. *J. Biol. Chem.* **2016**, *291*, 4779–4792. [CrossRef] [PubMed]
18. Li, X.; Tai, H.H. Activation of thromboxane A(2) receptors induces orphan nuclear receptor Nurr1 expression and stimulates cell proliferation in human lung cancer cells. *Carcinogenesis* **2009**, *30*, 1606–1613. [CrossRef] [PubMed]
19. Ricciotti, E.; FitzGerald, G.A. Prostaglandins and inflammation. *Arterioscler. Thromb. Vasc. Biol.* **2011**, *31*, 986–1000. [CrossRef] [PubMed]
20. Smith, W.L.; DeWitt, D.L.; Garavito, R.M. Cyclooxygenases: Structural, cellular, and molecular biology. *Annu. Rev. Biochem.* **2000**, *69*, 145–182. [CrossRef] [PubMed]
21. Zidar, N.; Odar, K.; Glavac, D.; Jerse, M.; Zupanc, T.; Stajer, D. Cyclooxygenase in normal human tissues—Is COX-1 really a constitutive isoform, and COX-2 an inducible isoform? *J. Cell. Mol. Med.* **2009**, *13*, 3753–3763. [CrossRef] [PubMed]
22. Kang, Y.J.; Mbonye, U.R.; DeLong, C.J.; Wada, M.; Smith, W.L. Regulation of intracellular cyclooxygenase levels by gene transcription and protein degradation. *Prog. Lipid Res.* **2007**, *46*, 108–125. [CrossRef] [PubMed]
23. Lutz, C.S.; Cornett, A.L. Regulation of genes in the arachidonic acid metabolic pathway by RNA processing and RNA-mediated mechanisms. *Wiley Interdiscip. Rev. RNA* **2013**, *4*, 593–605. [CrossRef] [PubMed]
24. Zhang, M.; Zhou, S.; Zhang, L.; Ye, W.; Wen, Q.; Wang, J. Role of cancer-related inflammation in esophageal cancer. *Crit. Rev. Eukaryot. Gene Expr.* **2013**, *23*, 27–35. [CrossRef] [PubMed]
25. Cheng, J.; Fan, X.M. Role of cyclooxygenase-2 in gastric cancer development and progression. *World J. Gastroenterol.* **2013**, *19*, 7361–7368. [CrossRef] [PubMed]
26. Cathcart, M.C.; O'Byrne, K.J.; Reynolds, J.V.; O'Sullivan, J.; Pidgeon, G.P. COX-derived prostanoid pathways in gastrointestinal cancer development and progression: Novel targets for prevention and intervention. *Biochim. Biophys. Acta* **2012**, *1825*, 49–63. [CrossRef] [PubMed]
27. Knab, L.M.; Grippo, P.J.; Bentrem, D.J. Involvement of eicosanoids in the pathogenesis of pancreatic cancer: The roles of cyclooxygenase-2 and 5-lipoxygenase. *World J. Gastroenterol.* **2014**, *20*, 10729–10739. [CrossRef] [PubMed]
28. Glover, J.A.; Hughes, C.M.; Cantwell, M.M.; Murray, L.J. A systematic review to establish the frequency of cyclooxygenase-2 expression in normal breast epithelium, ductal carcinoma in situ, microinvasive carcinoma of the breast and invasive breast cancer. *Br. J. Cancer* **2011**, *105*, 13–17. [CrossRef] [PubMed]
29. Parida, S.; Mandal, M. Inflammation induced by human papillomavirus in cervical cancer and its implication in prevention. *Eur. J. Cancer Prev.* **2014**, *23*, 432–448. [CrossRef] [PubMed]
30. Kaminska, K.; Szczylik, C.; Lian, F.; Czarnecka, A.M. The role of prostaglandin E2 in renal cell cancer development: Future implications for prognosis and therapy. *Future Oncol.* **2014**, *10*, 2177–2187. [CrossRef] [PubMed]
31. Shao, N.; Feng, N.; Wang, Y.; Mi, Y.; Li, T.; Hua, L. Systematic review and meta-analysis of COX-2 expression and polymorphisms in prostate cancer. *Mol. Biol. Rep.* **2012**, *39*, 10997–11004. [CrossRef] [PubMed]
32. Gakis, G. The role of inflammation in bladder cancer. *Adv. Exp. Med. Biol.* **2014**, *816*, 183–196. [CrossRef] [PubMed]
33. Elmets, C.A.; Ledet, J.J.; Athar, M. Cyclooxygenases: Mediators of UV-induced skin cancer and potential targets for prevention. *J. Investig. Dermatol.* **2014**, *134*, 2497–2502. [CrossRef] [PubMed]
34. Rundhaug, J.E.; Simper, M.S.; Surh, I.; Fischer, S.M. The role of the EP receptors for prostaglandin E2 in skin and skin cancer. *Cancer Metastasis Rev.* **2011**, *30*, 465–480. [CrossRef] [PubMed]
35. Mendes, R.A.; Carvalho, J.F.; van der Waal, I. An overview on the expression of cyclooxygenase-2 in tumors of the head and neck. *Oral Oncol.* **2009**, *45*, e124–e128. [CrossRef] [PubMed]
36. Ramon, S.; Woeller, C.F.; Phipps, R.P. The influence of Cox-2 and bioactive lipids on hematological cancers. *Curr. Angiogenes.* **2013**, *2*, 135–142. [CrossRef] [PubMed]
37. Nuvoli, B.; Galati, R. Cyclooxygenase-2, epidermal growth factor receptor, and aromatase signaling in inflammation and mesothelioma. *Mol. Cancer Ther.* **2013**, *12*, 844–852. [CrossRef] [PubMed]
38. Greenhough, A.; Smartt, H.J.; Moore, A.E.; Roberts, H.R.; Williams, A.C.; Paraskeva, C.; Kaidi, A. The COX-2/PGE2 pathway: Key roles in the hallmarks of cancer and adaptation to the tumour microenvironment. *Carcinogenesis* **2009**, *30*, 377–386. [CrossRef] [PubMed]

39. Harris, R.E. Cyclooxygenase-2 (cox-2) and the inflammogenesis of cancer. *Subcell. Biochem.* **2007**, *42*, 93–126. [CrossRef] [PubMed]
40. Dixon, D.A.; Blanco, F.F.; Bruno, A.; Patrignani, P. Mechanistic aspects of COX-2 expression in colorectal neoplasia. *Recent Results Cancer Res.* **2013**, *191*, 7–37. [CrossRef] [PubMed]
41. Cebola, I.; Peinado, M.A. Epigenetic deregulation of the COX pathway in cancer. *Prog. Lipid Res.* **2012**, *51*, 301–313. [CrossRef] [PubMed]
42. Fischer, S.M.; Hawk, E.T.; Lubet, R.A. Coxibs and other nonsteroidal anti-inflammatory drugs in animal models of cancer chemoprevention. *Cancer Prev. Res.* **2011**, *4*, 1728–1735. [CrossRef] [PubMed]
43. Gurpinar, E.; Grizzle, W.E.; Piazza, G.A. NSAIDs inhibit tumorigenesis, but how? *Clin. Cancer Res.* **2014**, *20*, 1104–1113. [CrossRef] [PubMed]
44. Rouzer, C.A.; Marnett, L.J. Cyclooxygenases: Structural and functional insights. *J. Lipid Res.* **2009**, *50*, S29–S34. [CrossRef] [PubMed]
45. Chulada, P.C.; Thompson, M.B.; Mahler, J.F.; Doyle, C.M.; Gaul, B.W.; Lee, C.; Tiano, H.F.; Morham, S.G.; Smithies, O.; Langenbach, R. Genetic disruption of Ptgs-1, as well as Ptgs-2, reduces intestinal tumorigenesis in Min mice. *Cancer Res.* **2000**, *60*, 4705–4708. [PubMed]
46. Tiano, H.F.; Loftin, C.D.; Akunda, J.; Lee, C.A.; Spalding, J.; Sessoms, A.; Dunson, D.B.; Rogan, E.G.; Morham, S.G.; Smart, R.C.; et al. Deficiency of either cyclooxygenase (COX)-1 or COX-2 alters epidermal differentiation and reduces mouse skin tumorigenesis. *Cancer Res.* **2002**, *62*, 3395–3401. [PubMed]
47. Okamoto, T.; Hara, A.; Hino, O. Down-regulation of cyclooxygenase-2 expression but up-regulation of cyclooxygenase-1 in renal carcinomas of the Eker (TSC2 gene mutant) rat model. *Cancer Sci.* **2003**, *94*, 22–25. [CrossRef] [PubMed]
48. Yu, Z.H.; Zhang, Q.; Wang, Y.D.; Chen, J.; Jiang, Z.M.; Shi, M.; Guo, X.; Qin, J.; Cui, G.H.; Cai, Z.M.; et al. Overexpression of cyclooxygenase-1 correlates with poor prognosis in renal cell carcinoma. *Asian Pac. J. Cancer Prev.* **2013**, *14*, 3729–3734. [CrossRef] [PubMed]
49. Osman, W.M.; Youssef, N.S. Combined use of COX-1 and VEGF immunohistochemistry refines the histopathologic prognosis of renal cell carcinoma. *Int. J. Clin. Exp. Pathol.* **2015**, *8*, 8165–8177. [PubMed]
50. Tang, J.Y.; Aszterbaum, M.; Athar, M.; Barsanti, F.; Cappola, C.; Estevez, N.; Hebert, J.; Hwang, J.; Khaimskiy, Y.; Kim, A.; et al. Basal cell carcinoma chemoprevention with nonsteroidal anti-inflammatory drugs in genetically predisposed PTCH1+/− humans and mice. *Cancer Prev. Res.* **2010**, *3*, 25–34. [CrossRef] [PubMed]
51. Müller-Decker, K. Cyclooxygenase-dependent signaling is causally linked to non-melanoma skin carcinogenesis: Pharmacological, genetic, and clinical evidence. *Cancer Metastasis Rev.* **2011**, *30*, 343–361. [CrossRef] [PubMed]
52. Erovic, B.M.; Woegerbauer, M.; Pammer, J.; Selzer, E.; Grasl, M.C.; Thurnher, D. Strong evidence for up-regulation of cyclooxygenase-1 in head and neck cancer. *Eur. J. Clin. Investig.* **2008**, *38*, 61–66. [CrossRef] [PubMed]
53. Mauro, A.; Lipari, L.; Leone, A.; Tortorici, S.; Burruano, F.; Provenzano, S.; Gerbino, A.; Buscemi, M. Expression of cyclooxygenase-1 and cyclooxygenase-2 in normal and pathological human oral mucosa. *Folia Histochem. Cytobiol.* **2010**, *48*, 555–563. [CrossRef] [PubMed]
54. Pannone, G.; Sanguedolce, F.; De Maria, S.; Farina, E.; Lo Muzio, L.; Serpico, R.; Emanuelli, M.; Rubini, C.; De Rosa, G.; Staibano, S.; et al. Cyclooxygenase isozymes in oral squamous cell carcinoma: A real-time RT-PCR study with clinic pathological correlations. *Int. J. Immunopathol. Pharmacol.* **2007**, *20*, 317–324. [CrossRef] [PubMed]
55. Erovic, B.M.; Al Habeeb, A.; Harris, L.; Goldstein, D.P.; Kim, D.; Ghazarian, D.; Irish, J.C. Identification of novel target proteins in sebaceous gland carcinoma. *Head Neck* **2013**, *35*, 642–648. [CrossRef] [PubMed]
56. Park, S.W.; Kim, H.S.; Hah, J.H.; Kim, K.H.; Heo, D.S.; Sung, M.W. Differential effects between cyclooxygenase-2 inhibitors and siRNA on vascular endothelial growth factor production in head and neck squamous cell carcinoma cell lines. *Head Neck* **2010**, *32*, 1534–1543. [CrossRef] [PubMed]
57. Park, S.W.; Kim, H.S.; Choi, M.S.; Kim, J.E.; Jeong, W.J.; Heo, D.S.; Sung, M.W. The influence of cyclooxygenase-1 expression on the efficacy of cyclooxygenase-2 inhibition in head and neck squamous cell carcinoma cell lines. *Anticancer Drugs* **2011**, *22*, 416–423. [CrossRef] [PubMed]

58. Akiyama, J.; Alexandre, L.; Baruah, A.; Buttar, N.; Chandra, R.; Clark, A.B.; Hart, A.R.; Hawk, E.; Kandioler, D.; Kappel, S.; et al. Strategy for prevention of cancers of the esophagus. *Ann. N. Y. Acad. Sci.* **2014**, *1325*, 108–126. [CrossRef] [PubMed]
59. Tsibouris, P.; Vlachou, E.; Isaacs, P.E. Role of chemoprophylaxis with either NSAIDs or statins in patients with Barrett's esophagus. *World J. Gastrointest. Pharmacol. Ther.* **2014**, *5*, 27–39. [CrossRef] [PubMed]
60. Morris, C.D.; Armstrong, G.R.; Bigley, G.; Green, H.; Attwood, S.E. Cyclooxygenase-2 expression in the Barrett's metaplasia–dysplasia–adenocarcinoma sequence. *Am. J. Gastroenterol.* **2001**, *96*, 990–996. [CrossRef] [PubMed]
61. Taddei, A.; Fabbroni, V.; Pini, A.; Lucarini, L.; Ringressi, M.N.; Fantappiè, O.; Bani, D.; Messerini, L.; Masini, E.; Bechi, P. Cyclooxygenase-2 and inflammation mediators have a crucial role in reflux-related esophageal histological changes and Barrett's esophagus. *Dig. Dis. Sci.* **2014**, *59*, 949–957. [CrossRef] [PubMed]
62. Von Rahden, B.H.; Stein, H.J.; Pühringer, F.; Koch, I.; Langer, R.; Piontek, G.; Siewert, J.R.; Höfler, H.; Sarbia, M. Coexpression of cyclooxygenases (COX-1, COX-2) and vascular endothelial growth factors (VEGF-A, VEGF-C) in esophageal adenocarcinoma. *Cancer Res.* **2005**, *65*, 5038–5044. [CrossRef] [PubMed]
63. Piazuelo, E.; Santander, S.; Cebrián, C.; Jiménez, P.; Pastor, C.; García-González, M.A.; Esteva, F.; Esquivias, P.; Ortego, J.; Lanas, A. Characterization of the prostaglandin E2 pathway in a rat model of esophageal adenocarcinoma. *Curr. Cancer Drug Targets* **2012**, *12*, 132–143. [CrossRef] [PubMed]
64. Esquivias, P.; Morandeira, A.; Escartín, A.; Cebrián, C.; Santander, S.; Esteva, F.; García-González, M.A.; Ortego, J.; Lanas, A.; Piazuelo, E. Indomethacin but not a selective cyclooxygenase-2 inhibitor inhibits esophageal adenocarcinogenesis in rats. *World J. Gastroenterol.* **2012**, *18*, 4866–4874. [CrossRef] [PubMed]
65. Zhang, S.; Zhang, X.Q.; Ding, X.W.; Yang, R.K.; Huang, S.L.; Kastelein, F.; Bruno, M.; Yu, X.J.; Zhou, D.; Zou, X.P. Cyclooxygenase inhibitors use is associated with reduced risk of esophageal adenocarcinoma in patients with Barrett's esophagus: A meta-analysis. *Br. J. Cancer* **2014**, *110*, 2378–2388. [CrossRef] [PubMed]
66. Janakiram, N.B.; Rao, C.V. The role of inflammation in colon cancer. *Adv. Exp. Med. Biol.* **2014**, *816*, 25–52. [CrossRef] [PubMed]
67. Arber, N.; Eagle, C.J.; Spicak, J.; Rácz, I.; Dite, P.; Hajer, J.; Zavoral, M.; Lechuga, M.J.; Gerletti, P.; Tang, J.; et al. PreSAP Trial Investigators. Celecoxib for the prevention of colorectal adenomatous polyps. *N. Engl. J. Med.* **2006**, *355*, 885–895. [CrossRef] [PubMed]
68. Kraus, S.; Naumov, I.; Arber, N. COX-2 active agents in the chemoprevention of colorectal cancer. *Recent Results Cancer Res.* **2013**, *191*, 95–103. [CrossRef] [PubMed]
69. Church, R.D.; Yu, J.; Fleshman, J.W.; Shannon, W.D.; Govindan, R.; McLeod, H.L. RNA profiling of cyclooxygenases 1 and 2 in colorectal cancer. *Br. J. Cancer* **2004**, *91*, 1015–1018. [CrossRef] [PubMed]
70. Von Rahden, B.H.; Brücher, B.L.; Langner, C.; Siewert, J.R.; Stein, H.J.; Sarbia, M. Expression of cyclo-oxygenase 1 and 2, prostaglandin E synthase and transforming growth factor beta1, and their relationship with vascular endothelial growth factors A and C, in primary adenocarcinoma of the small intestine. *Br. J. Surg.* **2006**, *93*, 1424–1432. [CrossRef] [PubMed]
71. Riehl, T.E.; George, R.J.; Sturmoski, M.A.; May, R.; Dieckgraefe, B.; Anant, S.; Houchen, C.W. Azoxymethane protects intestinal stem cells and reduces crypt epithelial mitosis through a COX-1 dependent mechanism. *Am. J. Physiol. Gastrointest. Liver Physiol.* **2006**, *291*, G1062–G1070. [CrossRef] [PubMed]
72. Takeda, H.; Sonoshita, M.; Oshima, H.; Sugihara, K.; Chulada, P.C.; Langenbach, R.; Oshima, M.; Taketo, M.M. Cooperation of cyclooxygenase 1 and cyclooxygenase 2 in intestinal polyposis. *Cancer Res.* **2003**, *63*, 4872–4877. [PubMed]
73. Smartt, H.J.; Greenhough, A.; Ordóñez-Morán, P.; Talero, E.; Cherry, C.A.; Wallam, C.A.; Parry, L.; Al Kharusi, M.; Roberts, H.R.; Mariadason, J.M.; et al. β-catenin represses expression of the tumour suppressor 15-prostaglandin dehydrogenase in the normal intestinal epithelium and colorectal tumour cells. *Gut* **2012**, *61*, 1306–13014. [CrossRef] [PubMed]
74. Li, H.; Zhu, F.; Chen, H.; Cheng, K.W.; Zykova, T.; Oi, N.; Lubet, R.A.; Bode, A.M.; Wang, M.; Dong, Z. 6-C-(E-phenylethenyl)-naringenin suppresses colorectal cancer growth by inhibiting cyclooxygenase-1. *Cancer Res.* **2014**, *74*, 243–252. [CrossRef] [PubMed]
75. Vona-Davis, L.; Rose, D.P. The obesity-inflammation-eicosanoid axis in breast cancer. *J. Mammary Gland Biol. Neoplasia* **2013**, *18*, 291–307. [CrossRef] [PubMed]

76. Hoellen, F.; Kelling, K.; Dittmer, C.; Diedrich, K.; Friedrich, M.; Thill, M. Impact of cyclooxygenase-2 in breast cancer. *Anticancer Res.* **2011**, *31*, 4359–4367. [PubMed]
77. Hwang, D.; Scollard, D.; Byrne, J.; Levine, E. Expression of cyclooxygenase-1 and cyclooxygenase-2 in human breast cancer. *J. Natl. Cancer Inst.* **1998**, *90*, 455–460. [CrossRef] [PubMed]
78. Fahlén, M.; Zhang, H.; Löfgren, L.; Masironi, B.; von Schoultz, E.; von Schoultz, B.; Sahlin, L. Expression of cyclooxygenase-1 and cyclooxygenase-2, syndecan-1 and connective tissue growth factor in benign and malignant breast tissue from premenopausal women. *Gynecol. Endocrinol.* **2017**, *33*, 353–358. [CrossRef] [PubMed]
79. Haakensen, V.D.; Bjøro, T.; Lüders, T.; Riis, M.; Bukholm, I.K.; Kristensen, V.N.; Troester, M.A.; Homen, M.M.; Ursin, G.; Børresen-Dale, A.L.; et al. Serum estradiol levels associated with specific gene expression patterns in normal breast tissue and in breast carcinomas. *BMC Cancer* **2011**, *11*, 332. [CrossRef] [PubMed]
80. Jeong, H.S.; Kim, J.H.; Choi, H.Y.; Lee, E.R.; Cho, S.G. Induction of cell growth arrest and apoptotic cell death in human breast cancer MCF-7 cells by the COX-1 inhibitor FR122047. *Oncol. Rep.* **2010**, *24*, 351–356. [CrossRef] [PubMed]
81. McFadden, D.W.; Riggs, D.R.; Jackson, B.J.; Cunningham, C. Additive effects of Cox-1 and Cox-2 inhibition on breast cancer in vitro. *Int. J. Oncol.* **2006**, *29*, 1019–1023. [CrossRef] [PubMed]
82. Kundu, N.; Fulton, A.M. Selective cyclooxygenase (COX)-1 or COX-2 inhibitors control metastatic disease in a murine model of breast cancer. *Cancer Res.* **2002**, *62*, 2343–2346. [PubMed]
83. Boccardo, E.; Lepique, A.P.; Villa, L.L. The role of inflammation in HPV carcinogenesis. *Carcinogenesis* **2010**, *31*, 1905–1912. [CrossRef] [PubMed]
84. Subbaramaiah, K.; Dannenberg, A.J. Cyclooxygenase-2 transcription is regulated by human papillomavirus 16 E6 and E7 oncoproteins: Evidence of a corepressor/coactivator exchange. *Cancer Res.* **2007**, *67*, 3976–3985. [CrossRef] [PubMed]
85. Young, J.L.; Jazaeri, A.A.; Darus, C.J.; Modesitt, S.C. Cyclooxygenase-2 in cervical neoplasia: A review. *Gynecol. Oncol.* **2008**, *109*, 140–145. [CrossRef] [PubMed]
86. Grabosch, S.M.; Shariff, O.M.; Wulff, J.L.; Helm, C.W. Non-steroidal anti-inflammatory agents to induce regression and prevent the progression of cervical intraepithelial neoplasia. *Cochrane Database Syst. Rev.* **2014**, CD004121. [CrossRef] [PubMed]
87. Sales, K.J.; Katz, A.A.; Howard, B.; Soeters, R.P.; Millar, R.P.; Jabbour, H.N. Cyclooxygenase 1 is up-regulated in cervical carcinomas: Autocrine/paracrine regulation of cyclooxygenase-2, prostaglandin E receptors and angiogenic factors by Cyclooxygenase-1. *Cancer Res.* **2002**, *62*, 424–432. [PubMed]
88. Sutherland, J.R.; Sales, K.J.; Jabbour, H.N.; Katz, A.A. Seminal plasma enhances cervical adenocarcinoma cell proliferation and tumour growth in vivo. *PLoS ONE* **2012**, *7*, e33848. [CrossRef] [PubMed]
89. Sales, K.J.; Sutherland, J.R.; Jabbour, H.N.; Katz, A.A. Seminal plasma induces angiogenic chemokine expression in cervical cancer cells and regulates vascular function. *Biochim. Biophys. Acta* **2012**, *1823*, 1789–1795. [CrossRef] [PubMed]
90. Radilova, H.; Libra, A.; Holasova, S.; Safarova, M.; Viskova, A.; Kunc, F.; Buncek, M. COX-1 is coupled with mPGES-1 and ABCC4 in human cervix cancer cells. *Mol. Cell. Biochem.* **2009**, *330*, 131–140. [CrossRef] [PubMed]
91. Jung, Y.W.; Kim, S.W.; Kim, S.; Kim, J.H.; Cho, N.H.; Kim, J.W.; Kim, Y.T. Prevalence and clinical relevance of cyclooxygenase-1 and -2 expression in stage IIB cervical adenocarcinoma. *Eur. J. Obstet. Gynecol. Reprod. Biol.* **2010**, *148*, 62–66. [CrossRef] [PubMed]
92. Athavale, R.; Clooney, K.; O'Hagan, J.; Shawki, H.; Clark, A.H.; Green, J.A. COX-1 and COX-2 expression in stage I and II invasive cervical carcinoma: Relationship to disease relapse and long-term survival. *Int. J. Gynecol. Cancer* **2006**, *16*, 1303–1308. [CrossRef] [PubMed]
93. Jeon, Y.T.; Song, Y.C.; Kim, S.H.; Wu, H.G.; Kim, I.H.; Park, I.A.; Kim, J.W.; Park, N.H.; Kang, S.B.; Lee, H.P.; et al. Influences of cyclooxygenase-1 and -2 expression on the radiosensitivities of human cervical cancer cell lines. *Cancer Lett.* **2007**, *256*, 33–38. [CrossRef] [PubMed]
94. Kim, H.S.; Kim, T.; Kim, M.K.; Suh, D.H.; Chung, H.H.; Song, YS. Cyclooxygenase-1 and -2: Molecular targets for cervical neoplasia. *J. Cancer Prev.* **2013**, *18*, 123–134. [CrossRef] [PubMed]
95. Ohno, S.; Ohno, Y.; Suzuki, N.; Inagawa, H.; Kohchi, C.; Soma, G.; Inoue, M. Multiple roles of cyclooxygenase-2 in endometrial cancer. *Anticancer Res.* **2005**, *25*, 3679–3687. [PubMed]

96. Nasir, A.; Boulware, D.; Kaiser, H.E.; Lancaster, J.M.; Coppola, D.; Smith, P.V.; Hakam, A.; Siegel, S.E.; Bodey, B. Cyclooxygenase-2 (COX-2) expression in human endometrial carcinoma and precursor lesions and its possible use in cancer chemoprevention and therapy. *In Vivo* **2007**, *21*, 35–43. [PubMed]
97. Hasegawa, K.; Torii, Y.; Ishii, R.; Oe, S.; Kato, R.; Udagawa, Y. Effects of a selective COX-2 inhibitor in patients with uterine endometrial cancers. *Arch. Gynecol. Obstet.* **2011**, *284*, 1515–1521. [CrossRef] [PubMed]
98. Sugimoto, T.; Koizumi, T.; Sudo, T.; Yamaguchi, S.; Kojima, A.; Kumagai, S.; Nishimura, R. Correlative expression of cyclooxygenase-1 (Cox-1) and human epidermal growth factor receptor type-2 (Her-2) in endometrial cancer. *Kobe J. Med. Sci.* **2007**, *53*, 177–187. [PubMed]
99. Déry, M.C.; Chaudhry, P.; Leblanc, V.; Parent, S.; Fortier, A.M.; Asselin, E. Oxytocin increases invasive properties of endometrial cancer cells through phosphatidylinositol 3-kinase/AKT-dependent up-regulation of cyclooxygenase-1, -2, and X-linked inhibitor of apoptosis protein. *Biol. Reprod.* **2011**, *85*, 1133–1142. [CrossRef] [PubMed]
100. Vaughan, S.; Coward, J.I.; Bast, R.C., Jr.; Berchuck, A.; Berek, J.S.; Brenton, J.D.; Coukos, G.; Crum, C.C.; Drapkin, R.; Etemadmoghadam, D.; et al. Rethinking ovarian cancer: Recommendations for improving outcomes. *Nat. Rev. Cancer* **2011**, *11*, 719–725. [CrossRef] [PubMed]
101. Shan, W.; Liu, J. Inflammation, a hidden path to breaking the spell of ovarian cancer. *Cell Cycle* **2009**, *8*, 3107–3111. [CrossRef] [PubMed]
102. Macciò, A.; Madeddu, C. Inflammation and ovarian cancer. *Cytokine* **2012**, *58*, 133–147. [CrossRef] [PubMed]
103. Lee, G.; Ng, H.T. Clinical evaluations of a new ovarian cancer marker, COX-1. *Int. J. Gynaecol. Obstet.* **1995**, *49*, S27–S32. [CrossRef]
104. Gupta, R.A.; Tejada, L.V.; Tong, B.J.; Das, S.K.; Morrow, J.D.; Dey, S.K.; DuBois, R.N. Cyclooxygenase-1 is overexpressed and promotes angiogenic growth factor production in ovarian cancer. *Cancer Res.* **2003**, *63*, 906–911. [PubMed]
105. Daikoku, T.; Wang, D.; Tranguch, S.; Morrow, J.D.; Orsulic, S.; DuBois, R.N.; Dey, S.K. Cyclooxygenase-1 is a potential target for prevention and treatment of ovarian epithelial cancer. *Cancer Res.* **2005**, *65*, 3735–3744. [CrossRef] [PubMed]
106. Daikoku, T.; Tranguch, S.; Trofimova, I.N.; Dinulescu, D.M.; Jacks, T.; Nikitin, A.Y.; Connolly, D.C.; Dey, S.K. Cyclooxygenase-1 is overexpressed in multiple genetically engineered mouse models of epithelial ovarian cancer. *Cancer Res.* **2006**, *66*, 2527–2531. [CrossRef] [PubMed]
107. Hales, D.B.; Zhuge, Y.; Lagman, J.A.; Ansenberger, K.; Mahon, C.; Barua, A.; Luborsky, J.L.; Bahr, J.M. Cyclooxygenases expression and distribution in the normal ovary and their role in ovarian cancer in the domestic hen (*Gallus domesticus*). *Endocrine* **2008**, *33*, 235–244. [CrossRef] [PubMed]
108. Urick, M.E.; Johnson, P.A. Cyclooxygenase 1 and 2 mRNA and protein expression in the *Gallus domesticus* model of ovarian cancer. *Gynecol. Oncol.* **2006**, *103*, 673–678. [CrossRef] [PubMed]
109. Eilati, E.; Pan, L.; Bahr, J.M.; Hales, D.B. Age dependent increase in prostaglandin pathway coincides with onset of ovarian cancer in laying hens. *Prostaglandins Leukot. Essent. Fat. Acids* **2012**, *87*, 177–184. [CrossRef] [PubMed]
110. Kino, Y.; Kojima, F.; Kiguchi, K.; Igarashi, R.; Ishizuka, B.; Kawai, S. Prostaglandin E2 production in ovarian cancer cell lines is regulated by cyclooxygenase-1, not cyclooxygenase-2. *Prostaglandins Leukot. Essent. Fat. Acids* **2005**, *73*, 103–111. [CrossRef] [PubMed]
111. Lau, M.T.; Wong, A.S.; Leung, P.C. Gonadotropins induce tumor cell migration and invasion by increasing cyclooxygenases expression and prostaglandin E(2) production in human ovarian cancer cells. *Endocrinology* **2010**, *151*, 2985–2993. [CrossRef] [PubMed]
112. Ali-Fehmi, R.; Semaan, A.; Sethi, S.; Arabi, H.; Bandyopadhyay, S.; Hussein, Y.R.; Diamond, M.P.; Saed, G.; Morris, R.T.; Munkarah, A.R. Molecular typing of epithelial ovarian carcinomas using inflammatory markers. *Cancer* **2011**, *117*, 301–309. [CrossRef] [PubMed]
113. Liu, M.; Matsumura, N.; Mandai, M.; Li, K.; Yagi, H.; Baba, T.; Suzuki, A.; Hamanishi, J.; Fukuhara, K.; Konishi, I. Classification using hierarchical clustering of tumor-infiltrating immune cells identifies poor prognostic ovarian cancers with high levels of COX expression. *Mod. Pathol.* **2009**, *22*, 373–384. [CrossRef] [PubMed]
114. Hamanishi, J.; Mandai, M.; Abiko, K.; Matsumura, N.; Baba, T.; Yoshioka, Y.; Kosaka, K.; Konishi, I. The comprehensive assessment of local immune status of ovarian cancer by the clustering of multiple immune factors. *Clin. Immunol.* **2011**, *141*, 338–347. [CrossRef] [PubMed]

115. Lee, J.Y.; Myung, S.K.; Song, Y.S. Prognostic role of cyclooxygenase-2 in epithelial ovarian cancer: A meta-analysis of observational studies. *Gynecol. Oncol.* **2013**, *129*, 613–619. [CrossRef] [PubMed]
116. Kim, H.J.; Yim, G.W.; Nam, E.J.; Kim, Y.T. Synergistic effect of COX-2 inhibitor on paclitaxel-induced apoptosis in the human ovarian cancer cell line OVCAR-3. *Cancer Res. Treat.* **2014**, *46*, 81–92. [CrossRef] [PubMed]
117. Guo, F.J.; Tian, J.Y.; Jin, Y.M.; Wang, L.; Yang, R.Q.; Cui, M.H. Effects of cyclooxygenase-2 gene silencing on the biological behavior of SKOV3 ovarian cancer cells. *Mol. Med. Rep.* **2015**, *11*, 59–66. [CrossRef] [PubMed]
118. Wilson, A.J.; Fadare, O.; Beeghly-Fadiel, A.; Son, D.S.; Liu, Q.; Zhao, S.; Saskowski, J.; Uddin, M.J.; Daniel, C.; Crews, B.; et al. Aberrant over-expression of COX-1 intersects multiple pro-tumorigenic pathways in high-grade serous ovarian cancer. *Oncotarget* **2015**, *6*, 21353–21368. [CrossRef] [PubMed]
119. Daikoku, T.; Tranguch, S.; Chakrabarty, A.; Wang, D.; Khabele, D.; Orsulic, S.; Morrow, J.D.; Dubois, R.N.; Dey, S.K. Extracellular signal-regulated kinase is a target of cyclooxygenase-1-peroxisome proliferator-activated receptor-delta signaling in epithelial ovarian cancer. *Cancer Res.* **2007**, *67*, 5285–5292. [CrossRef] [PubMed]
120. Sonnemann, J.; Hüls, I.; Sigler, M.; Palani, C.D.; Hong, L.T.T.; Völker, U.; Kroemer, H.K.; Beck, J.F. Histone deacetylase inhibitors and aspirin interact synergistically to induce cell death in ovarian cancer cells. *Oncol. Rep.* **2008**, *20*, 219–224. [CrossRef] [PubMed]
121. Cho, M.; Kabir, S.M.; Dong, Y.; Lee, E.; Rice, V.M.; Khabele, D.; Son, D.S. Aspirin blocks EGF-stimulated cell viability in a COX-1 dependent manner in ovarian cancer cells. *J. Cancer* **2013**, *4*, 671–678. [CrossRef] [PubMed]
122. Son, D.S.; Wilson, A.J.; Parl, A.K.; Khabele, D. The effects of the histone deacetylase inhibitor romidepsin (FK228) are enhanced by aspirin (ASA) in COX-1 positive ovarian cancer cells through augmentation of p21. *Cancer Biol. Ther.* **2010**, *9*, 928–935. [CrossRef] [PubMed]
123. Truffinet, V.; Donnard, M.; Vincent, C.; Faucher, J.L.; Bordessoule, D.; Turlure, P.; Trimoreau, F.; Denizot, Y. Cyclooxygenase-1, but not -2, in blast cells of patients with acute leukemia. *Int. J. Cancer* **2007**, *121*, 924–927. [CrossRef] [PubMed]
124. Fiancette, R.; Vincent-Fabert, C.; Guerin, E.; Trimoreau, F.; Denizot, Y. Lipid mediators and human leukemic blasts. *J. Oncol.* **2011**, *2011*, 389021. [CrossRef] [PubMed]
125. McCulloch, D.; Brown, C.; Iland, H. Retinoic acid and arsenic trioxide in the treatment of acute promyelocytic leukemia: Current perspectives. *Onco Targets Ther.* **2017**, *10*, 1585–1601. [CrossRef] [PubMed]
126. Zhou, G.B.; Li, G.; Chen, S.J.; Chen, Z. From dissection of disease pathogenesis to elucidation of mechanisms of targeted therapies: Leukemia research in the genomic era. *Acta Pharmacol. Sin.* **2007**, *28*, 1434–1449. [CrossRef] [PubMed]
127. Rocca, B.; Morosetti, R.; Habib, A.; Maggiano, N.; Zassadowski, F.; Ciabattoni, G.; Chomienne, C.; Papp, B.; Ranelletti, F.O. Cyclooxygenase-1, but not -2, is upregulated in NB4 leukemic cells and human primary promyelocytic blasts during differentiation. *Leukemia* **2004**, *18*, 1373–1379. [CrossRef] [PubMed]
128. Habib, A.; Hamade, E.; Mahfouz, R.; Nasrallah, M.S.; de Thé, H.; Bazarbachi, A. Arsenic trioxide inhibits ATRA-induced prostaglandin E2 and cyclooxygenase-1 in NB4 cells, a model of acute promyelocytic leukemia. *Leukemia* **2008**, *22*, 1125–1130. [CrossRef] [PubMed]
129. Lau, E.Y.; Ho, N.P.; Lee, T.K. Cancer stem cells and their microenvironment: Biology and therapeutic implications. *Stem Cells Int.* **2017**, *2017*, 3714190. [CrossRef] [PubMed]
130. Peitzsch, C.; Tyutyunnykova, A.; Pantel, K.; Dubrovska, A. Cancer stem cells: The root of tumor recurrence and metastases. *Semin. Cancer Biol.* **2017**, *44*, 10–24. [CrossRef] [PubMed]
131. Pang, L.Y.; Hurst, E.A.; Argyle, D.J. Cyclooxygenase-2: A role in cancer stem cell survival and repopulation of cancer cells during therapy. *Stem Cells Int.* **2016**, *2016*, 2048731. [CrossRef] [PubMed]
132. Goessling, W.; North, T.E.; Loewer, S.; Lord, A.M.; Lee, S.; Stoick-Cooper, C.L.; Weidinger, G.; Puder, M.; Daley, G.Q.; Moon, R.T.; et al. Genetic interaction of PGE2 and Wnt signaling regulates developmental specification of stem cells and regeneration. *Cell* **2009**, *136*, 1136–1147. [CrossRef] [PubMed]
133. Kanojia, D.; Zhou, W.; Zhang, J.; Jie, C.; Lo, P.K.; Wang, Q.; Chen, H. Proteomic profiling of cancer stem cells derived from primary tumors of HER2/Neu transgenic mice. *Proteomics* **2012**, *12*, 3407–3415. [CrossRef] [PubMed]
134. Lazennec, G.; Lam, P.Y. Recent discoveries concerning the tumor—Mesenchymal stem cell interactions. *Biochim. Biophys. Acta* **2016**, *1866*, 290–299. [CrossRef] [PubMed]

135. Roodhart, J.M.; Daenen, L.G.; Stigter, E.C.; Prins, H.J.; Gerrits, J.; Houthuijzen, J.M.; Gerritsen, M.G.; Schipper, H.S.; Backer, M.J.; van Amersfoort, M.; et al. Mesenchymal stem cells induce resistance to chemotherapy through the release of platinum-induced fatty acids. *Cancer Cell* **2011**, *20*, 370–383. [CrossRef] [PubMed]
136. Loftin, C.D.; Tiano, H.F.; Langenbanch, R. Phenotypes of the COX-deficient mice indicate physiological and pathophysiological roles for COX-1 and COX-2. *Prostaglandins Other Lipid Mediat.* **2002**, *68–69*, 177–185. [CrossRef]
137. Islam, A.B.; Dave, M.; Amin, S.; Jensen, R.V.; Amin, A.R. Genomic, lipidomic and metabolomic analysis of cyclooxygenase-null cells: Eicosanoid storm, cross talk, and compensation by COX-1. *Genom. Proteom. Bioinform.* **2016**, *14*, 81–93. [CrossRef] [PubMed]
138. Tortorella, M.D.; Zhang, Y.; Talley, J. Desirable Properties for 3rd Generation Cyclooxygenase-2 Inhibitors. *Mini Rev. Med. Chem.* **2016**, *16*, 1284–1289. [CrossRef] [PubMed]
139. Vitale, P.; Panella, A.; Scilimati, A.; Perrone, M.G. COX-1 inhibitors: Beyond structure toward therapy. *Med. Res. Rev.* **2016**, *36*, 641–671. [CrossRef] [PubMed]
140. Smith, C.J.; Zhang, Y.; Koboldt, C.M.; Muhammad, J.; Zweifel, B.S.; Shaffer, A.; Talley, J.J.; Masferrer, J.L.; Seibert, K.; Isakson, P.C. Pharmacological analysis of cyclooxygenase-1 in inflammation. *Proc. Natl. Acad. Sci. USA* **1998**, *95*, 13313–13318. [CrossRef] [PubMed]
141. Li, W.; Xu, R.J.; Lin, Z.Y.; Zhuo, G.C.; Zhang, H.H. Effects of a cyclooxygenase-1-selective inhibitor in a mouse model of ovarian cancer, administered alone or in combination with ibuprofen, a nonselective cyclooxygenase inhibitor. *Med. Oncol.* **2009**, *26*, 170–177. [CrossRef] [PubMed]
142. Li, W.; Ji, Z.L.; Zhuo, G.C.; Xu, R.J.; Wang, J.; Jiang, H.R. Effects of a selective cyclooxygenase-1 inhibitor in SKOV-3 ovarian carcinoma xenograft-bearing mice. *Med. Oncol.* **2010**, *27*, 98–104. [CrossRef] [PubMed]
143. Li, W.; Wang, J.; Jiang, H.R.; Xu, X.L.; Zhang, J.; Liu, M.L.; Zhai, L.Y. Combined effects of cyclooxygenase-1 and cyclooxygenase-2 selective inhibitors on ovarian carcinoma in vivo. *Int. J. Mol. Sci.* **2011**, *12*, 668–681. [CrossRef] [PubMed]
144. Li, W.; Liu, M.L.; Cai, J.H.; Tang, Y.X.; Zhai, L.Y.; Zhang, J. Effect of the combination of a cyclooxygenase-1 selective inhibitor and taxol on proliferation, apoptosis and angiogenesis of ovarian cancer in vivo. *Oncol. Lett.* **2012**, *4*, 168–174. [CrossRef] [PubMed]
145. Li, W.; Cai, J.H.; Zhang, J.; Tang, Y.X.; Wan, L. Effects of cyclooxygenase inhibitors in combination with taxol on expression of cyclin D1 and Ki-67 in a xenograft model of ovarian carcinoma. *Int. J. Mol. Sci.* **2012**, *13*, 9741–9753. [CrossRef] [PubMed]
146. Li, W.; Tang, Y.X.; Wan, L.; Cai, J.H.; Zhang, J. Effects of combining Taxol and cyclooxygenase inhibitors on the angiogenesis and apoptosis in human ovarian cancer xenografts. *Oncol. Lett.* **2013**, *5*, 923–928. [CrossRef] [PubMed]
147. Li, W.; Wan, L.; Zhai, L.Y.; Wang, J. Effects of SC-560 in combination with cisplatin or taxol on angiogenesis in human ovarian cancer xenografts. *Int. J. Mol. Sci.* **2014**, *5*, 19265–19280. [CrossRef] [PubMed]
148. Brenneis, C.; Maier, T.J.; Schmidt, R.; Hofacker, A.; Zulauf, L.; Jakobsson, P.J.; Scholich, K.; Geisslinger, G. Inhibition of prostaglandin E2 synthesis by SC-560 is independent of cyclooxygenase 1 inhibition. *FASEB J.* **2006**, *20*, 1352–1360. [CrossRef] [PubMed]
149. Saed, G.M. Immunohistochemical staining of cyclooxygenases with monoclonal antibodies. *Methods Mol. Biol.* **2008**, *477*, 219–228. [CrossRef] [PubMed]
150. Lee, J.P.; Hahn, H.S.; Hwang, S.J.; Choi, J.Y.; Park, J.S.; Lee, I.H.; Kim, T.J. Selective cyclooxygenase inhibitors increase paclitaxel sensitivity in taxane-resistant ovarian cancer by suppressing P-glycoprotein expression. *J. Gynecol. Oncol.* **2013**, *24*, 273–279. [CrossRef] [PubMed]
151. Huang, Y.; Ju, B.; Tian, J.; Liu, F.; Yu, H.; Xiao, H.; Liu, X.; Liu, W.; Yao, Z.; Hao, Q. Ovarian cancer stem cell-specific gene expression profiling and targeted drug prescreening. *Oncol. Rep.* **2014**, *31*, 1235–1248. [CrossRef] [PubMed]
152. Lee, J.K.; Havaleshko, D.M.; Cho, H.; Weinstein, J.N.; Kaldjian, E.P.; Karpovich, J.; Grimshaw, A.; Theodorescu, D. A strategy for predicting the chemosensitivity of human cancer and its application to drug discovery. *Proc. Natl. Acad. Sci. USA* **2007**, *104*, 13086–13091. [CrossRef] [PubMed]
153. Grösch, S.; Tegeder, I.; Niederberger, E.; Bräutigam, L.; Geisslinger, G. COX-2 independent induction of cell cycle arrest and apoptosis in colon cancer cells by the selective COX-2 inhibitor celecoxib. *FASEB J.* **2001**, *15*, 2742–2744. [CrossRef] [PubMed]

154. Wu, W.K.; Sung, J.J.; Wu, Y.C.; Li, H.T.; Yu, L.; Li, Z.J.; Cho, C.H. Inhibition of cyclooxygenase-1 lowers proliferation and induces macroautophagy in colon cancer cells. *Biochem. Biophys. Res. Commun.* **2009**, *382*, 79–84. [CrossRef] [PubMed]
155. Sheng, H.; Shao, J.; Kirkland, S.C.; Isakson, P.; Coffey, R.J.; Morrow, J.; Beauchamp, R.D.; DuBois, R.N. Inhibition of human colon cancer cell growth by selective inhibition of cyclooxygenase-2. *J. Clin. Investig.* **1997**, *99*, 2254–2259. [CrossRef] [PubMed]
156. Lee, E.; Choi, M.K.; Han, I.O.; Lim, S.J. Role of p21CIP1 as a determinant of SC560 response in human HCT116 colon carcinoma cells. *Exp. Mol. Med.* **2006**, *38*, 325–331. [CrossRef] [PubMed]
157. Sakoguchi-Okada, N.; Takahashi-Yanaga, F.; Fukada, K.; Shiraishi, F.; Taba, Y.; Miwa, Y.; Morimoto, S.; Iida, M.; Sasaguri, T. Celecoxib inhibits the expression of survivin via the suppression of promoter activity in human colon cancer cells. *Biochem. Pharmacol.* **2007**, *73*, 1318–1329. [CrossRef] [PubMed]
158. Jain, A.K.; Moore, S.M.; Yamaguchi, K.; Eling, T.E.; Baek, S.J. Selective nonsteroidal anti-inflammatory drugs induce thymosin beta-4 and alter actin cytoskeletal organization in human colorectal cancer cells. *J. Pharmacol. Exp. Ther.* **2004**, *311*, 885–891. [CrossRef] [PubMed]
159. Moon, Y. NSAID-activated gene 1 and its implications for mucosal integrity and intervention beyond NSAIDs. *Pharmacol. Res.* **2017**, *121*, 122–128. [CrossRef] [PubMed]
160. Wang, W.S.; Chen, P.M.; Hsiao, H.L.; Wang, H.S.; Liang, W.Y.; Su, Y. Overexpression of the thymosin beta-4 gene is associated with increased invasion of SW480 colon carcinoma cells and the distant metastasis of human colorectal carcinoma. *Oncogene* **2004**, *23*, 6666–6671. [CrossRef] [PubMed]
161. Piao, Z.; Hong, C.S.; Jung, M.R.; Choi, C.; Park, Y.K. Thymosin β4 induces invasion and migration of human colorectal cancer cells through the ILK/AKT/β-catenin signaling pathway. *Biochem. Biophys. Res. Commun.* **2014**, *452*, 858–864. [CrossRef] [PubMed]
162. Gemoll, T.; Strohkamp, S.; Schillo, K.; Thorns, C.; Habermann, J.K. MALDI-imaging reveals thymosin beta-4 as an independent prognostic marker for colorectal cancer. *Oncotarget* **2015**, *6*, 43869–43880. [CrossRef] [PubMed]
163. Lee, E.; Choi, M.K.; Youk, H.J.; Kim, C.H.; Han, I.O.; Yoo, B.C.; Lee, M.K.; Lim, S.J. 5-(4-chlorophenyl)-1-(4-methoxyphenyl)-3-trifluoromethylpyrazole acts in a reactive oxygen species-dependent manner to suppress human lung cancer growth. *J. Cancer Res. Clin. Oncol.* **2006**, *132*, 223–233. [CrossRef] [PubMed]
164. Ding, J.; Tsuboi, K.; Hoshikawa, H.; Goto, R.; Mori, N.; Katsukawa, M.; Hiraki, E.; Yamamoto, S.; Abe, M.; Ueda, N. Cyclooxygenase isozymes are expressed in human myeloma cells but not involved in anti-proliferative effect of cyclooxygenase inhibitors. *Mol. Carcinog.* **2006**, *45*, 250–259. [CrossRef] [PubMed]
165. Lampiasi, N.; Foderà, D.; D'Alessandro, N.; Cusimano, A.; Azzolina, A.; Tripodo, C.; Florena, A.M.; Minervini, M.I.; Notarbartolo, M.; Montalto, G.; et al. The selective cyclooxygenase-1 inhibitor SC-560 suppresses cell proliferation and induces apoptosis in human hepatocellular carcinoma cells. *Int. J. Mol. Med.* **2006**, *17*, 245–252. [CrossRef] [PubMed]
166. Goto, K.; Ochi, H.; Yasunaga, Y.; Matsuyuki, H.; Imayoshi, T.; Kusuhara, H.; Okumoto, T. Analgesic effect of mofezolac, a non-steroidal anti-inflammatory drug, against phenylquinone-induced acute pain in mice. *Prostaglandins Other Lipid Mediat.* **1998**, *56*, 245–254. [CrossRef]
167. Kusuhara, H.; Matsuyuki, H.; Matsuura, M.; Imayoshi, T.; Okumoto, T.; Matsui, H. Induction of apoptotic DNA fragmentation by nonsteroidal anti-inflammatory drugs in cultured rat gastric mucosal cells. *Eur. J. Pharmacol.* **1998**, *360*, 273–280. [CrossRef]
168. Kusuhara, H.; Komatsu, H.; Sumichika, H.; Sugahara, K. Reactive oxygen species are involved in the apoptosis induced by nonsteroidal anti-inflammatory drugs in cultured gastric cells. *Eur. J. Pharmacol.* **1999**, *383*, 331–337. [CrossRef]
169. Kitamura, T.; Kawamori, T.; Uchiya, N.; Itoh, M.; Noda, T.; Matsuura, M.; Sugimura, T.; Wakabayashi, K. Inhibitory effects of mofezolac, a cyclooxygenase-1 selective inhibitor, on intestinal carcinogenesis. *Carcinogenesis* **2002**, *23*, 1463–1466. [CrossRef] [PubMed]
170. Kitamura, T.; Itoh, M.; Noda, T.; Matsuura, M.; Wakabayashi, K. Combined effects of cyclooxygenase-1 and cyclooxygenase-2 selective inhibitors on intestinal tumorigenesis in adenomatous polyposis coli gene knockout mice. *Int. J. Cancer* **2004**, *109*, 576–580. [CrossRef] [PubMed]

171. Niho, N.; Kitamura, T.; Takahashi, M.; Mutoh, M.; Sato, H.; Matsuura, M.; Sugimura, T.; Wakabayashi, K. Suppression of azoxymethane-induced colon cancer development in rats by a cyclooxygenase-1 selective inhibitor, mofezolac. *Cancer Sci.* **2006**, *97*, 1011–1014. [CrossRef] [PubMed]
172. Miao, L.; Shiraishi, R.; Fujise, T.; Kuroki, T.; Kakimoto, T.; Sakata, Y.; Takashima, T.; Iwakiri, R.; Fujimoto, K.; Shi, R.; et al. Chemopreventive effect of mofezolac on beef tallow diet/azoxymethane-induced colon carcinogenesis in rats. *Hepatogastroenterology* **2011**, *58*, 81–88. [PubMed]
173. Tanaka, A.; Sakai, H.; Motoyama, Y.; Ishikawa, T.; Takasugi, H. Antiplatelet agents based on cyclooxygenase inhibition without ulcerogenesis. Evaluation and synthesis of 4,5-bis(4-methoxyphenyl)-2-substituted-thiazoles. *J. Med. Chem.* **1994**, *37*, 1189–1199. [CrossRef] [PubMed]
174. Ochi, T.; Motoyama, Y.; Goto, T. The analgesic effect profile of FR122047, a selective cyclooxygenase-1 inhibitor, in chemical nociceptive models. *Eur. J. Pharmacol.* **2000**, *391*, 49–54. [CrossRef]
175. Ochi, T.; Goto, T. Differential effect of FR122047, a selective cyclo-oxygenase-1 inhibitor, in rat chronic models of arthritis. *Br. J. Pharmacol.* **2002**, *135*, 782–788. [CrossRef] [PubMed]
176. Ochi, T.; Ohkubo, Y.; Mutoh, S. Role of cyclooxygenase-2, but not cyclooxygenase-1, on type II collagen-induced arthritis in DBA/1J mice. *Biochem. Pharmacol.* **2003**, *66*, 1055–1060. [CrossRef]
177. Jeong, H.S.; Choi, H.Y.; Lee, E.R.; Kim, J.H.; Jeon, K.; Lee, H.J.; Cho, S.G. Involvement of caspase-9 in autophagy-mediated cell survival pathway. *Biochim. Biophys. Acta* **2011**, *1813*, 80–90. [CrossRef] [PubMed]
178. Boccarelli, A.; Pannunzio, A.; Coluccia, M. The Challenge of Establishing Reliable Screening Tests for Selecting Anticancer Metal Compounds. In *Bioinorganic Medicinal Chemistry*; Alessio, E., Ed.; Wiley-VCH Verlag GmbH & Co., KGaA: Weinheim, Germany, 2011; pp. 175–196. ISBN 978-3-527-32631-0.
179. Lin, J.H.; Cocchetto, D.M.; Duggan, D.E. Protein binding as a primary determinant of the clinical pharmacokinetic properties of non-steroidal anti-inflammatory drugs. *Clin. Pharmacokinet.* **1987**, *12*, 402–432. [CrossRef] [PubMed]
180. Duan, W.; Zhang, L. Cyclooxygenase inhibitors not inhibit resting lung cancer A549 cell proliferation. *Prostaglandins Leukot. Essent. Fat. Acids.* **2006**, *74*, 317–321. [CrossRef] [PubMed]
181. Cancer Cell Line Encyclopedia (CCLE). Available online: http://www.broadinstitute.org/ccle (accessed on 4 September 2018).
182. Domcke, S.; Sinha, R.; Levine, D.A.; Sander, C.; Schultz, N. Evaluating cell lines as tumour models by comparison of genomic profiles. *Nat. Commun.* **2013**, *4*, 2126. [CrossRef] [PubMed]
183. Bray, M.A.; Singh, S.; Han, H.; Davis, C.T.; Borgeson, B.; Hartland, C.; Kost-Alimova, M.; Gustafsdottir, S.M.; Gibson, C.C.; Carpenter, A.E. Cell Painting a high-content image-based assay for morphological profiling using multiplexed fluorescent dyes. *Nat. Protoc.* **2016**, *11*, 1757–1774. [CrossRef] [PubMed]
184. Grösch, S.; Maier, T.J.; Schiffmann, S.; Geisslinger, G. Cyclooxygenase-2 (COX-2)-independent anticarcinogenic effects of selective COX-2 inhibitors. *J. Natl. Cancer Inst.* **2006**, *98*, 736–747. [CrossRef] [PubMed]
185. National Center for Biotechnology Information. PubChem BioAssay Database, AID=624141. Available online: https://pubchem.ncbi.nlm.nih.gov/bioassay/624141 (accessed on 4 September 2018).

pharmaceuticals

MDPI

Review

Antibody-Drug Conjugates for Cancer Therapy: Chemistry to Clinical Implications

Nirnoy Dan, Saini Setua, Vivek K. Kashyap, Sheema Khan, Meena Jaggi, Murali M. Yallapu * and Subhash C. Chauhan *

Department of Pharmaceutical Sciences and Cancer Research Center, University of Tennessee Health Science Center, Memphis, TN 38163, USA; ndan@uthsc.edu (N.D.); ssetua@uthsc.edu (S.S.); vkashya1@uthsc.edu (V.K.K.); skhan14@uthsc.edu (S.K.); mjaggi@uthsc.edu (M.J.)

* Correspondence: myallapu@uthsc.edu (M.M.Y.); schauha1@uthsc.edu (S.C.C.); Tel.: +1-901-448-1536 (M.M.Y.); +1-901-448-2175 (S.C.C.)

Received: 15 February 2018; Accepted: 3 April 2018; Published: 9 April 2018

Abstract: Chemotherapy is one of the major therapeutic options for cancer treatment. Chemotherapy is often associated with a low therapeutic window due to its poor specificity towards tumor cells/tissues. Antibody-drug conjugate (ADC) technology may provide a potentially new therapeutic solution for cancer treatment. ADC technology uses an antibody-mediated delivery of cytotoxic drugs to the tumors in a targeted manner, while sparing normal cells. Such a targeted approach can improve the tumor-to-normal tissue selectivity and specificity in chemotherapy. Considering its importance in cancer treatment, we aim to review recent efforts for the design and development of ADCs. ADCs are mainly composed of an antibody, a cytotoxic payload, and a linker, which can offer selectivity against tumors, anti-cancer activity, and stability in systemic circulation. Therefore, we have reviewed recent updates and principal considerations behind ADC designs, which are not only based on the identification of target antigen, cytotoxic drug, and linker, but also on the drug-linker chemistry and conjugation site at the antibody. Our review focuses on site-specific conjugation methods for producing homogenous ADCs with constant drug-antibody ratio (DAR) in order to tackle several drawbacks that exists in conventional conjugation methods.

Keywords: antibody; drug conjugation; chemical linker; drug delivery; and cancer therapy

1. Introduction

Cancer, responsible for about 8.2 million deaths per year globally, is the second most common deadly disease which severely affects the human health worldwide [1]. Current treatment options for cancer include surgery, chemotherapy, radiation, and immunotherapy. Modern approaches to combat cancer include stem cell therapy, hyperthermia, photodynamic therapy, laser treatment, etc. Among these therapeutic interventions, chemotherapy, either alone or in combination with surgery or radiation therapy, is the most widely used therapeutic option. Neoadjuvant chemotherapy is used to shrink tumors before surgery or radiation. Adjuvant chemotherapy is employed after surgery or radiation to kill remaining cancer cells. Conventional chemotherapy is often associated with a low therapeutic window due to poor pharmacokinetic properties of the drugs used. Additionally, chemotherapeutic agents are not specific to tumor cells and they can affect normal cells with high mitotic rates. This can lead to life-threatening side effects in cancer patients. The severity of such uninvited side effects can be reduced by conjugating different types of highly potent un-targeted drugs such as tubulin polymerization inhibitors, DNA damaging agents conjugated to a monoclonal antibody (mAb). Another proven approach to minimize chemotherapy side effects is nanotechnology. This approach gives the ability to load drug molecules in polymer/metal nanoparticles, liposomes, micelles, self-assemblies, and nanogels. Nanotechnolgy enhances passive delivery of chemotherapeutics to malignant cells (due to leaky vasculature) [2]. However, the existence of abundant stromal/fibrosis (desmoplasia) in tumors, leads to inefficient drug delivery and emergence of drug resistance [3]. All these unmet needs imply the importance to consider alternative approaches for successful therapeutic intervention in cancer.

A site-specific targeted delivery of cytotoxic drugs is proving to be a better option for efficient drug delivery. This can be achieved by conjugating cytotoxic drugs to a suitable and validated mAb. ADC strategy not only enhances the therapeutic window of potent cytotoxic drugs, but also minimizes chemo-associated side effects. ADCs attain the idea of a "magic bullet" conceptualized by Paul Ehrlich [4]. The concept of ADC in drug development was well recognized following the Food and Drug Administration (FDA) approval for Adcetris® (brentuximab vedotin) in 2011 and Kadcyla® (trastuzumab emtansine) in 2013. These successes prompted enormous interest among antibody guided therapeutic researchers from both academia and industry. This is evident from a sharp increase in related publication in PubMed (Figure 1a) and registered clinical trials in different phases of various types of ADCs (Figure 1b).

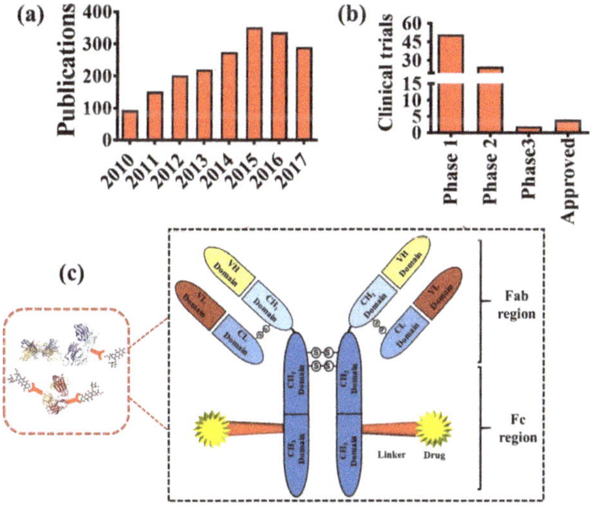

Figure 1. (**a**) Yearly peer-reviewed articles on ADCs based on PubMed search; (**b**) Registered clinical trials of ADCs based on Clinicaltrials.gov database; (**c**) Key components of an ADC.

ADCs are typically comprised of a fully humanized mAb targeting an antigen specifically/preferentially expressed on tumor cells, a cytotoxic payload, and a suitable linker (Figure 1c). This composition mainstay preserves cytotoxicity of drugs, targeting characteristics, and stability of ADCs in systemic circulation. The right combination of selection is key in developing a succeessful ADC. To acheive specific delivery of a cytotoxic payload, the target antigen must be highly expressed on the surface of the tumor cells rather than the normal cells. Conjugating a mAb to highly potent cytotoxic payloads facilitates site-specific delivery of the payload to the target cells, thus minimizing the chances of off target cytotoxicity. Upon binding to the specific antigen, the antibody gets absorbed through rapid internalization followed by lysosomal degradation, and subsequently releasing the cytotoxic drug inside the cell (Figure 2a). This way, ADCs can be used to deliver cytotoxic drugs to cancer cells [5].

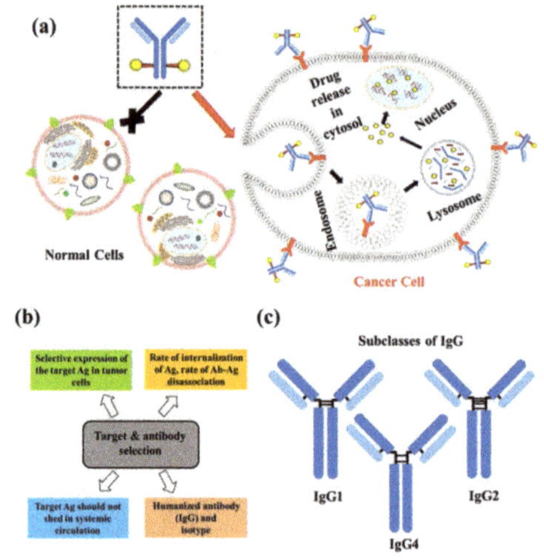

Figure 2. (**a**) Schematic representation of ADC uptake in cells expressing target antigen followed by release of the payload; (**b**) Key considerations while choosing target and antibody isotype for ADC developments; and (**c**) subclasses of IgG.

Over the past 30 years of ADC research, several new linkers, and conjugation strategies have been discovered. However, very few of them have reached to the clinic. This shows the degree of difficulty in optimizing key parameters of ADC such as choosing a potent cytotoxic payload, a suitable target, a stable linker, the conjugation site to the mAb, and the conjugation technology. Therefore, in this review, we attempt to discuss various advancements and challenges in ADC technologies with a special focus on linkers and conjugation methods.

2. Composition of ADCs

2.1. *Target and Antibody*

The conjugation of potent cytotoxic drug molecules to mAbs demonstrates a promising approach for the development of targeted cancer therapy. The selection of mAbs for specific targeting and harnessing the therapeutic drug molecule(s) with mAbs represents ADCs precision acting only on cancer cells, increasing the therapeutic index while minimizing the off-target effects (Figure 2b). Therefore, determining which antigen to target is the first major step in ADC development. The target antigen should be overexpressed on tumor cells surface homogenously with relatively low to no expression on healthy cells to ensure site-specific targeting delivery of cytotoxic payloads [6]. Immunohistochemistry, flow cytometry, tissue microarrays, reverse transcription polymerase chain reaction (RT-PCR), messenger RNA (mRNA) profiling are commonly used to anlyze tumor expression of the target antigen in patient tissue samples [7]. Upon confirming antigen overexpression, mAbs against this particular antigen are generated through Hybridoma Technology (a method for producing monoclonal antibodies). The hybridoma cells are immortalized by fusing antibody producing B cells from mice and mouse myeloma cells, then they are further cultured to generate monoclonal antibodies of interest [8]. Selection of mAbs for generation of ADCs is based on their tumor penetrating ability and binding affinity (Kd $<$ 10 nM) [5]. MAbs with strong binding on antigens were found to be confined in perivascular spaces, whereas as low binding affinity mAbs can internalize well inside the tumor [9]. Thus, a balance between internaliztion and disassociation rates of the antigen-antibody (Ab-Ag) complexes governs effective delivery of the payload to the tumor space. Sometimes shedding of a target antigen from tumor tissues or the presence of a circulating antigen in systemic circulation, in a considerable amount, can alter the potency and pharmacokinetics of the ADCs. In these circumstances a significant amount of the payload on ADCs will be lost in systemic circulation and cleared by the liver [10,11]. Studies on drug conjugates with shedding antigens, like tumor-associated carbohydrate antigen CanAg (a glycoform of mucin 1) and carcinoma antigen 125 (CA-125), showed no decrease in therapeutic efficacy [11,12]. The mAbs used for drug cross-linking are of the IgG isotype (Figure 2c) specifically IgG1, because of their inherent ability to trigger immune-mediated effector functions. This includes antibody-dependent cellular cytoxicity (ADCC) and complement-dependent cytotoxicity (CDC) by binding to Fcγ receptors and complement C1q protein complex, respectively [13]. Independent functions of mAbs can be an added advantage over the cell killing potency of the ADC warhead but they can contribute to toxicity sometimes [14]. For instance, anti-HER2 trastuzumab, in trastuzumab-emtansine (DM1) contributes to the antitumor efficacy of the ADC by mediating antibody-dependent cell-mediated cytotoxicity (ADCC) [15]. IgG2 and IgG4 isotypes can be used in ADCs but are less efficient in modulating effector functions and delivery in comparison to IgG1 [7,13]. IgG3 isotypes have a lower half-life, exteneded hinge region compraed to other isotypes and they are prone to polymorphisms and immunogenic reactions. Immunogenicity caused by previouly used murine and chimeric mAbs is countered by converting them to humanized mAbs. In humanized mAbs, the Fc region is from the human source and complementarity determining region are from non-human (rat/mouse) sources [16].

2.2. Linker

One of main challenges in developing ADCs is to incorporate a linker that will maintain the stability of the ADC in systemic circulation for a prolonged period and release the payload after internalization at the target site. The site of conjugation and choice of linker play a critical role in the stability, the pharmacokinetic properties of ADCs. Attachment sites in antibody mAb can also be engineered via several ways for incorporation of a linker and subsequently the drug. Based on release mechanism, linkers are generally divided as cleavable (Figure 3a) and non-cleavable linkers (Figure 3b).

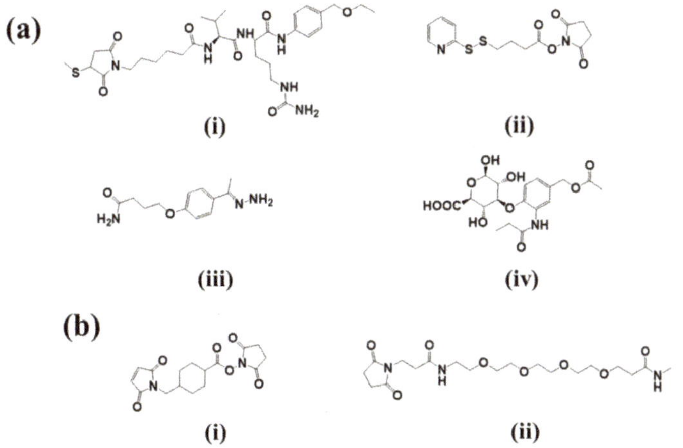

Figure 3. Chemical structures of linkers used in ADCs development. (**a**) Key cleavable linkers: (i) Lysosomal protease sensitive Val-Cit dipeptide linker; (ii) Glutathione sensitive SPDB linker; (iii) Acid Sensitive AcBut linker; and (iv) β-Glucuronidase sensitive linker; and (**b**) non-cleavable linkers: (i) SMCC linker; and (ii) PEG4Mal linkers.

2.2.1. Cleavable Linkers

- *Acid-sensitive linkers*: Acid-sensitive hydrazone groups in acid-labile linkers remains stable in systemic circulation (pH 7.5) and gets hydrolyzed in lysosomal (pH 4.8) and endosomal (pH 5–6) acidic tumor micro-environment upon internalization in the targeted cells [17]. Withdrawal of gemtuzumab ozogamicin (Mylotarg®) in 2010, an anti-CD33 ADC for treatment of acute myeloid lymphoma, raises concern over the stability of this linker [18]. The heterogeneous nature of the drug conjugate contributed to premature release of payload, which in turn may have contributed to its remarkable toxicity compared to conventional chemotherapy. Currently, inotuzumab ozogamicin and milatuzumab doxorubicin, that are developed with a hydrazone linker.
- *Glutathione-sensitive disulfide linkers: Another common example of cleavable linkers is glutathione-sensitive* disulfide linkers. Glutathione is a low molecular weight thiol which is present in the cytoplasm (0.5–10 mmol/L) and extracellular environment (2–20 μmol/L in plasma) [19]. In tumor cells elevated levels of thiols are found during stress conditions such as hypoxia [20]. The difference in glutathione concentration in cytoplasm and extracellular environment can be implemented as a selective delivery of the drug payload to target tumor via breakdown of disulfide linkers [21]. Besides glutathione, intercellular protein disulfide isomerase (PDI) is also capable to reduce disulfide bonds. Two cysteine residues in the active site of this enzyme governs the thiol-disulfide exchange reactions with or within substrates [22]. Maytansinoid drug conjugates have been widely employed for disulfide bonds with an average DAR of 3–4 [23].
- *Lysosomal protease-sensitive peptide linkers*: Tumor cells have higher expression of lysosomal proteases like cathepsin B than normal cells. Cathepsin B-sensitive peptide linker conjugated ADCs selectively binds to and get internalized into tumor cells via receptor mediated endocytosis [24]. Proteases are inactivated in serum in presence of a high pH and different serum protease inhibitors [24]. This makes the peptide linker stable in systemic circulation and only to be cleaved upon internalization in tumors. In case of the FDA approved Adecetris®, cathepsin B-sensitive valine-citruline linker is found to be superior to hydrazone linker. The valine-citruline linker connects the bridge between *p*-aminobenzylcarbamate-monomethyl auristatin E (MMAE) and anti-CD30-mAb [5].
- *β-glucuronide linker*: β-Glucuronidase-sensitive linkers have been successfully used in a handful of glucuronide prodrugs [25]. Lysosomes and tumor necrotic areas are rich in β-glucuronidase which is active at lysosomal pH and inactive at physiological pH [26]. This selective site of action allows for a selective release of cytotoxic payloads through cleavage of the glycosidic bond of β-glucuronidase-sensitive β-glucuronide linkers. Further, the hydrophilic nature of this linker provides aqueous solubility for hydrophobic payloads and decreases aggregation of ADCs [27]. A highly hydrophobic CBI payload was conjugated to h1F6 and cAC10 mAbs utilizing β-glucuronide linker with an average DAR ~4–5 [27]. Such ADC compositions were found to be mostly monomeric in nature compared to extremely aggregated PABC-dipeptide based CBI conjugates [27]. Psymberin/irciniastatin A, a phenolic cytotoxic payload-based ADC was developed with *N,N′*-dimethylethylene diamine self-immolative spacers and a β-glucuronide linker for targeting CD-30-positive and CD-70-positive malignancies [28]. This development led to the possibility of developing phenolic warhead-based ADCs as many anti-cancer drugs have phenol functional groups. Another β-glucuronidase-sensitive linker based ADC has recently been developed utilizing tertiary amine functional group of payloads (tubulysins and auristatin E) as the conjugation site to the linker [29]. Tertiary-ammonium based linkers provide an excellent strategy for conjugating payloads without affecting their activity [29].

2.2.2. Non-Cleavable Linkers

ADCs with non-cleavable thioether linkers have better plasma stability. Higher plasma stability decreases the non-specific drug release of ADCs as compared to cleavable linkers [30]. The linker is attached to the amino acid residues of the mAb through a nonreducible bond, accounting for high plasma stability. Following internalization, the drug is released from these conjugates due to lysosomal proteolytic degradation of the mAb. The drug-linker-amino acid residue itself must retain the activity of the drug [31]. FDA approved trastuzumab emtansine (Kadcyla®/T-DM1) uses a non-cleavable SMCC (*N*-succinimidyl-4-(maleimidomethyl) cyclohexane-1-carboxylate) linker to crosslink the warhead DM1 to lysine residues of anti-HER2 mAb trastuzumab. The intercellular metabolite lysine-MCC-DM1 complex was found to be as active as the parent drug, DM1, after lysosomal degradation of trastuzumab [32]. The hydrophobic nature of lysine-MCC-DM1 metabolites restricted the bystander effect and caused aggregation leading to immunogenicity. Polarity of the DM1 conjugates was increased with a tetramer PEG4Mal linker. Lysine-PEGMal-DM1 metabolites were found to be more potent, effectively retaining in MDR1 expressing cancer cells compared to lysine-MCC-DM1 metabolites [33]. Monomethyl auristatin F (MMAF) conjugates with non-reducible thioether linker were found to be highly stable with equal potency as compared to valine-citrulline conjugates [34].

2.2.3. Rational Linker Design to Overcome Resistance

Increasing occurrence of resistance in cancer patients, is a major challenge in anti-cancer drug discovery. Resistance to ADCs can be inherent or acquired and can be caused by several reasons including overexpression of efflux transporter proteins, downregulation or altered expression of target antigen, activation of different signaling pathways, blocked binding site at the target antigen etc. [35]. Commonly used cytotoxic payloads in ADC, such as calicheamicin, auristatins, maytansines, taxnes, and doxorubicin are well-known substrates of efflux transporter of P-gp, which pumps out the drug from intracellular space. This commonly observed phenomenon is key to the development of multi drug resistance (MDR), where patients fail to respond to several chemotherapies [36]. Clinically approved gemtuzumab ozogamicin was found to be less effective in acute myeloid leukemia patients with high expression of MDR proteins [37]. However, effective linker design can help to overcome multidrug resistance. Hydrophobic compounds are found to be more sensitive towards MDR1 efflux transporter. In a study with the hydrophilic DM1 payload, incorporation of a hydrophobic PEG4Mal linker enhanced potency of the ADC in MDR1 containing xenograft models [33]. When compared to SMCC linker, lysine-PEG4Mal-DM1 metabolites were more accumulated in MDR expressing COLO 205 cells than lysine-SMCC-DM1 metabolites [33]. In cleavable linkers, the payload gets more sensitive after it is released from the linker whereas, payloads with non-cleavable linkers are found to be less susceptible towards efflux proteins, where the mAb is digested but the linker-payload metabolite remains active [38]. Further, Zhao and co-workers showed that incorporation of a non-charged PEG group or negative charged α-sulphonic acid group increased hydrophilicity of commonly available hydrophobic SPDP, SMCC linkers as well as provided better therapeutic window for maytansine conjugates against MDR1 expressing cell lines in vitro and in vivo [39].

2.3. Payloads

Clinically approved chemotherapeutics with known clinical profiles like doxorubicin, methotrexate, and 5-flurouracil (Figure 4a) were commonly used as payloads in ADCs [40].

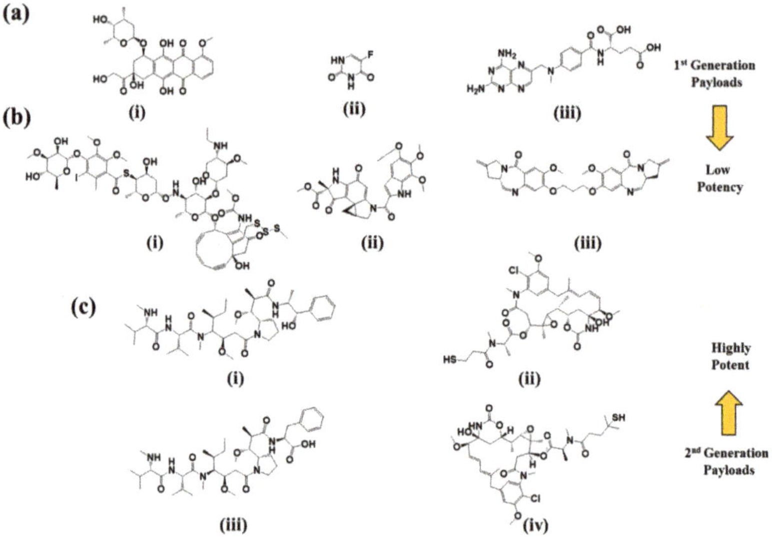

Figure 4. Chemical structures of first and second generation payloads used in ADCs. (**a**) 1st generation ADC payloads: (i) doxorubicin; (ii) 5-fluorouracil; and (iii) methotrexate; (**b**) DNA damaging agents: (i) calicheamicin γ1; (ii) duocarmycin A; and (iii) SJG-136 PDB dimer; and (**c**) tubulin polymerization inhibitors: (i) monomethyl auristatin E (MMAE); (ii) mertansine (DM1), monomethylauristatin F (MMAF), and ravtansine (DM4).

The clinically approved topoisomerase II inhibitor doxorubicin conjugated is to the hinge region cysteine residues of BR96 humanized mAb through an acid sensitive hydrazone linker is one of the 1st generation ADCs targeting the Lewis Y antigen, found to be overexpressed in different cancers [41]. The effective dose of BR96-doxorubicin in in vivo studies was found to be very high due to low potency of the payload (IC_{50} 0.1–0.2 μM) although with a high DAR value of 8. Despite such promising preclinical data, the BR96-doxorubicin conjugates failed to show enough efficacy in clinical trials, while patients experienced significant gastrointestinal toxicity due to the presence of Lewis Y in the gut [42]. Lessons from the story of BR96-doxorubicin established the use of more potent cytotoxic payloads, preferably with IC_{50} values in the sub-nanomolar range, as there is only a certain amount of payload that can be delivered via ADCs. Antibody conjugated delivery of highly potent chemotherapeutic drugs can increase tumor specificity, therapeutic index as well as decrease systemic toxicity. The cytotoxic payloads used in ADCs development can be divided in two classes based on their mechanism of action, DNA damaging agents (Figure 4b) and tubulin inhibitors (Figure 4c).

2.3.1. DNA Damaging Agents

Calicheamicins are naturally occurring highly potent DNA damaging agents isolated from the fermentation broth of a soil microorganism *Micromonospora echinospora* ssp. *Calichensis* [43]. Upon binding at the minor grove of the DNA they are reduced by cellular thiols to form a 1,4-dehydrobenzene radical intermediate, which then removes hydrogen from the deoxyribose ring and breaks the DNA strand [44] through a reaction commonly known as Bergman cyclization [45]. Calicheamicin was found to alter the expression of different key cell elements at the transcriptional level such as ribosomal proteins, nuclear proteins, and proteins accountable for stress response, different genes involved in DNA repair/synthesis, as well as metabolic and biosynthetic genes [46]. Calicheamicin is being investigated as payload in several ADCs; gemtuzumab ozogamicin and inotuzumab ozogamicin are noteworthy among them. Gemtuzumab ozogamicin incorporates a hydrazide derivative of calicheamicin, *N*-acetyl-γ-calicheamicin dimethyl hydrazide. CD-22 selective inotuzumab ozogamicin also incorporates *N*-acetyl-γ-calicheamicin dimethyl hydrazide as a payload [47]. Duocarmycins and pyrrolobenzodiazepines (PBD) are other notable chemotherapeutics in this class which are now in early stages of clinical development for payloads in ADCs [44]. Duocarmycins (DNA minor groove binders) exerts their cytotoxicity by alkylating adenine residues at the N3 position of DNA strands. SYD983, a duocarmycin-trastuzumab ADC was recently developed [48]. Of note, potent PBDs are naturally produced by *actinomycetes*. They covalently bind to a particular sequence in DNA minor groove and form an amine bond in-between C11 of PBD and N2 of guanine bases [49]. Although they do not disrupt the DNA structure considerably, formation of DNA-PBD adduct impedes key DNA functions like transcription and translation [50]. Several ADCs currently under clinical trial (SGN-CD70A, SGN-CD 33A and SGN-CD123A from Seattle Genetics) employ a PBD dimer SGD-1882 as their payload [51]. ADCs with PDB dimers are also found to be involved in bystander killing [50].

2.3.2. Tubulin Polymerization Inhibitors

Tubulin polymerization inhibitors (auristatins and maytansinoids) are widely employed as cytotoxic payloads [44]. Auristatins are water-soluble synthetic analogs of a marine natural product (dolastatin 10) isolated form the extract of a sea hare, *Dolabella auricularia*. The parent compound was also found in cyanobacteria *Symploca hydnoides* and *Lyngbya majuscula*, which are nourishment to the sea hare [52,53]. Dolastatin 10, a series of linear peptides comprised of dolavaline, valine, dolaisoleuine, dolaproine amino acid residues and a complex primary amine (dolaphenine) is found to be active against a wide range of cancer cell lines and solid tumors at very low concentrations (average IC_{50} value is in sub nanomolar range) [52,54]. It shares the same tubulin-binding site as vinca alkaloids and inhibits tubulin polymerization and tubulin-dependent GTP hydrolysis that causes cell cycle arrest in the G2/M phase, eventually leading to cell death [55]. Seattle Genetics has developed two auristatin derivatives (MMAE and MMAF), which are currently being used as payloads in several ADCs by linking to the cysteine residues of the mAb [56–58]. Bentuximab vedotin, a FDA approved ADC, incorporates MMAE which is linked to the cysteine residues of anti-CD30 antibody by a protease sensitive valine-citrulline dipeptide linker with an average 4 drug molecules per antibody [56]. Bentuximab vedotin is taken up in-to cytosol via cell-mediated endocytosis, where the linker is selectively cleaved in the presence of elevated lysosomal protease cathepsin B [59]. MMAE can penetrate the cell membrane, and as a result it can prompt bystander killing where it diffuses through nearby cells independent of antigen expression; by contrast, MMAF is impermeable to cell membrane [60]. This is because MMAF is more hydrophilic, less potent, and less toxic than MMAE. The presence of a charged phenylalanine moiety at the C-terminus of MMAF structure perturbs its cell membrane permeability [34]. Maytansiniod derivatives DM1 and DM4 are another type of microtubule polymerization inhibitors that are developed by Immunogen. Maytansine, an ansa antimitotic isolated from the bark of Ethiopian shrubs *Maytenus ovatus* and *Maytenus serrata* shares the same tubulin binding site and mechanism of action as vinca alkaloids and destabilizes microtubule assembly resulting cell cycle arrest in G2/M phase [61–63]. DM1 and DM4 are maytansinoids with methyl disulfide substitutions at the C3 *N*-acyl-*N*-methyl-L-alanyl ester side chain of maytansine [64]. Clinically approved Kadcyla® uses DM1 as a payload with an average DAR of 3.5 for treatment of HER2+ metastatic breast cancers [32]. SAR3419, a CD-19 targeted ADC with DM4 payload is in phase II clinical trial for the treatment of B-cell malignancies. DM4 is linked to the lysine residues of the mAbs with a thiol sensitive *N*-succinimidyl-4-(2-pyridyldithio) butyrate (SPDB) linker yielding an average DAR of 3.5 [65].

α-Amanitin, a RNA polymerase II inhibitor, is a highly water-soluble mushroom derived octapeptide, which is currently being investigated as a payload in pre-clinical ADCs [66]. In proof of concept studies α-amanitin was efficiently delivered to the target cells through an anti-HER2 mAb and the IC_{50} values were found to be in pico molar range [67]. An anti-EpCAM ADC conjugated with α-Amanitin payload via a protease/esterase sensitive glutamate linker was also found to be highly effective in EpCAM expressing tumor models [68]. Recently, anti-PSMA-α-amanitin ADCs were successfully employed to reduce tumor growth in preclinical prostate cancer model with stable and cleavable linker [69].

3. Conjugation

Mylotarg™ was the first ADC to be approved by the FDA, first marketed in 2000 until it's voluntary withdrawal in 2010 due to lack of significantly improved clinical benefits. The heterogeneous nature of drug conjugates and hydrazine linker instability were thought be accountable for the failure of this ADC. Thus, there was an urgent need for developing new strategies for producing homogenous drug antibody conjugation methods. Several strategies have been employed for cross-linking the antibody to drug by a linker using solvent reachable reactive amino acids with nucleophilic groups in antibody side chains. Side chain cysteine (SH group) and lysine (NH_2 group) have been extensively used for conjugation (Table 1). The main problem with these conventional conjugation methods is the heterogeneous nature of the end products with different DAR values [70]. The conjugation strategy must not alter any key blocks of an antibody that are responsible for its binding to the target antigens.

Table 1. Comparison between different side chain conjugation methods.

Conjugation	Reactive Groups	Advantages
Cysteine Residues	Maleimides, haloacetyls, other Michael acceptors	Simple and reproducible method Used in FDA approved Adcetris, widely employed in pipeline candidates, DAR ~0–8 Comparatively less heterogeneous by products than lysine conjugation Easier to characterize pharmacokinetically
Lysine Residues	Activated ester functional groups like *N*-hydroxysuccinimide esters	Though highly heterogeneous, this method is employed in FDA approved Kadcyla®, Mylotarg™, DAR ~3.5 (Kadcyla®), ~2.5 (Mylotarg™) Mostly used to crosslink via non-reducible linkers.

3.1. Via Side Chain Cystine Residues

Conjugation via side chain cysteines is a widely utilized and accepted technology in conjugation chemistry of ADCs. Seattle Genetics' ADC brentuximab vedotin utilizes this method to conjugate MMAE with the anti-CD30 mAb (cAC10) via an enzymatically cleavable dipeptide linker [71]. Cysteines are engaged in interchain and intrachain disulfide bridges in an antibody, which did not contribute to the building blocks of an antibody. In an IgG1 antibody, there are four interchain disulfide bonds [72,73]. It was also found that interchain disulfide bonds are more susceptible to reduction than intrachain disulfide bonds, which allow for a controlled reduction of the four interchain disulfide bonds with dithiothreitol (DTT) or tris(2-carboxyethyl)phosphine (TCEP) while keeping intrachain disulfide bond intact. This can yield up to eight reactive sulfhydryl groups, facilitating drug conjugation with DAR values of 0–8 [70,74]. These reactive sulfhydryl groups which are nucleophilic in nature, can be reacted with electrophiles like maleimides, haloacetyls for crosslinking proteins [75]. Conjugation via cysteine produces more uniform products than lysine conjugation that are easier to purify and characterize pharmacokinetically. Previously mentioned problems with non-specific conjugation methods established a need for more specific methods for conjugation.

3.2. Via Side Chain Lysine Residues

Mylotarg™ had utilized side-chain reactive lysine residues of a humanized anti-CD33 mAb for conjugating the drug calicheamicin by a bifunctional acid sensitive hydrazone linker [76]. However, Pfizer voluntarily withdrew this product in 2010 [77]. Ado-trastuzumab-emtansine (Kadcyla®), one of four approved ADCs in the market utilizing side chain lysines for conjugating the potent tubulin inhibitor emtansine to mAb trastuzumab (Herceptin®) [32]. An ESI-TOF MS method confirms that 40 out of 86 lysine residues of humanized monoclonal IgG1 huN901-antibody are available for conjugation to DM1 molecules. Peptide mapping further showed conjugation sites present in both the heavy and light chain [78].

3.3. Drug Antibody Ratio (DAR)

DAR is defined as the number of drug molecules per mAb. DAR plays a definitive role in developing ADCs, as it determines the dose needed to produce the desired effect in patients. There is a limited number of drug molecules that can be efficiently delivered to the target site and drug loading significantly contributes to the pharmacokinetic profile of ADC. Hamblett and co-workers showed that the effect of drug distribution on the different properties like therapeutic window, pharmacokinetic properties, and maximum tolerated dose of cAC10-MMAE conjugates. Decreasing the DAR resulted in a superior therapeutic window of cAC10-MMAE conjugates, proving that drug loading as a decisive parameter for designing ADCs. Although cAC10-MMAE conjugates with DAR ~2–4 were less active in in vitro studies, but their results in in vivo studies were found to be equivalently potent (DAR~4) and better tolerated than the conjugate with higher DAR ~8. Similar observations were found with regards to pharmacokinetic properties [70]. If fewer drug molecules are conjugated per mAb, the ADC system will not be effective clinically. On the other hand, conjugating too many drug molecules per mAb will make the ADC unstable, toxic and may lead to aggregation and immunogenic reactions [79,80]. Hydrophobic MMAE conjugates using interchain cysteines with higher DAR are found to be physically unstable [79]. Normally ADCs contain different species with differing DAR values and every species has its own distinct pharmacokinetics. ADCs with heavily loaded drugs are more rapidly cleared from the system. In general, an average DAR of 3–4 is used to achieve optimum effect in ADCs, depending upon potency of the payload [70,81]. However, a recently developed poly-1-hydroxymethylethylene hydroxymethylformal (PHF) polymer-based ADC with a higher DAR of ~20 challenged this conventional concept. With vinca alkaloid as the payload and trastuzumab as the targeting mAb, the newly developed platform not only showed promising activity in xenograft tumor models, but also demonstrated good pharmacokinetic properties [82]. Conjugations through side-chain lysine residues are highly heterogeneous leading to inconsistent DAR values and different conjugation sites in the antibody. In case of Kadcyla® where the drug DM1 was conjugated with the trastuzumab through the side chain lysine residues, an average DAR was found to be ~3.5 [83]. Side chain cysteine conjugation employs a controlled reduction of four intrachain disulfide bonds that allows conjugation of 0–8 drug molecules per antibody [84]. Common analytical methods for determining DAR are UV-Vis spectroscopy, hydrophobic interaction chromatography (HIC), LC-ESI-MS and rpHPLC. UV visible spectroscopy exploits the dissimilarities in maximum wave length absorbance of payload and mAb for determining respective concentrations [85]. UV-Vis spectroscopic method is widely employed to characterize huN901-DM1, 791T/36-methotrexate and cAC10-MMAE conjugates [70,86,87]. HIC uses a column consisting of a hydrophobic stationary phase and a mobile phase with gradient salt concentration to separate ADC species based on hydrophobic interactions. Mostly the ADC payloads are hydrophobic in nature, and hydrophobic conjugated species are retained in the column, whereas unconjugated species elute first in neutral pH and non-denaturizing conditions [88]. This method is more compatible with ADCs with cysteine conjugation sites on mAb, while LC-ESI-MS method was developed for characterizing lysine-conjugated ADCs [89,90]. LC-MS is advantageous over HIC or UV-Vis spectroscopic characterization as it not only gives information on DAR or drug distribution but also gives crucial structural insights of ADCs at the molecular level [91]. Wagner-Rousset and co-workers designed a simple and fast method of DAR determination based on antibody-fluorophore conjugates (AFCs) with the same linker and conjugation chemistry as ADCs. Instead of toxic payloads, a non-toxic dansyl sulfonamide ethyl amine payload was used. AFCs were subjected to digestion by *Streptococcus pyogenes* (IdeS) accompanied by DTT reduction, which generated seven easily ionizable fragments (Fd0, Fd1, Fd2, Fd3. L0, L1, Fc/2) of ~25 kDa. These resultant fragments were analyzed by

LC-ESI-TOF-MS method. This method is advantageous over single step reduction as it not only gives routine information like DAR and drug distribution but also provides crucial structural details like *N*-glycosylation profiling, C-terminal lysine truncation, pyroglutamylation, oxidation and degradation products [92].

3.4. Site Specific Conjugation

The most common problems with conventional conjugation technologies are heterogeneous byproducts with different drug distributions per mAb, un-conjugated and overly conjugated mAbs. These phenomena are attributed to poor pharmacokinetic properties and instability of ADCs in systemic circulation [70]. Un-conjugated antibodies occupy the site of attachment, competing with drug-conjugated antibodies and block the site for internalization for the targeting mAb. On the other hand, overly conjugated mAbs are more rapidly cleared as well as can cause immunogenic reactions and toxicity. Engineering of the conjugation site may lead to a more homogenous product with defined and uniform drug stoichiometry (Table 2).

Table 2. Comparison between different site-specific conjugation technologies.

Method of Conjugation	Reactive Groups	Advantages	Developer
Engineered side chain cysteine residues (ThioMAb) [93]	Maleimides	Improved clinical safety, tolerability and therapeutic index over conventional conjugates. Controlled and reproducible DAR 2. Compatible for producing in large scale.	Genentech
Incorporation of un-natural amino acids (unAA) [94]	Alkoxy-amine	Highly stable and extended half-life in systemic circulation. Improved pharmacological profile compared to conventional ADCs. Ketone group present in unAA provided conjugation site for different alternative payloads like kinase inhibitors, proteasome inhibitors.	Ambrx
Enzymatic Site-Specific Conjugation Process [95]	Amine, Indole	DAR 2-4, More stable conjugates than yielded by ThioMAb and oxime ligation. Controlled conjugation site of the payload on the mAb. Better pharmacokinetic profile over conventional conjugates.	Innate Pharma, Glycos, Pfizer. Inc.

3.4.1. Engineering of Side Chain Cysteine Residues

The first site-specific conjugation method for cysteine residues was developed at Genentech [93]. In this method, potential sites, which do not contribute to pivotal functions of the mAb like antigen folding or binding were identified and mutated with cysteine residues to generate a novel platform, called Thiomab™. A phage display-based biochemical assay (Phage ELISA for Selection of Reactive Thiols, PHESELECTOR) was employed to identify tolerated reactive cysteine residues from fab region of the mAb [96]. Resultant Thiomabs are subjected to controlled reduction in presence of DTT or TCEP to produce free thiols from cysteines. Previously reduced interchain disulfides are reinstated by an oxidation process with copper sulfate or dehydroascorbic acid, while the engineered cysteines are kept in a reduced form. Thus, only the reduced cysteines were available for site-specific conjugation. In the proof of concept study, nearly homogenous (92%) anti-MUC16-Thiomab™-MC-vc-PAB-MMAE conjugates with a DAR ~2 retained activity, improved therapeutic window and were better tolerated in preclinical studies on Sprague-Dawley rats and cynomolgus monkeys when compared to conventional ADCs with higher average DAR [93]. In a different study, Thiomab™-trastuzumab-BMPEO-DM1 conjugates were also found to be better tolerated at the same dose than the conventional trastuzumab-MCC-DM1 conjugates [97]. Engineered cysteine residues at the A114C position were used for conjugation and thus site-specific conjugation at those sites lead to better linker stability, therapeutic window, and more homogenous Thiomab™ ADCs. Another site-specific conjugation approach via modifying cysteine is disulfide rebridging, where interchain disulfide bonds were reduced first and then reinstated by a bis-alkylation process to form a three carbon bridge. Resulting conjugates were found to be more stable than the maleamide conjugates in serum and high albumin concentrations [98].

3.4.2. Incorporation of Unnatural Amino Acids (unAA)

Another powerful approach to the site-specific conjugation was developed via incorporation of unnatural amino acids (unAA) as the 21st amino acid with a reactive handle on different side chains of the mAb. It allowed selective conjugation of different classes of payloads that have not been able to be conjugated because of the limitations of conventional conjugation methods. This method also allowed conjugation ofcombination of payloads with different mechanism of action [99]. The most common method for unAA insertion employs t-RNA/amino-acyl t-RNA synthetase pair which incorporates the un-natural amino acid at the place of the amber stop codon (TAG) encoded in the gene of interest [100]. Nearly homogenous trastuzumab-MMAF conjugates with an average DAR ~2 were synthesized utilizing a site specifically introduced *p*-acetylphenylalanie unAA. The ketone group present in the *p*-acetylphenylalanie unAA formed a stable oxime linkage with the alkoxy-amine-MMAF payloads. Resulting conjugates were found to be highly stable and with a similar pharmacokinetic profile of the naked mAb [94]. In a similar study hydroxylamine-MMAD payloads conjugated to the site-specifically incorporated *p*-acetylphenylalanine residue of the 5-T4/anti-HER2 mAb via a non-cleavable linker were found to be superior to the corresponding ADCs with interchain cysteine or engineered cysteine residues as conjugation site [101].

3.4.3. Enzymatic Site-Specific Conjugation Processes

Reactive functional groups for site-specific conjugation of the drug payloads were also introduced to the antibodies by several enzymes like transglutaminase and glycotransferase. Bacterial transglutamiase from *Streptoverticillium mobaraense* forms a stable isopeptide bond in-between an amine group and g-carboxamide moiety from a glutamine tag engineered in the flexible region of the deglycosylated mAbs but not from the naturally available glutamines [95,102]. Strop and co-workers introduced a short glutamine tag LLQG into 90 different regions of an anti-EGFR antibody, among them 12 were fit for drug crosslinking. Then two (LLQGA in heavy chain and GGLLQGA in light chain) out of the 12 glutamine tags were chosen for conjugating amine containing MMAD derivatives with both the cleavable and non-cleavable linker in presence of transglutaminase. Resulting ADCs were found to be highly stable, monomeric and with an average DAR ~1.9 and better pharmacokinetic profile compared to the conventional ADCs [103]. Similar conjugates were synthesized by this method using anti-M1S1-C16 (Clone 16) mAb and an anti-Her2 mAb. A recently developed anti-Trop2 ADC, with a LLQGA glutamine tag for site-specific conjugation with an undisclosed microtubule inhibitor showed promising efficacy in preclinical studies [104]. Another additional approach for enzyme-mediated conjugation is SmartTags (Specific Modifiable Aldehyde Recombinant Tag) technology using CxPxR recognizing formyl glycine generating enzyme, which converts cysteines to formylglycine with a reactive aldehyde group [105]. Pictet−Spengler ligation chemistry allowed bio conjugation of indole based payloads to the aldehyde group of the modified mAb [106]. A modified version of Pictet-Spengler reaction is Hydrazino-Pictet-Spengler Ligation, which not only provides an effective, quick and one step conjugation as well as found to be advantageous over oxime ligation conjugation [107].

4. Clinical Trials

The number of ADCs in clinical trial is rapidly increasing with two of the recently approved ADCs (Besponsa®, re-approved Mylotarg™). Currently there are more than 50 ADCs, which are in different phases of clinical trial as monotherapy as well as in combination with other chemotherapeutic drugs for treatment of different types of cancer and showing promising results. Most of the ADCs under clinical trial uses common type of payload-linker motifs although they differ in the mAb to target different types of malignancies (Figure 5).

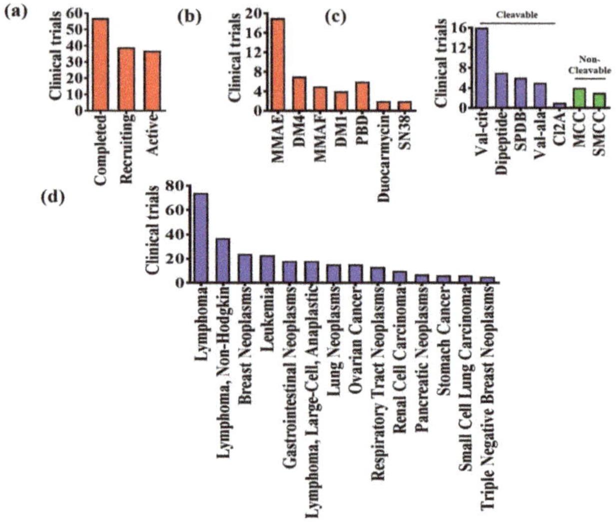

Figure 5. (**a**) Status of clinical trials on ADCs; (**b**) Different ADC payloads in clinical trials; (**c**) Different ADC linkers in clinical trials; (**d**) Clinical trials of ADCs for different type of oncologic indications based on clinicaltrials.gov database search.

Among them three candidates are in phase III of clinical trials. Several ADCs are in preclinical development. In this section, we discuss about development of sacituzumab govitecan (IMMU-132), mirvetuximab soravtansine (IMGN-853), and inotuzumab ozogamicin (CMC-544), which are now investigated in phase III clinical trial.

Sacituzumab Govitecan (IMMU-132): This is a moderately toxic topoisomerase I inhibitor SN38, metabolite of prodrug irinotecan conjugated to a humanized anti-Trop2 mAb by a pH sensitive CL2A linker [108]. The average DAR (7.6) of this ADC is comparatively high because of the moderately toxic payload. A short PEG spacer incorporated in-between the linker and the payload enhances the aqueous solubility of the payload. However, IMMU-132 delivers more SN-38 (active metabolite of irinotecan) to the tumor tissue than the prodrug formulation irinotecan [109]. The target trop-2 (trophoblast cell surface antigen) is over expressed in different types of cancer like breast, lung, pancreatic, colorectal, prostate and cervical [109]. Trop2 is an attractive target for triple negative breast cancer (TNBC). In phase II clinical trial, 8–10 mg/kg dose of IMMU-132 showed promising activity with manageable grade 3–4 side effects like diarrhea, neutropenia, fatigue, and anemia. No occurrence of immunogenicity was reported [110], thus a phase III trial for this drug has been initiated (NCT02574455) for refractory/relapsed TNBC patients. IMMU-132 earned Breakthrough Therapy designation from the FDA for the treatment of TNBC, small cell lung cancer, and non-small cell lung cancer.

Mirvetuximab Soravtansine (IMGN-853): It uses a humanized anti-folate receptor-α (FR-α) mAb conjugated to the maytansine payload DM-4 through a cleavable sulpho-SPDB linker. FR-α comes under class of glycoproteins that govern endocytosis mediated uptake of folates [111]. FR-α has limited expression in healthy tissues, whereas it is elevated in several malignancies [112]. A hydrophilic sulpho-SPDB linker established the bridge between the lysine residues of the mAb and the microtubule-disrupting payload DM4. After lysosomal degradation, one of the metabolites S-methyl-DM4, which is lipophilic in nature induced bystander killing in neighboring cells irrespective of the antigen expression [112,113]. Mirvetuximab soravtansine is reported to be upregulating effects of conventional chemo drugs like carboplatin in ovarian cancer [114]. In phase I dose escalation study, patients received doses from 0.15 to 7.0 mg/kg once in a three week. From the phase I study, the encouraging potency of IGMN-853 was noted for epithelial ovarian cancer with a favorable toxicity profile. From the phase I, trial results a dose of 6 mg/kg once in a three weeks was chosen for phase II clinical studies [115]. In the phase II study on patients with platinum-resistant ovarian cancer, IMGN-853 was found to be active mostly in less heavily treated individuals with a reasonable toxicity profile. Grade 2 side effects like diarrhea, nausea, blurred vision were reported [116]. Phase III clinical trial (NCT02631876) of this drug is started in patients with FR-α expressing epithelial ovarian cancer, primary peritoneal cancer or fallopian tube cancer along with a choice of chemotherapy of the investigator.

Inotuzumab Ozogamicin (Besponsa™): Pfizer, Wyeth and University of California, Berkeley jointly developed this ADC. It entered phase III clinical trial with frontline chemotherapy in young adult patients with B Acute Lymphoblastic Leukemia (NCT03150693). It is consisted of an humanized anti-CD22 mAb G5/44 (IgG4 isotype) with a DNA damaging *N*-acetyl-γ-calicheamicin dimethyl hydrazide derivative as payload connected through an acid-sensitive 4-(4-acetylphenoxy) butanoic acid (AcBut) linker [47]. The target CD22 is a B-acute lymphoblastic leukemia (B-ALL) specific antigen with restricted expression in the surface of full-grown B cells [117]. An investigation on adult acute lymphoid leukemia patients confirmed abundance of CD22 expression [118]. Inotuzumab ozogamicin in preclinical models established it's superiority over non-targeted conventional combination chemotherapy comprised of cyclophosphamide, vincristine and prednisone (CVP) or doxorubicin (CHOP) in in vitro studies as well as in vivo human B-cell lymphoma xenograft mice models. When it is used together with CVP, it exerted more potency but with CHOP resulted in toxicity in mice models. However, dose-dense study with 2 dosages of inotuzumab ozogamicin and CHOP found to be potent with no toxicities [119]. From the phase I study, of inotuzumab ozogamicin, MTD was found to be 1.8 mg/m^2 with side effects like thrombocytopenia (major), asthenia, nausea and neutropenia B-cell non-hodgkin's lymphoma [120]. Phase II clinical trial (NCT01134575) of this drug was conducted at MD Anderson Cancer Center with an adult I.V. dose 1.8 mg/m^2 and a pediatrics I.V. dose 1.3 mg/m^2. This drug was administered in 49 refractory and relapsed B-ALL patients with a median age of 36 years. The complete response rate from this study was 57% with an overall median survival rate of 7.9 months in responders [121]. Clinical trials (NCT01564784) of inotuzumab ozogamicin with investigator's choice of chemotherapy further proved its superiority over standard chemotherapy and was approved by FDA to treat adult patients with relapsed/refractory B-cell precursor acute lymphoblastic leukemia in August 2017.

5. Future Directions

Conventional chemotherapy accounted for consequential toxicities and low therapeutic window for the treatment of malignancies. In the era of personalized medicines, pharmacogenetic testing of the patients followed by ADC treatment can be an excellent alternative over the conventional chemotherapies (Figure 6). For patient selection, a threshold expression of the target antigen must be defined during preclinical development. ADCs also serve as a target-guided tool for the delivery for highly potent cytotoxic drug(s) that cannot be administered as a monotherapy.

A considerable rise in this field has been observed following the success and FDA approval for Adcetris® in 2011, Kadcyla® in 2013, Besponsa™ in 2017 and reapproval of Mylotarg™. These recent successes have bolstered ADC developments and presently ~50 ADCs are in pipeline for the treatment of hematologic and solid tumor malignancies. The choice of target, mAb isotype, the linker, the conjugation site and the cytotoxic payload plays crucial part in ADC design. Better understanding of all ADC components may lead to successful generation of an effective ADC. Conventionally, ADC employs a heavily cytotoxic drug as payload (such as calicheamicins, duocarmycins, auristatins, and maytansinoids) however, site specific conjugated ADCs like milatuzumab-Dox, IMMU132, IMMU-130 with moderately cytotoxic payloads like doxorubicin, camptothecin analog SN-38 were also found to be promising, thus redefining the conventional ADC concept. The main challenge remains to optimize the bio-conjugation process to produce homogenous antibody drug conjugates. A better understanding of the role of linker and method of conjugation to the clinical profile of the ADC have led to development of several state of art site-specific conjugation methods for homogenous antibody conjugate production. Table 3 incorporates noteworthy overview(s) on ADCs development through review articles.

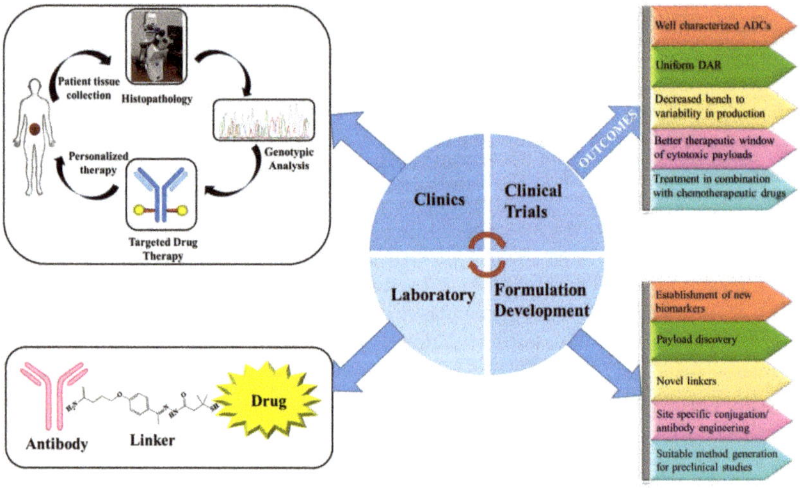

Figure 6. Schematic diagram showing transition of ADCs from laboratory to clinic.

Table 3. List of some of the key review articles on ADCs.

Name of the Review Article	Focus of the Review	Year of Publication
Antibody-Drug Conjugates for Cancer Therapy [7]	This article is focused on different key issues like choosing an appropriate target, expression of the target, selecting right mAb isotype.	2008
Antibody Conjugate Therapeutics: Challenges and Potential [122]	The key consideration behind choosing an appropriate target for ADC developments.	2011
Pharmacokinetic Considerations for Antibody Drug Conjugates [10]	Different pharmacokinetic considerations to characterize ADCs as well as PK-PD modellings for development of ADCs	2012
Site-Specific Antibody–Drug Conjugates: The Nexus of Biorthogonal Chemistry, Protein Engineering, and Drug Development [75]	Focuses on methods to synthesize site-specific homogenous ADCs with details of bio-orthogonal chemistries.	2014
Antibody-Drug Conjugates: Design, Formulation and Physicochemical Stability [123]	Physiochemical characterization, formulation considerations, and factors involved in process control.	2015
Methods to Design and Synthesize Antibody-Drug Conjugates (ADCs) [98]	Accounts for different conjugation methods and the chemistry behind in the field of ADCs.	2016
Mechanisms of Resistance to Antibody–Drug Conjugates [35]	Resistance of various ADCs and possible mechanism.	2016
Antibodies and associates: Partners in targeted drug delivery [124]	Engineering antibodies and their subsequent use in different targeted drug delivery systems.	2017

Site conjugation processes like Thiomab®, enzymatic conjugation, incorporation of unnatural amino acid (unAA) has been used to install reactive handle on the mAb for facilitating a homogenous conjugation process without disrupting the mAb functions. The most common mechanism reported regarding resistances of ADC therapy is attributed to the MDR protein. However, this problem is countered with replacing P-gp substrate drugs with several new naturally occurring toxins, ADC prodrugs as well structural altercations in the drug-linker [38]. A significant effort is also directed towards developing suitable preclinical model to evaluate ADCs therapeutic efficacy.

Xenograft bearing mice models does not replicate human conditions genetically in proper way, but genetically engineered mice models are more reliable for evaluating ADCs as they can bear relevant target oncogenes. Another important challenge is to produce cost effective and affordable ADC medications. At present ADCs are quite expansive, for example yearly brentuximab vedotin treatment regimen costs ~$100,000 [125]. In our review, we have put together up-to-date advances in the field of payload discovery, their mechanism of action as well as linker and conjugation technologies. However, regardless of different challenges, recent success in this field can shift the paradigm of cancer therapy to personalized ADCs treatments.

Acknowledgments: This work was supported by the National Institutes of Health Research Project Grant Program (R01 CA210192, R01 CA206069, and CA204552) to SCC. This research was supported by National Institute of Health/National Cancer Center's Career Development Award (K22CA174841) and AREA grant (CA213232) to MMY. UTHSC-CORNET, NEW GRANT and College of Pharmacy-Dean's Seed Grant to S.C.C., M.J., M.M.Y is also acknowledged. Authors acknowledge Sonam Kumari, Andrew Massey, and Kyle Doxtater for proof reading this manuscript.

Author Contributions: N.D., M.M.Y., S.C.C. conceived the idea, reviewed literature/data, and crucially involved throughout the writing of this manuscript. N.D., M.M.Y., S.C.C., M.J., S.S., V.K.K., S.K., have participated in discussion, edited and reviewed the manuscript.

Conflicts of Interest: The authors declare no conflict of interest.

References

1. WHO: Cancer World Health Organization. Available online: http://www.who.int/mediacentre/factsheets/fs297/en/ (accessed on 5 April 2018).
2. Peer, D.; Karp, J.M.; Hong, S.; Farokhzad, O.C.; Margalit, R.; Langer, R. Nanocarriers as an emerging platform for cancer therapy. *Nat. Nanotechnol.* **2007**, *2*, 751–760. [CrossRef] [PubMed]
3. Gottesman, M.M.; Fojo, T.; Bates, S.E. Multidrug resistance in cancer: Role of atp-dependent transporters. *Nat. Rev. Cancer* **2002**, *2*, 48–58. [CrossRef] [PubMed]
4. Strebhardt, K.; Ullrich, A. Paul ehrlich's magic bullet concept: 100 years of progress. *Nat. Rev. Cancer* **2008**, *8*, 473–480. [CrossRef] [PubMed]
5. Panowski, S.; Bhakta, S.; Raab, H.; Polakis, P.; Junutula, J.R. Site-specific antibody drug conjugates for cancer therapy. *mAbs* **2014**, *6*, 34–45. [CrossRef] [PubMed]
6. Chari, R.V.J.; Miller, M.L.; Widdison, W.C. Antibody–drug conjugates: An emerging concept in cancer therapy. *Angew. Chem. Int. Ed.* **2014**, *53*, 3796–3827. [CrossRef] [PubMed]
7. Carter, P.J.; Senter, P.D. Antibody-drug conjugates for cancer therapy. *Cancer J.* **2008**, *14*, 154–169. [CrossRef] [PubMed]
8. Milstein, G.K.C. Continuous cultures of fused cells secreting antibody of predefined specificity. *Nature* **1975**, *256*, 495–497.
9. Rudnick, S.I.; Lou, J.; Shaller, C.C.; Tang, Y.; Klein-Szanto, A.J.P.; Weiner, L.M.; Marks, J.D.; Adams, G.P. Influence of affinity and antigen internalization on the uptake and penetration of anti-her2 antibodies in solid tumors. *Cancer Res.* **2011**, *71*, 2250–2259. [CrossRef] [PubMed]
10. Lin, K.; Tibbitts, J. Pharmacokinetic considerations for antibody drug conjugates. *Pharm. Res.* **2012**, *29*, 2354–2366. [CrossRef] [PubMed]
11. Tolcher, A.W.; Ochoa, L.; Hammond, L.A.; Patnaik, A.; Edwards, T.; Takimoto, C.; Smith, L.; de Bono, J.; Schwartz, G.; Mays, T.; et al. Cantuzumab mertansine, a maytansinoid immunoconjugate directed to the canag antigen: A phase I, pharmacokinetic, and biologic correlative study. *J. Clin. Oncol.* **2003**, *21*, 211–222. [CrossRef] [PubMed]
12. Pastuskovas, C.V.; Mallet, W.; Clark, S.; Kenrick, M.; Majidy, M.; Schweiger, M.; Van Hoy, M.; Tsai, S.P.; Bennett, G.; Shen, B.-Q. Effect of immune complex formation on the distribution of a novel antibody to the ovarian tumor antigen CA125. *Drug Metab. Dispos.* **2010**, *38*, 2309–2319. [CrossRef] [PubMed]
13. Jiang, X.-R.; Song, A.; Bergelson, S.; Arroll, T.; Parekh, B.; May, K.; Chung, S.; Strouse, R.; Mire-Sluis, A.; Schenerman, M. Advances in the assessment and control of the effector functions of therapeutic antibodies. *Nat. Rev. Drug Discov.* **2011**, *10*, 101–111. [CrossRef] [PubMed]

14. Sapra, P.; Hooper, A.T.; O'Donnell, C.J.; Gerber, H.P. Investigational antibody drug conjugates for solid tumors. *Expert Opin. Investig. Drugs* **2011**, *20*, 1131–1149. [CrossRef] [PubMed]
15. Junttila, T.T.; Li, G.; Parsons, K.; Phillips, G.L.; Sliwkowski, M.X. Trastuzumab-DM1 (T-DM1) retains all the mechanisms of action of trastuzumab and efficiently inhibits growth of lapatinib insensitive breast cancer. *Breast Cancer Res. Treat.* **2011**, *128*, 347–356. [CrossRef] [PubMed]
16. Sharkey, R.M.; Goldenberg, D.M. Targeted therapy of cancer: New prospects for antibodies and immunoconjugates. *CA-A Cancer J. Clin.* **2006**, *56*, 226–243. [CrossRef]
17. Pillay, C.S.; Elliott, E.; Dennison, C. Endolysosomal proteolysis and its regulation. *Biochem. J.* **2002**, *363*, 417–429. [CrossRef] [PubMed]
18. Alley, S.C.; Okeley, N.M.; Senter, P.D. Antibody-drug conjugates: Targeted drug delivery for cancer. *Curr. Opin. Chem. Biol.* **2010**, *14*, 529–537. [CrossRef] [PubMed]
19. Griffith, O.W. Biologic and pharmacologic regulation of mammalian glutathione synthesis. *Free Radic. Biol. Med.* **1999**, *27*, 922–935. [CrossRef]
20. Balendiran, G.K.; Dabur, R.; Fraser, D. The role of glutathione in cancer. *Cell Biochem. Funct.* **2004**, *22*, 343–352. [CrossRef] [PubMed]
21. Wu, G.; Fang, Y.-Z.; Yang, S.; Lupton, J.R.; Turner, N.D. Glutathione metabolism and its implications for health. *J. Nutr.* **2004**, *134*, 489–492. [CrossRef] [PubMed]
22. Appenzeller-Herzog, C.; Ellgaard, L. The human pdi family: Versatility packed into a single fold. *BBA-Mol. Cell. Res.* **2008**, *1783*, 535–548. [CrossRef] [PubMed]
23. Chari, R.V.J. Targeted cancer therapy: Conferring specificity to cytotoxic drugs. *Acc. Chem. Res.* **2008**, *41*, 98–107. [CrossRef] [PubMed]
24. Dubowchik, G.M.; Firestone, R.A. Cathepsin b-sensitive dipeptide prodrugs. 1. A model study of structural requirements for efficient release of doxorubicin. *Bioorg. Med. Chem. Lett.* **1998**, *8*, 3341–3346. [CrossRef]
25. Tranoy-Opalinski, I.; Legigan, T.; Barat, R.; Clarhaut, J.; Thomas, M.; Renoux, B.; Papot, S. Beta-glucuronidase-responsive prodrugs for selective cancer chemotherapy: An update. *Eur. J. Med. Chem.* **2014**, *74*, 302–313. [CrossRef] [PubMed]
26. Michelle de, G.; Epie, B.; Hans, W.S.; Hidde, J.H.; Herbert, M.P. Beta-glucuronidase-mediated drug release. *Curr. Pharm. Des.* **2002**, *8*, 1391–1403.
27. Jeffrey, S.C.; Andreyka, J.B.; Bernhardt, S.X.; Kissler, K.M.; Kline, T.; Lenox, J.S.; Moser, R.F.; Nguyen, M.T.; Okeley, N.M.; Stone, I.J.; et al. Development and properties of β-glucuronide linkers for monoclonal antibody−drug conjugates. *Bioconj. Chem.* **2006**, *17*, 831–840. [CrossRef] [PubMed]
28. Jeffrey, S.C.; De Brabander, J.; Miyamoto, J.; Senter, P.D. Expanded utility of the β-glucuronide linker: ADCs that deliver phenolic cytotoxic agents. *ACS Med. Chem. Lett.* **2010**, *1*, 277–280. [CrossRef] [PubMed]
29. Burke, P.J.; Hamilton, J.Z.; Pires, T.A.; Setter, J.R.; Hunter, J.H.; Cochran, J.H.; Waight, A.B.; Gordon, K.A.; Toki, B.E.; Emmerton, K.K.; et al. Development of novel quaternary ammonium linkers for antibody–drug conjugates. *Mol. Cancer Ther.* **2016**, *15*, 938–945. [CrossRef] [PubMed]
30. Senter, P.D.; Sievers, E.L. The discovery and development of brentuximab vedotin for use in relapsed hodgkin lymphoma and systemic anaplastic large cell lymphoma. *Nat. Biotechnol.* **2012**, *30*, 631–637. [CrossRef] [PubMed]
31. Diamantis, N.; Banerji, U. Antibody-drug conjugates—An emerging class of cancer treatment. *Br. J. Cancer* **2016**, *114*, 362–367. [CrossRef] [PubMed]
32. LoRusso, P.M.; Weiss, D.; Guardino, E.; Girish, S.; Sliwkowski, M.X. Trastuzumab emtansine: A unique antibody-drug conjugate in development for human epidermal growth factor receptor 2–positive cancer. *Clin. Cancer Res.* **2011**, *17*, 6437–6447. [CrossRef] [PubMed]
33. Kovtun, Y.V.; Audette, C.A.; Mayo, M.F.; Jones, G.E.; Doherty, H.; Maloney, E.K.; Erickson, H.K.; Sun, X.; Wilhelm, S.; Ab, O.; et al. Antibody-maytansinoid conjugates designed to bypass multidrug resistance. *Cancer Res.* **2010**, *70*, 2528–2537. [CrossRef] [PubMed]
34. Doronina, S.O.; Mendelsohn, B.A.; Bovee, T.D.; Cerveny, C.G.; Alley, S.C.; Meyer, D.L.; Oflazoglu, E.; Toki, B.E.; Sanderson, R.J.; Zabinski, R.F.; et al. Enhanced activity of monomethylauristatin f through monoclonal antibody delivery: Effects of linker technology on efficacy and toxicity. *Bioconj. Chem.* **2006**, *17*, 114–124. [CrossRef] [PubMed]
35. Loganzo, F.; Sung, M.; Gerber, H.-P. Mechanisms of resistance to antibody–drug conjugates. *Mol. Cancer Ther.* **2016**, *15*, 2825–2834. [CrossRef] [PubMed]

36. Parslow, A.; Parakh, S.; Lee, F.-T.; Gan, H.; Scott, A. Antibody–drug conjugates for cancer therapy. *Biomedicines* **2016**, *4*, 14. [CrossRef] [PubMed]
37. Linenberger, M.L.; Hong, T.; Flowers, D.; Sievers, E.L.; Gooley, T.A.; Bennett, J.M.; Berger, M.S.; Leopold, L.H.; Appelbaum, F.R.; Bernstein, I.D. Multidrug-resistance phenotype and clinical responses to gemtuzumab ozogamicin. *Blood* **2001**, *98*, 988–994. [CrossRef] [PubMed]
38. Shefet-Carasso, L.; Benhar, I. Antibody-targeted drugs and drug resistance–challenges and solutions. *Drug Resist. Updates* **2015**, *18*, 36–46. [CrossRef] [PubMed]
39. Zhao, R.Y.; Wilhelm, S.D.; Audette, C.; Jones, G.; Leece, B.A.; Lazar, A.C.; Goldmacher, V.S.; Singh, R.; Kovtun, Y.; Widdison, W.C.; et al. Synthesis and evaluation of hydrophilic linkers for antibody-maytansinoid conjugates. *J. Med. Chem.* **2011**, *54*, 3606–3623. [CrossRef] [PubMed]
40. Ducry, L.; Stump, B. Antibody−drug conjugates: Linking cytotoxic payloads to monoclonal antibodies. *Bioconj. Chem.* **2010**, *21*, 5–13. [CrossRef] [PubMed]
41. Trail, P.; Willner, D.; Lasch, S.; Henderson, A.; Hofstead, S.; Casazza, A.; Firestone, R.; Hellstrom, I.; Hellstrom, K. Cure of xenografted human carcinomas by Br96-doxorubicin immunoconjugates. *Science* **1993**, *261*, 212–215. [CrossRef] [PubMed]
42. Tolcher, A.W.; Sugarman, S.; Gelmon, K.A.; Cohen, R.; Saleh, M.; Isaacs, C.; Young, L.; Healey, D.; Onetto, N.; Slichenmyer, W. Randomized phase ii study of br96-doxorubicin conjugate in patients with metastatic breast cancer. *J. Clin. Oncol.* **1999**, *17*, 478–484. [CrossRef] [PubMed]
43. Maiese, W.M.; Lechevalier, M.P.; Lechevalier, H.A.; Korshalla, J.; Kuck, N.; Fantini, A.; Wildey, M.J.; Thomas, J.; Greenstein, M. Calicheamicins, a novel family of antitumor antibiotics: Taxonomy, fermentation and biological properties. *J. Antibiot.* **1989**, *42*, 558–563. [CrossRef] [PubMed]
44. Polakis, P. Antibody drug conjugates for cancer therapy. *Pharmacol. Rev.* **2016**, *68*, 3–19. [CrossRef] [PubMed]
45. Jones, R.R.; Bergman, R.G. P-benzyne. Generation as an intermediate in a thermal isomerization reaction and trapping evidence for the 1,4-benzenediyl structure. *J. Am. Chem. Soc.* **1972**, *94*, 660–661. [CrossRef]
46. Watanabe, C.M.; Supekova, L.; Schultz, P.G. Transcriptional effects of the potent enediyne anti-cancer agent calicheamicin gamma(i)(1). *Chem. Biol.* **2002**, *9*, 245–251. [CrossRef]
47. De Vries, J.F.; Zwaan, C.M.; De Bie, M.; Voerman, J.S.; den Boer, M.L.; van Dongen, J.J.; van der Velden, V.H. The novel calicheamicin-conjugated CD22 antibody inotuzumab ozogamicin (CMC-544) effectively kills primary pediatric acute lymphoblastic leukemia cells. *Leukemia* **2012**, *26*, 255–264. [CrossRef] [PubMed]
48. Elgersma, R.C.; Coumans, R.G.; Huijbregts, T.; Menge, W.M.; Joosten, J.A.; Spijker, H.J.; de Groot, F.M.; van der Lee, M.M.; Ubink, R.; van den Dobbelsteen, D.J.; et al. Design, synthesis, and evaluation of linker-duocarmycin payloads: Toward selection of HER2-targeting antibody-drug conjugate SYD985. *Mol. Pharm.* **2015**, *12*, 1813–1835. [CrossRef] [PubMed]
49. Li, W.; Khullar, A.; Chou, S.; Sacramo, A.; Gerratana, B. Biosynthesis of sibiromycin, a potent antitumor antibiotic. *Appl. Environ. Microbiol.* **2009**, *75*, 2869–2878. [CrossRef] [PubMed]
50. Bouchard, H.; Viskov, C.; Garcia-Echeverria, C. Antibody-drug conjugates—A new wave of cancer drugs. *Bioorg. Med. Chem. Lett.* **2014**, *24*, 5357–5363. [CrossRef] [PubMed]
51. Mantaj, J.; Jackson, P.J.; Rahman, K.M.; Thurston, D.E. From anthramycin to pyrrolobenzodiazepine (PBD)-containing antibody-drug conjugates (ADCs). *Angew. Chem. Int. Ed. Engl.* **2017**, *56*, 462–488. [CrossRef] [PubMed]
52. Amador, M.L.; Jimeno, J.; Paz-Ares, L.; Cortes-Funes, H.; Hidalgo, M. Progress in the development and acquisition of anticancer agents from marine sources. *Ann. Oncol.* **2003**, *14*, 1607–1615. [CrossRef] [PubMed]
53. Pettit, G.R.; Srirangam, J.K.; Barkoczy, J.; Williams, M.D.; Boyd, M.R.; Hamel, E.; Pettit, R.K.; Hogan, F.; Bai, R.; Chapuis, J.C.; et al. Antineoplastic agents 365. Dolastatin 10 sar probes. *Anticancer Drug Des.* **1998**, *13*, 243–277. [PubMed]
54. Pettit, R.K.; Pettit, G.R.; Hazen, K.C. Specific activities of dolastatin 10 and peptide derivatives against cryptococcus neoformans. *Antimicrob. Agents Chemother.* **1998**, *42*, 2961–2965. [PubMed]
55. Bai, R.L.; Pettit, G.R.; Hamel, E. Binding of dolastatin 10 to tubulin at a distinct site for peptide antimitotic agents near the exchangeable nucleotide and vinca alkaloid sites. *J. Biol. Chem.* **1990**, *265*, 17141–17149. [PubMed]
56. Katz, J.; Janik, J.E.; Younes, A. Brentuximab vedotin (SGN-35). *Clin. Cancer Res.* **2011**, *17*, 6428–6436. [CrossRef] [PubMed]

57. Liu, J.F.; Moore, K.N.; Birrer, M.J.; Berlin, S.; Matulonis, U.A.; Infante, J.R.; Wolpin, B.; Poon, K.A.; Firestein, R.; Xu, J.; et al. Phase I study of safety and pharmacokinetics of the anti-MUC16 antibody-drug conjugate DMUC5754A in patients with platinum-resistant ovarian cancer or unresectable pancreatic cancer. *Ann. Oncol.* **2016**, *27*, 2124–2130. [CrossRef] [PubMed]
58. Tai, Y.T.; Mayes, P.A.; Acharya, C.; Zhong, M.Y.; Cea, M.; Cagnetta, A.; Craigen, J.; Yates, J.; Gliddon, L.; Fieles, W.; et al. Novel anti-b-cell maturation antigen antibody-drug conjugate (GSK2857916) selectively induces killing of multiple myeloma. *Blood* **2014**, *123*, 3128–3138. [CrossRef] [PubMed]
59. Francisco, J.A.; Cerveny, C.G.; Meyer, D.L.; Mixan, B.J.; Klussman, K.; Chace, D.F.; Rejniak, S.X.; Gordon, K.A.; DeBlanc, R.; Toki, B.E.; et al. cAC10-vcMMAE, an anti-CD30-monomethyl auristatin E conjugate with potent and selective antitumor activity. *Blood* **2003**, *102*, 1458–1465. [CrossRef] [PubMed]
60. Li, F.; Emmerton, K.K.; Jonas, M.; Zhang, X.; Miyamoto, J.B.; Setter, J.R.; Nicholas, N.D.; Okeley, N.M.; Lyon, R.P.; Benjamin, D.R.; et al. Intracellular released payload influences potency and bystander-killing effects of antibody-drug conjugates in preclinical models. *Cancer Res.* **2016**, *76*, 2710–2719. [CrossRef] [PubMed]
61. Kupchan, S.M.; Komoda, Y.; Court, W.A.; Thomas, G.J.; Smith, R.M.; Karim, A.; Gilmore, C.J.; Haltiwanger, R.C.; Bryan, R.F. Maytansine, a novel antileukemic ansa macrolide from maytenus ovatus. *J. Am. Chem. Soc.* **1972**, *94*, 1354–1356. [CrossRef] [PubMed]
62. Kupchan, S.M.; Komoda, Y.; Branfman, A.R.; Sneden, A.T.; Court, W.A.; Thomas, G.J.; Hintz, H.P.; Smith, R.M.; Karim, A.; Howie, G.A.; et al. The maytansinoids. Isolation, structural elucidation, and chemical interrelation of novel ansa macrolides. *J. Org. Chem.* **1977**, *42*, 2349–2357. [CrossRef] [PubMed]
63. Mandelbaum-Shavit, F.; Wolpert-DeFilippes, M.K.; Johns, D.G. Binding of maytansine to rat brain tubulin. *Biochem. Biophys. Res. Commun.* **1976**, *72*, 47–54. [CrossRef]
64. Widdison, W.C.; Wilhelm, S.D.; Cavanagh, E.E.; Whiteman, K.R.; Leece, B.A.; Kovtun, Y.; Goldmacher, V.S.; Xie, H.; Steeves, R.M.; Lutz, R.J.; et al. Semisynthetic maytansine analogues for the targeted treatment of cancer. *J. Med. Chem.* **2006**, *49*, 4392–4408. [CrossRef] [PubMed]
65. Blanc, V.; Bousseau, A.; Caron, A.; Carrez, C.; Lutz, R.J.; Lambert, J.M. Sar3419: An anti-CD19-maytansinoid immunoconjugate for the treatment of B-cell malignancies. *Clin. Cancer Res.* **2011**, *17*, 6448–6458. [CrossRef] [PubMed]
66. Lindell, T.J.; Weinberg, F.; Morris, P.W.; Roeder, R.G.; Rutter, W.J. Specific inhibition of nuclear RNA polymerase II by alpha-amanitin. *Science* **1970**, *170*, 447–449. [CrossRef] [PubMed]
67. Anderl, J.; Müller, C.; Heckl-Östreicher, B.; Wehr, R. Abstract 3616: Highly potent antibody-amanitin conjugates cause tumor-selective apoptosis. *Cancer Res.* **2011**, *71*, 3616. [CrossRef]
68. Moldenhauer, G.; Salnikov, A.V.; Luttgau, S.; Herr, I.; Anderl, J.; Faulstich, H. Therapeutic potential of amanitin-conjugated anti-epithelial cell adhesion molecule monoclonal antibody against pancreatic carcinoma. *J. Natl. Cancer Inst.* **2012**, *104*, 622–634. [CrossRef] [PubMed]
69. Hechler, T.; Kulke, M.; Mueller, C.; Pahl, A.; Anderl, J. Abstract 664: Amanitin-based antibody-drug conjugates targeting the prostate-specific membrane antigen. *Cancer Res.* **2014**, *74*. [CrossRef]
70. Hamblett, K.J.; Senter, P.D.; Chace, D.F.; Sun, M.M.; Lenox, J.; Cerveny, C.G.; Kissler, K.M.; Bernhardt, S.X.; Kopcha, A.K.; Zabinski, R.F.; et al. Effects of drug loading on the antitumor activity of a monoclonal antibody drug conjugate. *Clin. Cancer Res.* **2004**, *10*, 7063–7070. [CrossRef] [PubMed]
71. Doronina, S.O.; Toki, B.E.; Torgov, M.Y.; Mendelsohn, B.A.; Cerveny, C.G.; Chace, D.F.; DeBlanc, R.L.; Gearing, R.P.; Bovee, T.D.; Siegall, C.B.; et al. Development of potent monoclonal antibody auristatin conjugates for cancer therapy. *Nat. Biotechnol.* **2003**, *21*, 778–784. [CrossRef] [PubMed]
72. McAuley, A.; Jacob, J.; Kolvenbach, C.G.; Westland, K.; Lee, H.J.; Brych, S.R.; Rehder, D.; Kleemann, G.R.; Brems, D.N.; Matsumura, M. Contributions of a disulfide bond to the structure, stability, and dimerization of human igg1 antibody ch3 domain. *Protein Sci.* **2008**, *17*, 95–106. [CrossRef] [PubMed]
73. Sun, M.M.; Beam, K.S.; Cerveny, C.G.; Hamblett, K.J.; Blackmore, R.S.; Torgov, M.Y.; Handley, F.G.; Ihle, N.C.; Senter, P.D.; Alley, S.C. Reduction-alkylation strategies for the modification of specific monoclonal antibody disulfides. *Bioconj. Chem.* **2005**, *16*, 1282–1290. [CrossRef] [PubMed]
74. Schroeder, D.D.; Tankersley, D.L.; Lundblad, J.L. A new preparation of modified immune serum globulin (human) suitable for intravenous administration. I. Standardization of the reduction and alkylation reaction. *Vox Sang.* **1981**, *40*, 373–382. [CrossRef] [PubMed]

75. Agarwal, P.; Bertozzi, C.R. Site-specific antibody–drug conjugates: The nexus of bioorthogonal chemistry, protein engineering, and drug development. *Bioconj. Chem.* **2015**, *26*, 176–192. [CrossRef] [PubMed]
76. Hamann, P.R.; Hinman, L.M.; Hollander, I.; Beyer, C.F.; Lindh, D.; Holcomb, R.; Hallett, W.; Tsou, H.R.; Upeslacis, J.; Shochat, D.; et al. Gemtuzumab ozogamicin, a potent and selective anti-CD33 antibody-calicheamicin conjugate for treatment of acute myeloid leukemia. *Bioconjug. Chem.* **2002**, *13*, 47–58. [CrossRef] [PubMed]
77. Burnett, A.K.; Hills, R.K.; Milligan, D.; Kjeldsen, L.; Kell, J.; Russell, N.H.; Yin, J.A.; Hunter, A.; Goldstone, A.H.; Wheatley, K. Identification of patients with acute myeloblastic leukemia who benefit from the addition of gemtuzumab ozogamicin: Results of the mrc aml15 trial. *J. Clin. Oncol.* **2011**, *29*, 369–377. [CrossRef] [PubMed]
78. Luo, Q.; Chung, H.H.; Borths, C.; Janson, M.; Wen, J.; Joubert, M.K.; Wypych, J. Structural characterization of a monoclonal antibody-maytansinoid immunoconjugate. *Anal. Chem.* **2016**, *88*, 695–702. [CrossRef] [PubMed]
79. Adem, Y.T.; Schwarz, K.A.; Duenas, E.; Patapoff, T.W.; Galush, W.J.; Esue, O. Auristatin antibody drug conjugate physical instability and the role of drug payload. *Bioconj. Chem.* **2014**, *25*, 656–664. [CrossRef] [PubMed]
80. Moussa, E.M.; Panchal, J.P.; Moorthy, B.S.; Blum, J.S.; Joubert, M.K.; Narhi, L.O.; Topp, E.M. Immunogenicity of therapeutic protein aggregates. *J. Pharm. Sci.* **2016**, *105*, 417–430. [CrossRef] [PubMed]
81. McDonagh, C.F.; Turcott, E.; Westendorf, L.; Webster, J.B.; Alley, S.C.; Kim, K.; Andreyka, J.; Stone, I.; Hamblett, K.J.; Francisco, J.A.; et al. Engineered antibody-drug conjugates with defined sites and stoichiometries of drug attachment. *Protein Eng. Des. Sel.* **2006**, *19*, 299–307. [CrossRef] [PubMed]
82. Yurkovetskiy, A.V.; Yin, M.; Bodyak, N.; Stevenson, C.A.; Thomas, J.D.; Hammond, C.E.; Qin, L.; Zhu, B.; Gumerov, D.R.; Ter-Ovanesyan, E.; et al. A polymer-based antibody–vinca drug conjugate platform: Characterization and preclinical efficacy. *Cancer Res.* **2015**, *75*, 3365–3372. [CrossRef] [PubMed]
83. Krop, I.; Winer, E.P. Trastuzumab emtansine: A novel antibody-drug conjugate for HER2-positive breast cancer. *Clin. Cancer Res.* **2014**, *20*, 15–20. [CrossRef] [PubMed]
84. Tsuchikama, K.; An, Z. Antibody-drug conjugates: Recent advances in conjugation and linker chemistries. *Protein Cell* **2018**, *9*, 33–46. [CrossRef] [PubMed]
85. Chen, Y. Drug-to-antibody ratio (DAR) by UV/vis spectroscopy. *Methods Mol. Med.* **2013**, *1045*, 267–273.
86. Wang, L.; Amphlett, G.; Blättler, W.A.; Lambert, J.M.; Zhang, W. Structural characterization of the maytansinoid–monoclonal antibody immunoconjugate, HUN901–DM1, by mass spectrometry. *Protein Sci.* **2005**, *14*, 2436–2446. [CrossRef] [PubMed]
87. Hudecz, F.; Garnett, M.C.; Khan, T.; Baldwin, R.W. The influence of synthetic conditions on the stability of methotrexate-monoclonal antibody conjugates determined by reversed phase high performance liquid chromatography. *Biomed. Chromatogr.* **1992**, *6*, 128–132. [CrossRef] [PubMed]
88. Ouyang, J. Drug-to-antibody ratio (DAR) and drug load distribution by hydrophobic interaction chromatography and reversed phase high-performance liquid chromatography. *Methods Mol. Biol.* **2013**, *1045*, 275–283. [PubMed]
89. Chen, T.; Zhang, K.; Gruenhagen, J.; Medley, C.D.; Hydrophobic interaction chromatography for antibody drug conjugate drug distribution analysis. *Am. Pharm. Rev.* 2015. Available online: https://www.americanpharmaceuticalreview.com/Featured-Articles/177927-Hydrophobic-Interaction-Chromatography-for-Antibody-Drug-Conjugate-Drug-Distribution-Analysis/ (accessed on 3 April 2018).
90. Basa, L. Drug-to-antibody ratio (DAR) and drug load distribution by lc-esi-ms. *Methods Mol. Biol.* **2013**, *1045*, 285–293. [PubMed]
91. Huang, R.Y.C.; Chen, G. Characterization of antibody–drug conjugates by mass spectrometry: Advances and future trends. *Drug Discov. Today* **2016**, *21*, 850–855. [CrossRef] [PubMed]
92. Wagner-Rousset, E.; Janin-Bussat, M.C.; Colas, O.; Excoffier, M.; Ayoub, D.; Haeuw, J.F.; Rilatt, I.; Perez, M.; Corvaia, N.; Beck, A. Antibody-drug conjugate model fast characterization by lc-ms following ides proteolytic digestion. *mAbs* **2014**, *6*, 273–285. [CrossRef] [PubMed]
93. Junutula, J.R.; Raab, H.; Clark, S.; Bhakta, S.; Leipold, D.D.; Weir, S.; Chen, Y.; Simpson, M.; Tsai, S.P.; Dennis, M.S.; et al. Site-specific conjugation of a cytotoxic drug to an antibody improves the therapeutic index. *Nat. Biotechnol.* **2008**, *26*, 925–932. [CrossRef] [PubMed]

94. Axup, J.Y.; Bajjuri, K.M.; Ritland, M.; Hutchins, B.M.; Kim, C.H.; Kazane, S.A.; Halder, R.; Forsyth, J.S.; Santidrian, A.F.; Stafin, K.; et al. Synthesis of site-specific antibody-drug conjugates using unnatural amino acids. *Proc. Natl. Acad. Sci. USA* **2012**, *109*, 16101–16106. [CrossRef] [PubMed]
95. Jeger, S.; Zimmermann, K.; Blanc, A.; Grunberg, J.; Honer, M.; Hunziker, P.; Struthers, H.; Schibli, R. Site-specific and stoichiometric modification of antibodies by bacterial transglutaminase. *Angew. Chem. Int. Ed. Engl.* **2010**, *49*, 9995–9997. [CrossRef] [PubMed]
96. Junutula, J.R.; Bhakta, S.; Raab, H.; Ervin, K.E.; Eigenbrot, C.; Vandlen, R.; Scheller, R.H.; Lowman, H.B. Rapid identification of reactive cysteine residues for site-specific labeling of antibody-fabs. *J. Immunol. Methods* **2008**, *332*, 41–52. [CrossRef] [PubMed]
97. Junutula, J.R.; Flagella, K.M.; Graham, R.A.; Parsons, K.L.; Ha, E.; Raab, H.; Bhakta, S.; Nguyen, T.; Dugger, D.L.; Li, G.; et al. Engineered thio-trastuzumab-dm1 conjugate with an improved therapeutic index to target human epidermal growth factor receptor 2-positive breast cancer. *Clin. Cancer Res.* **2010**, *16*, 4769–4778. [CrossRef] [PubMed]
98. Yao, H.; Jiang, F.; Lu, A.; Zhang, G. Methods to design and synthesize antibody-drug conjugates (adcs). *Int. J. Mol. Sci.* **2016**, *17*, 194. [CrossRef] [PubMed]
99. Hallam, T.J.; Smider, V.V. Unnatural amino acids in novel antibody conjugates. *Future Med. Chem.* **2014**, *6*, 1309–1324. [CrossRef] [PubMed]
100. Liu, C.C.; Schultz, P.G. Adding new chemistries to the genetic code. *Annu. Rev. Biochem.* **2010**, *79*, 413–444. [CrossRef] [PubMed]
101. Tian, F.; Lu, Y.; Manibusan, A.; Sellers, A.; Tran, H.; Sun, Y.; Phuong, T.; Barnett, R.; Hehli, B.; Song, F.; et al. A general approach to site-specific antibody drug conjugates. *Proc. Natl. Acad. Sci. USA* **2014**, *111*, 1766–1771. [CrossRef] [PubMed]
102. Yokoyama, K.; Nio, N.; Kikuchi, Y. Properties and applications of microbial transglutaminase. *Appl. Microbiol. Biotechnol.* **2004**, *64*, 447–454. [CrossRef] [PubMed]
103. Strop, P.; Liu, S.H.; Dorywalska, M.; Delaria, K.; Dushin, R.G.; Tran, T.T.; Ho, W.H.; Farias, S.; Casas, M.G.; Abdiche, Y.; et al. Location matters: Site of conjugation modulates stability and pharmacokinetics of antibody drug conjugates. *Chem. Biol.* **2013**, *20*, 161–167. [CrossRef] [PubMed]
104. Strop, P.; Tran, T.T.; Dorywalska, M.; Delaria, K.; Dushin, R.; Wong, O.K.; Ho, W.H.; Zhou, D.; Wu, A.; Kraynov, E.; et al. RN927C, a site-specific trop-2 antibody-drug conjugate (ADC) with enhanced stability, is highly efficacious in preclinical solid tumor models. *Mol. Cancer Ther.* **2016**, *15*, 2698–2708. [CrossRef] [PubMed]
105. Carrico, I.S.; Carlson, B.L.; Bertozzi, C.R. Introducing genetically encoded aldehydes into proteins. *Nat. Chem. Biol.* **2007**, *3*, 321–322. [CrossRef] [PubMed]
106. Agarwal, P.; van der Weijden, J.; Sletten, E.M.; Rabuka, D.; Bertozzi, C.R. A pictet-spengler ligation for protein chemical modification. *Proc. Natl. Acad. Sci. USA* **2013**, *110*, 46–51. [CrossRef] [PubMed]
107. Agarwal, P.; Kudirka, R.; Albers, A.E.; Barfield, R.M.; de Hart, G.W.; Drake, P.M.; Jones, L.C.; Rabuka, D. Hydrazino-pictet-spengler ligation as a biocompatible method for the generation of stable protein conjugates. *Bioconj. Chem.* **2013**, *24*, 846–851. [CrossRef] [PubMed]
108. Starodub, A.N.; Ocean, A.J.; Shah, M.A.; Vahdat, L.T.; Chuang, E.; Guarino, M.J.; Picozzi, V.J.; Thomas, S.S.; Maliakal, P.P.; Govindan, S.V.; et al. Abstract CT206: SN-38 antibody-drug conjugate (ADC) targeting Trop-2, IMMU-132, as a novel platform for the therapy of diverse metastatic solid cancers: Initial clinical results. *Cancer Res.* **2014**, *74*, CT206. [CrossRef]
109. Goldenberg, D.M.; Cardillo, T.M.; Govindan, S.V.; Rossi, E.A.; Sharkey, R.M. Trop-2 is a novel target for solid cancer therapy with sacituzumab govitecan (immu-132), an antibody-drug conjugate (ADC). *Oncotarget* **2015**, *6*, 22496–22512. [CrossRef] [PubMed]
110. Bardia, A.; Vahdat, L.T.; Diamond, J.R.; Starodub, A.; Moroose, R.L.; Isakoff, S.J.; Ocean, A.J.; Berlin, J.; Messersmith, W.A.; Thomas, S.S.; et al. Therapy of refractory/relapsed metastatic triple-negative breast cancer (TNBC) with an anti-Trop-2-SN-38 antibody-drug conjugate (ADC), sacituzumab govitecan (IMMU-132): Phase I/II clinical experience. *J. Clin. Oncol.* **2015**, *33*, 1016. [CrossRef]
111. Elnakat, H.; Ratnam, M. Distribution, functionality and gene regulation of folate receptor isoforms: Implications in targeted therapy. *Adv. Drug Deliv. Rev.* **2004**, *56*, 1067–1084. [CrossRef] [PubMed]
112. Ab, O.; Whiteman, K.R.; Bartle, L.M.; Sun, X.; Singh, R.; Tavares, D.; LaBelle, A.; Payne, G.; Lutz, R.J.; Pinkas, J.; et al. Imgn853, a folate receptor-α (FRα)-targeting antibody-drug conjugate, exhibits potent

targeted antitumor activity against fralpha-expressing tumors. *Mol. Cancer Ther.* **2015**, *14*, 1605–1613. [CrossRef] [PubMed]
113. Erickson, H.K.; Park, P.U.; Widdison, W.C.; Kovtun, Y.V.; Garrett, L.M.; Hoffman, K.; Lutz, R.J.; Goldmacher, V.S.; Blattler, W.A. Antibody-maytansinoid conjugates are activated in targeted cancer cells by lysosomal degradation and linker-dependent intracellular processing. *Cancer Res.* **2006**, *66*, 4426–4433. [CrossRef] [PubMed]
114. Ponte, J.F.; Ab, O.; Lanieri, L.; Lee, J.; Coccia, J.; Bartle, L.M.; Themeles, M.; Zhou, Y.; Pinkas, J.; Ruiz-Soto, R. Mirvetuximab soravtansine (IMGN853), a folate receptor alpha-targeting antibody-drug conjugate, potentiates the activity of standard of care therapeutics in ovarian cancer models. *Neoplasia* **2016**, *18*, 775–784. [CrossRef] [PubMed]
115. Moore, K.N.; Borghaei, H.; O'Malley, D.M.; Jeong, W.; Seward, S.M.; Bauer, T.M.; Perez, R.P.; Matulonis, U.A.; Running, K.L.; Zhang, X.; et al. Phase 1 dose-escalation study of mirvetuximab soravtansine (IMGN853), a folate receptor alpha-targeting antibody-drug conjugate, in patients with solid tumors. *Cancer* **2017**, *123*, 3080–3087. [CrossRef] [PubMed]
116. Moore, K.N.; Martin, L.P.; O'Malley, D.M.; Matulonis, U.A.; Konner, J.A.; Perez, R.P.; Bauer, T.M.; Ruiz-Soto, R.; Birrer, M.J. Safety and activity of mirvetuximab soravtansine (IMGN853), a folate receptor alpha-targeting antibody-drug conjugate, in platinum-resistant ovarian, fallopian tube, or primary peritoneal cancer: A phase i expansion study. *J. Clin. Oncol.* **2017**, *35*, 1112–1118. [CrossRef] [PubMed]
117. Tedder, T.F.; Tuscano, J.; Sato, S.; Kehrl, J.H. Cd22, a B lymphocyte-specific adhesion molecule that regulates antigen receptor signaling. *Annu. Rev. Immunol.* **1997**, *15*, 481–504. [CrossRef] [PubMed]
118. Piccaluga, P.P.; Arpinati, M.; Candoni, A.; Laterza, C.; Paolini, S.; Gazzola, A.; Sabattini, E.; Visani, G.; Pileri, S.A. Surface antigens analysis reveals significant expression of candidate targets for immunotherapy in adult acute lymphoid leukemia. *Leuk. lymphoma* **2011**, *52*, 325–327. [CrossRef] [PubMed]
119. DiJoseph, J.F.; Dougher, M.M.; Evans, D.Y.; Zhou, B.-B.; Damle, N.K. Preclinical anti-tumor activity of antibody-targeted chemotherapy with CMC-544 (inotuzumab ozogamicin), a CD22-specific immunoconjugate of calicheamicin, compared with non-targeted combination chemotherapy with cvp or chop. *Cancer Chemother. Pharmacol.* **2011**, *67*, 741–749. [CrossRef] [PubMed]
120. Advani, A.; Coiffier, B.; Czuczman, M.S.; Dreyling, M.; Foran, J.; Gine, E.; Gisselbrecht, C.; Ketterer, N.; Nasta, S.; Rohatiner, A.; et al. Safety, pharmacokinetics, and preliminary clinical activity of inotuzumab ozogamicin, a novel immunoconjugate for the treatment of B-cell non-hodgkin's lymphoma: Results of a phase i study. *J. Clin. Oncol.* **2010**, *28*, 2085–2093. [CrossRef] [PubMed]
121. Goy, A.; Forero, A.; Wagner-Johnston, N.; Christopher Ehmann, W.; Tsai, M.; Hatake, K.; Ananthakrishnan, R.; Volkert, A.; Vandendries, E.; Ogura, M. A phase 2 study of inotuzumab ozogamicin in patients with indolent b-cell non-hodgkin lymphoma refractory to rituximab alone, rituximab and chemotherapy, or radioimmunotherapy. *Br. J. Haematol.* **2016**, *174*, 571–581. [CrossRef] [PubMed]
122. Teicher, B.A.; Chari, R.V. Antibody conjugate therapeutics: Challenges and potential. *Clin. Cancer Res.* **2011**, *17*, 6389–6397. [CrossRef] [PubMed]
123. Singh, S.K.; Luisi, D.L.; Pak, R.H. Antibody-drug conjugates: Design, formulation and physicochemical stability. *Pharm. Res.* **2015**, *32*, 3541–3571. [CrossRef] [PubMed]
124. Kennedy, P.J.; Oliveira, C.; Granja, P.L.; Sarmento, B. Antibodies and associates: Partners in targeted drug delivery. *Pharmacol. Ther.* **2017**, *177*, 129–145. [CrossRef] [PubMed]
125. Zolot, R.S.; Basu, S.; Million, R.P. Antibody-drug conjugates. *Nat. Rev. Drug Discov.* **2013**, *12*, 259–260. [CrossRef] [PubMed]

MDPI
St. Alban-Anlage 66
4052 Basel
Switzerland
Tel. +41 61 683 77 34
Fax +41 61 302 89 18
www.mdpi.com

Pharmaceuticals Editorial Office
E-mail: pharmaceuticals@mdpi.com
www.mdpi.com/journal/pharmaceuticals

www.ingramcontent.com/pod-product-compliance
Lightning Source LLC
LaVergne TN
LVHW071944080526
838202LV00064B/6677
* 9 7 8 3 0 3 9 2 1 5 8 6 7 *